# Emergency Headache

## Diagnosis and Management

# Emergency Headache

## Diagnosis and Management

Edited by

**Serena L. Orr MD MSc**
University of Ottawa and Children's Hospital of Eastern Ontario, Ottawa, ON, Canada

**Benjamin W. Friedman MD MS**
Albert Einstein College of Medicine, Montefiore Medical Center, Bronx, NY, USA

**David W. Dodick MD**
Mayo Clinic College of Medicine, Department of Neurology, Phoenix, AZ, USA

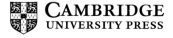

CAMBRIDGE
UNIVERSITY PRESS

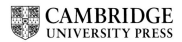

Shaftesbury Road, Cambridge CB2 8EA, United Kingdom

One Liberty Plaza, 20th Floor, New York, NY 10006, USA

477 Williamstown Road, Port Melbourne, VIC 3207, Australia

314–321, 3rd Floor, Plot 3, Splendor Forum, Jasola District Centre, New Delhi – 110025, India

103 Penang Road, #05–06/07, Visioncrest Commercial, Singapore 238467

Cambridge University Press is part of Cambridge University Press & Assessment,
a department of the University of Cambridge.

We share the University's mission to contribute to society through the pursuit of
education, learning and research at the highest international levels of excellence.

www.cambridge.org
Information on this title: www.cambridge.org/9781009592659

DOI: 10.1017/9781316819388

First published 2017
First paperback edition 2025

*A catalogue record for this publication is available from the British Library*

*Library of Congress Cataloging-in-Publication data*
Names: Orr, Serena L., editor. | Friedman, Benjamin W., editor. | Dodick, David, editor.
Title: Emergency headache : diagnosis and management /
edited by Serena L. Orr, Benjamin W. Friedman, David W. Dodick.
Description: Cambridge, United Kingdom ; New York, NY : Cambridge University Press, 2017. |
Includes bibliographical references and index.
Identifiers: LCCN 2017032479 | ISBN 9781107177208 (hardback)
Subjects: | MESH: Headache Disorders – diagnosis | Headache Disorders – therapy |
Headache – etiology | Emergency Treatment
Classification: LCC RB128 | NLM WL 342 | DDC 616.8/491025–dc23
LC record available at https://lccn.loc.gov/2017032479

ISBN     978-1-107-17720-8     Hardback
ISBN     978-1-009-59265-9     Paperback

# Contents

*List of Contributors*    *page* vi
*Preface*    viii

1  **Introduction**    1
   Serena L. Orr and David W. Dodick

2  **Epidemiology of Headache in the Emergency Department**    4
   Serena L. Orr and David W. Dodick

3  **Approach to History Taking and the Physical Examination**    15
   Suzanne Christie and Garth Dickinson

4  **Approach to Investigations**    26
   Meir H. Scheinfeld and Benjamin W. Friedman

5  **Thunderclap Headache in the Emergency Department**    43
   James Ducharme

6  **Other Secondary Headaches in the Emergency Department**    50
   Michael J. Marmura and Benjamin W. Friedman

7  **The Migraine Patient in the Emergency Department**    65
   Serena L. Orr and Brian H. Rowe

8  **The Patient with a Trigeminal Autonomic Cephalalgia in the Emergency Department**    80
   Anne Ducros

9  **Other Primary Headache Disorders That Can Present to the Emergency Department**    88
   Yasmin Idu Jion and Brian M. Grosberg

10  **Medication Overuse Headache in the Emergency Department**    99
    Chia-Chun Chiang, Todd J. Schwedt, Shuu-Jiun Wang and David W. Dodick

11  **Approach to the Pediatric Patient with Headache in the Emergency Department**    110
    Serena L. Orr and David Sheridan

12  **Approach to Pregnant or Lactating Patients with Headache in the Emergency Department**    125
    Sylvia Lucas and Esther Rawner

13  **Approach to the Elderly Patient with Headache in the Emergency Department**    141
    Fabio Frediani and Gennaro Bussone

14  **Preventing Emergency Department Visits in Primary Headache Patients and Prevention of Bounce-Backs to the Emergency Department**    149
    Wm. Jeptha Davenport

*Index*    159

# Contributors

**Gennaro Bussone**
Founder and Director Emeritus, Center for
Headache, Carlo Besta Neurological Institute,
Milan, Italy

**Chia-Chun Chiang** MD
Department of Neurology, Mayo Clinic, Phoenix,
AZ, USA

**Suzanne Christie** MD FRCPC
Ottawa Headache Centre, Nepean, ON, Canada;
Assistant Professor of Neurology and Medicine,
University of Ottawa, Ottawa, ON, Canada

**Wm. Jeptha Davenport** MD FRCPC (Neurology)
Clinical Associate Professor, Division of Neurology,
Departments of Clinical Neurosciences and Medical
Genetics, Hotchkiss Brain Institute, Cumming
School of Medicine, University of Calgary, Calgary,
AB, Canada

**Garth Dickinson** MD FRCPC FIFEM
Associate Professor, Department of Emergency
Medicine, University of Ottawa, Ottawa, ON, Canada

**David W. Dodick** MD
Mayo Clinic College of Medicine, Department of
Neurology, Phoenix, AZ, USA

**James Ducharme** MD CM FRCP(c)
Clinical Professor of Medicine, Division of
Emergency Medicine, McMaster University,
Hamilton, ON, Canada; Emergency Physician,
Humber River Hospital, Toronto, ON, Canada

**Anne Ducros**
Department of Neurology, Montpellier University
and Montpellier Hospital, Montpellier, France

**Fabio Frediani**
Headache Center, Neurology and Stroke Unit
Division, ASST Santi Paolo e Carlo, S. Carlo
Borromeo Hospital, Milan, Italy

**Benjamin W. Friedman** MD MS
Associate Professor of Emergency Medicine, Albert
Einstein College of Medicine, Montefiore Medical
Center, Bronx, NY, USA

**Brian M. Grosberg** MD FAHS
Director, Hartford Healthcare Headache Program,
Department of Neurology, University of Connecticut
School of Medicine, Farmington, CT, USA

**Yasmin Idu Jion** MD
Department of Neurology, National Neuroscience
Institute, Singapore

**Sylvia Lucas** MD PhD
University of Washington Medical Center, Seattle,
WA, USA; Harborview Medical Center, Seattle,
WA, USA

**Michael J. Marmura** MD
Assistant Professor of Neurology, Jefferson Headache
Center, Thomas Jefferson University Hospital,
Philadelphia, PA, USA

**Serena L. Orr** MD MSc
University of Ottawa and Children's Hospital of
Eastern Ontario, Ottawa, ON, Canada

**Esther Rawner** MD
Northwest Hospital, Seattle, WA, USA

**Brian H. Rowe** MD MSc CCFP(EM) FCCP FCAHS
Scientific Director, Institute of Circulatory and
Respiratory Health (ICRH), Canadian Institutes of
Health Research, Ottawa, ON, Canada; Tier I Canada
Research Chair in Evidence-Based Emergency Medicine
and Professor, Department of Emergency Medicine,
University of Alberta, Edmonton, AB, Canada

**Meir H. Scheinfeld** MD PhD
Associate Professor of Radiology, Albert Einstein
College of Medicine, Montefiore Medical Center,
Bronx, NY, USA

**Todd J. Schwedt** MD
Department of Neurology, Mayo Clinic, Phoenix, AZ, USA

**David Sheridan** MD
Oregon Health and Science University, Doernbecher Children's Hospital, Department of Emergency Medicine, Portland, OR, USA

**Shuu-Jiun Wang** MD
Department of Neurology, Taipei Veterans General Hospital, Taipei, Taiwan

# Preface

Headache is one of the most common reasons for emergency department visits. The patient with headache presents a challenge to the emergency clinician, given the very long list of diagnostic possibilities. The emergency clinician must be able to recognize life-threatening causes of acute headache and generate a judicious differential diagnosis. Investigations should be ordered with discernment, balancing the importance of identifying life-threatening causes of headache with resource utilization and cost considerations, given the ubiquity of headache in this setting.

There is a lack of accessible, evidence-based literature that provides an approach to the diagnosis and management of headaches in the emergency department. The dearth of resources, coupled with the complexity of headache as a presenting symptom, renders it challenging for clinicians to provide timely access to best-practice care in this setting. We hope to bridge this gap with this book. As clinicians with experience in evaluating and managing patients who present to the emergency department with headache, we recognize the need to rapidly make an accurate diagnosis. This book has been designed to assist the busy clinician with this objective. It is the result of collaborative work between a large number of headache experts, with representation of specialists from both Neurology and Emergency Medicine. In this way, the book strives not only to provide an evidence-based approach to headache in the emergency department, but also to provide a balanced approach considering the perspective of both the neurologist and the emergency physician. In addition, although the primary aim of this work is to provide clinicians with evidence-based information, there are scenarios in which the headache literature provides little guidance on how to approach patient management. Where these scenarios arise, we have drawn on expert opinion to provide guidance to the clinician who must manage the patient despite the lack of an available base of evidence.

The book opens with an introduction to the problem of headache in the emergency department. We then summarize pertinent epidemiological facts about headache in this setting. The next two chapters provide readers with a practical approach to the history and physical examination as well as investigations for headache while highlighting clinical pearls and how to target the assessment to the patient scenario. We then aim to provide an overview of secondary headaches in the emergency department and give a detailed review of the primary headache disorders in the emergency department, given their high prevalence in this setting. Several subsequent chapters provide practical guidance on how to approach special patient populations that present to the emergency department with headache. Finally, we review evidence for strategies to prevent headache recurrence in patients with primary headache disorders who have presented to the emergency department, as well as guidance on preventing initial and return visits.

We are very grateful to all of the authors who contributed their clinical expertise, knowledge of the literature, and invaluable time to create comprehensive, reader-friendly, and evidence-based chapters for this book. We would also like to acknowledge the collaborative nature of the work required to write this book, seeing it was carefully written and reviewed by a large number of experts from Neurology and Emergency Medicine. In this way, we are confident that it will provide emergency clinicians with a practical, accessible, balanced, and evidence-based resource to assist in delivering the highest level of patient care.

# Introduction

Serena L. Orr
David W. Dodick

Headache is one of the most common presenting symptoms in the emergency department (ED). It has been found to be the fifth most common reason for visiting the ED in the United States [1] and a variety of studies have shown that it accounts for a significant percentage of ED visits [2–4]. Unsurprisingly, given its prevalence, the cost of headache care in the ED is substantial. It has been estimated that the cost of ED visits for headache amounts to $520 million per year in the United States [5].

Not only is it common, but the management of headache in the ED is also very complex. Headache is a relatively non-specific symptom and it is associated with myriad potential diagnoses. When approaching the differential diagnosis of headache, it is important to have an organized approach. The most crucial aspect of headache diagnosis is determining whether the patient has a primary or a secondary headache. Secondary headaches are those with recognized underlying causes, while primary headache disorders are neurological diseases unto themselves. The International Classification of Headache Disorders, currently in its third edition (beta version), provides an exhaustive list of both primary and secondary headaches [6]. Subsequent chapters will address the most common primary and secondary headaches presenting to the ED. As will be described in detail in Chapter 2, secondary headaches represent the majority of headaches in the pediatric ED, whereas primary headaches comprise the majority of headaches in the adult ED.

There are several important management issues that arise with headache in the ED, all of which will be addressed in detail throughout the next few chapters. The most critical issue is to make the correct diagnosis. In order to do so, one must obtain a targeted history and collect data from the physical exam that will allow for the generation of a focused differential diagnosis. The importance of the history and physical exam cannot be overstated. Without high-quality initial data, the clinician may be misled in their decision-making regarding investigations, consultations, and further management. Knowing the high-yield questions to ask and the physical exam maneuvers to perform in the common headache scenarios will result in more timely and accurate diagnoses, with fewer unnecessary investigations.

Once a list of potential diagnoses has been established, the judicious use of investigations for ED headache is very important. First, the clinician must consider all possible secondary headache diagnoses and collect information from the history and physical exam that hints at headache red flags – key indicators of an underlying serious secondary cause. If any red flags are present or if specific secondary headaches are being considered based on the history and physical exam, then the clinician must know the appropriate investigations to carry out. In many cases, there will be several investigation options at the clinician's disposal, but it is important, where possible, to adhere to evidence-based guidelines. For example, there are several guidelines [7–9] that prescribe a sequence of diagnostic tests for suspected subarachnoid hemorrhage. Patients with suspected subarachnoid hemorrhage are to be screened with a computed tomography (CT) scan of the head. Where the CT scan is negative, a lumbar puncture is often carried out in order to search for red blood cells or cerebrospinal fluid xanthochromia. The case of subarachnoid hemorrhage illustrates that, where evidence is available, a reasoned and evidence-based approach to the diagnostic work-up for headache is expected of the treating clinician. Throughout this book, the latest evidence-based strategies for headache diagnosis and investigations will be reviewed.

Once a diagnosis has been established, the optimal course of management may be unclear. This is especially true with primary headaches, given a multitude of therapeutic options, a lack of high-quality evidence in the literature [10,11], and a lack of awareness and familiarity among clinicians regarding the use of evidence-based therapies. For example, studies have shown that evidence-based therapies are often not used first-line in patients presenting to the ED with migraine. Several US-based studies have found that patients commonly receive opioids rather than evidence-based therapies, and in many cases the majority of patients are not being treated in an evidence-based fashion [12,13]. This is also true in Canada [14,15]. Practice variation also appears to be a problem in the management of pediatric migraine, according to a multicenter study carried out in Canadian EDs [16]. Finally, there is evidence that patients presenting to the ED with headache may be undertreated. One US study found that just over one-third of patients visiting the emergency department for headache received neither an intravenous line nor any medication, and that only 21.8 percent of the patients were headache-free at discharge [17]. Thus, there is significant room for improvement on current headache management in the ED, especially as pertains to the management of primary headaches.

The lack of appropriate treatment for headache in the ED can have significant consequences not only for patients with secondary headaches, but also for those with primary headaches. The case of treating migraine with opioids, which is discouraged by the American Academy of Neurology in their Choosing Wisely recommendations [18], illustrates this well. The overuse of opioids to treat migraine in the ED appears to not only lead to worse short-term outcomes [14,19,20], but may have lasting long-term consequences for the patient. The ED may be the initial setting where the patient is exposed to opioids that may influence future opioid overuse. Additionally, patients using opioids tend to visit the ED more frequently for their headaches [21]. In the upcoming chapters, we will provide a review of the most appropriate evidence-based strategies for the management of the various headache disorders in the ED.

Patients presenting to the ED with headache have a variety of expectations and concerns. In many cases, if they have not already been diagnosed with a primary headache disorder, they may be concerned about the prospect of an underlying sinister cause for their head pain. There is often a significant amount of associated anxiety and it is imperative that the physician recognizes and acknowledges this as it can confound the clinical picture. Patients who are already aware of the fact that they have a primary headache disorder will often have different expectations and reasons for visiting the ED, although in one US study, one-third of patients visiting the ED for migraine were concerned about a life-threatening condition or had been referred to the ED by a physician [22]. One small study based in an ED in France found that the vast majority of patients presenting to the emergency headache service with migraine were visiting because of increasing headache frequency and/or severity. Only a small proportion of this selected patient group presented for diagnostic clarification [23]. Wherever possible, the emergency physician can best serve the patient by understanding the expectations and goals the patient has established for the visit.

This book aims to provide clinicians working in the ED with a comprehensive, accessible, and evidence-based review of essential topics pertaining to headaches in the ED. Given how common they are in the ED, an emphasis is placed on the approach to primary headaches in this setting. The book will begin with a review of headache epidemiology in the ED. Subsequently, a practical approach to the history, physical exam, and investigation of emergency headaches is described. Next, an overview of secondary headaches in the ED setting is provided. Several chapters are devoted to a detailed review of primary headaches in the ED, followed by chapters dealing with special populations presenting to the ED with headache. Finally, the book will conclude with a broader discussion on how to prevent ED visits for primary headaches and how to optimally treat primary headaches in this setting, with the goal of avoiding headache recurrence and return visits to the ED.

## References

1. Smitherman TA, Burch R, Sheikh H, Loder E. The prevalence, impact, and treatment of migraine and severe headaches in the United States: a review of statistics from national surveillance studies. *Headache.* 2013;53(3):427–36.

2. Lucado J, Paez K, Elixhauser A. Headaches in US Hospitals and Emergency Departments, 2008: Statistical Brief #111. *Healthcare Cost and Utilization Project (HCUP) Statistical Briefs.* 2011;24:1–12.

3. Barton CW. Evaluation and treatment of headache patients in the emergency department: a survey. *Headache.* 1994;34(2):91–4.

4. De Carli GF, Fabbri L, Cavazzuti L, et al. The epidemiology of migraine: a retrospective study in Italian emergency departments. *Headache*. 1998;38(9):697–704.

5. Hawkins K, Wang S, Rupnow M. Direct cost burden among insured US employees with migraine. *Headache*. 2008;48(4):553–63.

6. Headache Classification Committee of the International Headache Society (IHS). The International Classification of Headache Disorders, 3rd edition (beta version). *Cephalalgia*. 2013;33(9):629–808.

7. Vivancos J, Gilo F, Frutos R, et al. Clinical management guidelines for subarachnoid haemorrhage: diagnosis and treatment. *Neurologia*. 2014;29(6):353–70.

8. Steiner T, Juvela S, Unterberg A, et al. European Stroke Organization guidelines for the management of intracranial aneurysms and subarachnoid haemorrhage. *Cerebrovasc Dis*. 2013;35(2):93–112.

9. Connolly ES, Rabinstein AA, Carhuapoma JR, et al. Guidelines for the management of aneurysmal subarachnoid hemorrhage: a guideline for healthcare professionals from the American Heart Association/American Stroke Association. *Stroke*. 2012;43(6):1711–37.

10. Orr SL, Aubé M, Becker WJ, et al. Canadian Headache Society systematic review and recommendations on the treatment of migraine pain in emergency settings. *Cephalalgia*. 2015;35(3):271–84.

11. Weinman D, Nicastro O, Akala O, Friedman BW. Parenteral treatment of episodic tension-type headache: a systematic review. *Headache*. 2014;54(2):260–8.

12. Vinson DR. Treatment patterns of isolated benign headache in US emergency departments. *Ann Emerg Med*. 2002;39(3):215–22.

13. Vinson DR, Hurtado TR, Vandenberg JT, Banwart L. Variations among emergency departments in the treatment of benign headache. *Ann Emerg Med*. 2003;41(1):90–7.

14. Colman I, Rothney A, Wright S, Zilkalns B, Rowe BH. Use of narcotic analgesics in the emergency department treatment of migraine headache. *Neurology*. 2004;62(10):1695–700.

15. Nijjar SS, Pink L, Gordon AS. Examination of migraine management in emergency departments. *Pain Res Manag*. 2011;16(3):183–6.

16. Richer LP, Laycock K, Millar K, et al. Treatment of children with migraine in emergency departments: national practice variation study. *Pediatrics*. 2010;126(1):e150–5.

17. Gupta MX, Silberstein SD, Young WB, et al. Less is not more: underutilization of headache medications in a university hospital emergency department. *Headache*. 2007;47(8):1125–33.

18. Langer-Gould AM, Anderson WE, Armstrong MJ, et al. The American Academy of Neurology's top five choosing wisely recommendations. *Neurology*. 2013;81(11):1004–11.

19. McCarthy LH, Cowan RP. Comparison of parenteral treatments of acute primary headache in a large academic emergency department cohort. *Cephalalgia*. 2015;35(9):807–15.

20. Friedman B, Kapoor A, Friedman M, Hochberg M, Rowe B. The relative efficacy of meperidine for the treatment of acute migraine: a meta-analysis of randomized controlled trials. *Ann Emerg Med*. 2008;52(6):705–13.

21. Buse DC, Pearlman SH, Reed ML, et al. Opioid use and dependence among persons with migraine: results of the AMPP study. *Headache*. 2012;52(1):18–36.

22. Minen MT, Loder E, Friedman B. Factors associated with emergency department visits for migraine: an observational study. *Headache*. 2014;54(10):1611–18.

23. Ducros A. Emergency treatment of migraine. *Cephalalgia*. 2008;28(Suppl. 2):9–13.

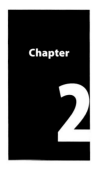

# Epidemiology of Headache in the Emergency Department

Serena L. Orr

David W. Dodick

## Abstract

Headache is one of the most common chief complaints in the emergency department (ED). Several demographic and other factors are associated with the propensity to visit the ED with headache. Whereas primary headaches are the most common cause of headache in the adult ED, secondary, non-life-threatening causes, such as headaches associated with viral illnesses, underlie most headaches in the pediatric ED. Costs associated with ED headache visits are high, partly due to the rising use of neuroimaging in this patient population. Several strategies could help to mitigate the cost of headache care in the ED, primarily by aiming to improve community-based care for patients with primary headaches. In this chapter, a detailed overview of the epidemiology of headache in the ED is provided.

## Prevalence of Headache in the Emergency Department

### The Prevalence of Headache Visits to the ED

Headache accounts for a large proportion of visits to the ED. In the United States, approximately 1.7–2.4 percent of all ED visits are due to headache [1,2]. Headache has been identified as the fifth most common reason for visiting the ED in the United States, accounting for somewhere between three and five million ED visits per year [1,3]. Interestingly, these numbers translate into 989 ED visits for headache per 100,000 individuals per day in the United States, reflecting the commonality of the problem [1].

The prevalence of headache in the ED differs significantly both at the regional level and from country to country. For example, within the United States there is a wide range of variability in the frequency

of ED visits for headache, with the midwestern and southernmost states having the highest rates, and the western and northeastern states having the lowest rates [1]. One example of between-country differences is found when comparing the United States to Greece: in Greece, the prevalence of ED visits for headache of any cause has been estimated at 1.3 percent [4]. One study carried out in England found an even lower rate, with only 0.36 percent of all ED visits attributed to headache [5]. Italian data suggest that the prevalence of headache visits in Italian EDs is anywhere from 0.6 to 1.2 percent [6,7] when secondary headaches are excluded. A study of healthcare units in Brazil, which provide front-line acute care services, found that 9.3 percent of patients presented with headache as their chief complaint [8]. This rate seems relatively high, and may reflect differences in the structure of the healthcare system in Brazil as compared to other countries. Although the differences in prevalence are due in part to factors such as access to healthcare, structure of healthcare systems, and other socioeconomic factors that vary from country to country and region to region, differences in study design likely inflate the variability in prevalence rates. What is consistent is the fact that headache is one of the most common chief complaints presenting to the ED, regardless of region or country.

## Individual Factors Affecting Prevalence of Emergency Department Visits for Headache

Several demographic characteristics are associated with a higher likelihood of visiting the ED with headache (Figure 2.1). Women appear to be more likely to present with headache. US-based population data revealed that women were 2.7 times more likely than men to visit the ED with headache of any cause, and 4.6 times more likely to visit the ED with migraine.

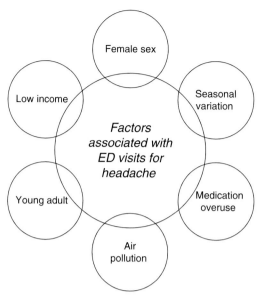

**Figure 2.1** Factors associated with ED visits for headache.

This gender disparity is much more significant than that seen for all ED visits: overall, women are only 1.2 times more likely to present to the ED for any reason [1]. The majority of the sex difference is likely due to migraine, which accounts for a large proportion of ED headache visits and has a well-established female predominance.

Young adults, aged 18 to 44 years, constitute the most common age demographic presenting to the ED with headache. Again, the age pattern mirrors the epidemiology of migraine, which is most prevalent among young adults. Children and adolescents appear to visit the ED much less frequently than the other age groups, at a rate of 345 per 100,000 individuals compared to 1626 per 100,000 individuals age 18 to 44 years [1].

There appears to be an inverse relationship between income and ED visits for headache, at least in the United States. People in the lowest income bracket have the most ED visits for headache, and with each income bracket the proportion of ED visits for headache decreases, with those in the highest income bracket having the lowest proportion of ED visits for headache. This trend is reflective of the relationship between income and ED visits of all causes [1]. Given that the data originate from the United States, the trend might reflect important differences in health insurance based on income, and ensuing differential access to healthcare services in the community.

Interestingly, among primary headache patients, a small proportion of patients account for a large proportion of ED visits. In one study, 50 percent of the ED visits for primary headache occurred among only 10 percent of the patients. These patients had a high prevalence of acute headache medication overuse (MO), with opioids being the most commonly used medication in this subset of patients with frequent ED visits [9]. Therefore, there is a small proportion of primary headache patients that use a disproportionate amount of ED health services. Also, MO is associated with more frequent ED visits among patients with primary headaches [9].

## Other Factors Affecting Trends of Emergency Department Visits for Headache

Environmental factors are known to impact the trend of visits to the ED for headache.

Studies based in Canada have demonstrated a robust association between air pollution and visits to the ED for headache. One study carried out in five different Canadian cities found an association between higher concentrations of air pollutants, such as nitrogen oxide and particulate matter, and ED visits for headache [10]. The same group also found an association between sulfur dioxide levels and visits to the ED for migraine in Vancouver [11], as well as associations between multiple air pollutants and ED visits for headache in Edmonton [12] and Ottawa [13]. The pathophysiology linking air pollution with increased incidence of headache is poorly understood. It is possible that air pollutants trigger neurogenic dural inflammation among migraine patients, but this association is purely speculative [10].

Seasonal variation in the incidence of ED visits for headache has been well documented. In a US-based study, ED visits for headache among all age groups were highest from June to September, with the lowest rates being in February and December [1]. A different pattern has been observed in the pediatric setting after exclusion of most severe secondary headache etiologies. In children and adolescents, the lowest proportion of visits appears to occur during the summer months [14,15], with the highest proportion of visits observed during the first few months of the academic year, from September to November [14] and in January [15]. The pattern displayed among pediatric patients is likely heavily influenced by the primary headache disorders, when the frequency of headaches is typically higher during the academic year. This likely relates to the role of stress in triggering migraine and tension-type headache. The peak in January could relate to viral season and a higher incidence of headache secondary to viral illness.

## Causes of Emergency Department Visits for Headache

The determination of headache etiology requires one to differentiate between primary and secondary headaches. Primary headaches are very common, both in the clinic setting as well as in the ED. However, due to the life-threatening nature of some secondary headaches, there has been a disproportionate focus on management algorithms for suspected secondary headaches in the ED, despite the fact that, at least in the adult population, primary headaches account for the majority of ED visits for headache.

In the pediatric literature, studies have differed significantly in their findings on the distribution of headache etiologies across different EDs. Pediatric ED studies have shown that 10.0–56.7 percent of headache visits are accounted for by primary headaches, with the majority being due to migraine or unspecified primary headache [16–19]. Of the secondary headaches, most appear to be due to minor infections. Anywhere from 28.5 to 60.4 percent of headaches in the pediatric ED can be explained by minor infections

[16–21], with viral infections and upper respiratory tract infections predominating. Neurologic causes of headache, such as brain tumor, meningitis, and cerebrovascular disease, occur in 6–45.2 percent of cases, with the higher estimates stemming from studies that included post-traumatic headache in this category [16–21]. These estimates of the various headache etiologies all share a large amount of imprecision, which is likely explained by differences in study design, selection bias in the studies, diagnostic errors leading to headache misclassification, and geographic variations. Figure 2.2 illustrates the distribution of headache etiologies uncovered from the pediatric studies.

Headache etiologies are considerably different in the adult ED population as compared to the pediatric ED population (Table 2.1 and Figure 2.3). Primary headaches comprise the majority of headaches seen in the adult ED, with anywhere from 32 to 79.3 percent of headaches ultimately attributed to a primary headache disorder [4,5,8,22–24]. The variability in estimates of the proportion of headache visits accounted for by primary headaches is explained by several factors: these studies were conducted in a variety of countries with different healthcare systems and access to care for primary headache patients; the EDs sampled in these studies varied in their setting (i.e., anywhere from academic tertiary care hospitals to primary care health units); the study designs were vulnerable to bias (e.g., selection bias); and random error

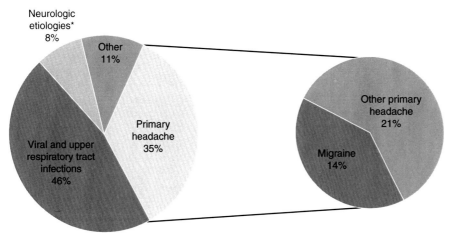

**Figure 2.2** Etiology of headache in the pediatric ED.
* Neurologic etiologies include meningitis, brain tumor, post-traumatic headache, seizure, cerebrovascular diseases and ventriculoperitoneal shunt-related headaches.
** The percentages displayed were generated by pooling together results from the referenced studies [16–21].

**Table 2.1** Table of studies assessing headache etiology in the adult ED

| Parameter | Dermitzakis et al., 2010 [4] | Bigal et al., 2000 [8] | Fodden et al., 1989 [5] | Leicht, 1980 [22] | Locker, 2004 [23] | Luda et al., 1995 [24] |
|---|---|---|---|---|---|---|
| Location of ED | Greece | Brazil | England | United States | England | Italy |
| Number of patients | 851 | 561 | 130 | 485 | 353 | 215 |
| All primary headaches (%) | 77.9 | 55.6 | 32 | 54.5 | 79.3 | 56 |
| Migraine (%) | 15.4 | 45.1 | 19 | 22.3 | 30 | 28.8 |
| Tension-type headache (%) | 33.6 | 7.3 | 13 | 32.2 | 14.7 | 24.6 |
| Cluster headache (%) | 1.2 | – | – | – | 1.7 | 2.8 |
| Primary headache not specified (%) | 27.7 | – | 26 | – | 32.9 | – |
| All secondary headaches (%) | 22.1 | 44.3 | 31.5 | 38.1 | 18.4 | 43.7 |
| Secondary systemic causes (%) | – | 39.4 | 26 | 32.6 | 13 | 15.8 |
| Secondary neurologic causes (%) | – | 5 | 15 | 5.5 | 5.4 | 27.9* |
| Severe underlying secondary causes (%)** | – | 2.1 | 13 | 4.5 | 5.4 | 8.4 |
| Other (%) | – | – | – | 7.4 | 2.3 | – |

*  Includes post-traumatic headaches.
** Comprised a variety of different disease processes in each study, including but not limited to: intracerebral hemorrhage, subarachnoid hemorrhage, brain tumors, brain abscesses, and meningitis.

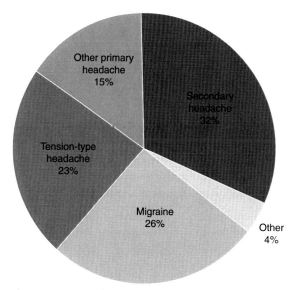

**Figure 2.3** Etiology of headache in the adult ED.
* The percentages displayed were generated by pooling together results from the referenced studies [4,5,8,22–24].

being relatively rare, accounting for less than 3 percent of all ED visits for headache. Secondary systemic causes are less common than in the pediatric population. Neurologic causes account for 5–15 percent of headache cases [4,5,8,22,23], with a higher percentage resulting when post-traumatic headaches are included in this category. Approximately 2.1–13 percent of adult patients presenting to the ED with headache have a serious underlying secondary etiology, such as meningitis, intracranial hemorrhage, or elevated intracranial pressure [5]. A detailed breakdown of headache etiology for each study is provided in Table 2.1. In Figure 2.3, results from the studies were pooled to generate estimates of the proportions for each headache category.

A common phenomenon related to classifying headaches in the ED deserves mention. There is a tendency to label a large proportion of primary headache patients with a diagnosis of "headache not otherwise specified." In one large academic center in the United States, 73.2 percent of patients presenting to the ED with a primary headache received a discharge diagnosis of headache not otherwise specified. Those patients were more likely to be given opioids, and the administration of opioids was associated with longer lengths of stay [25]. Although most estimates of the proportion of patients diagnosed with headache not otherwise

likely also accounts for a proportion of the differences. Of the primary headaches in the ED, migraine is the most common, with tension-type headache accounting for a significant proportion and cluster headache specified have been lower, it appears that at least one-third of primary headaches in the ED are ultimately given this ambiguous label [4,5,23]. Although it can be challenging, ED clinicians should always strive to make a specific headache diagnosis, as identifying the specific headache disorder is more likely to lead to more specific and optimal management and outcomes.

# Frequency of ED Visits Among Patients with Primary Headache Disorders

## Frequency of ED Visits Among Patients with Migraine

Patients with migraine commonly present to the ED and are more likely to use ED services than the general population. Migraine patients from a US health maintenance organization were more likely than controls to have visited an ED in the past 12 months (20.7 percent vs. 17.6 percent) [26]. In addition, although tension-type headache is more prevalent, migraine accounts for a larger proportion of ED visits for headache (see Figure 2.3) and patients with migraine are much more likely to present to the ED than those with tension-type headache [27]. This very likely reflects the higher pain intensity associated with migraine, but may also be related to other factors such as the relatively lower socioeconomic status of migraine patients and the higher prevalence of psychiatric comorbidities among migraine patients as compared to patients with tension-type headache.

It is difficult to obtain precise estimates regarding the proportion of migraine patients that use the ED for migraine, and the numbers vary considerably from country to country. A study of resource utilization in a cross-sectional sample of European migraine patients demonstrated that 2–16 percent of the cohort had visited the ED in the past three months, with the frequency varying based on country of residence [28]. Other studies have found that Canada, the United States, and Australia have a higher proportion of migraine patients using ED services relative to European countries [29], and that Latin American countries tend to exceed North American countries in terms of the proportion of migraine patients using ED services [30]. The precise reasons for the country-to-country variability are unknown, but likely reflect significant differences in healthcare access and the structure of healthcare systems between the countries.

For example, migraine patients residing in the United States appear to be less likely to have visited a primary care provider for migraine, but more likely to have used the ED for migraine care as compared to migraine patients in other countries [29]. Therefore, in some instances the ED may be utilized as a replacement for primary care when access is limited. This is corroborated by findings suggesting that uninsured US migraine patients receive a greater proportion of their migraine care in the ED as compared to their insured counterparts [31].

Several factors impact the likelihood of ED use among migraine patients. These factors are described in detail in Chapter 7. Briefly, patients with a more severe baseline headache disorder [27], those with chronic migraine [27], those with a history of opioid use [32], those using the ED frequently for other health conditions [27], those with low socioeconomic status [27] and those with psychiatric comorbidities [33] are more likely to visit the ED for migraine. Dissatisfaction with outpatient migraine treatment appears to be another predictor of more frequent ED visits [34]. The use of migraine prophylactic medications [35] and triptans [36] is inversely related to the frequency of ED visits for migraine. In one study, the addition of migraine prophylactic medications to a regimen of sumatriptan for acute migraine relief resulted in an 81.8 percent decrease in ED migraine visits [35].

## Frequency of ED Visits Among Patients with Tension-Type Headache

There are less data to describe and characterize the ED presence of tension-type headache. As described above, patients with tension-type headache use the ED less frequently for headache management than their counterparts with migraine. Data from the American Migraine Prevalence and Prevention Study (AMPP) found that, among a US cohort of severe headache sufferers, only 3 percent of the patients with episodic tension-type headache had visited the ED in the past year, as compared to 7.3 percent of the patients with episodic migraine. When comparing the two groups of episodic headache patients, those with tension-type headache were 60 percent less likely to have visited the ED in the past year as compared to those with migraine (OR = 0.4, 95 percent CI 0.3–0.6) [27]. This 3 percent figure likely overestimates the actual proportion of episodic tension-type headache patients using the ED, given that the AMPP study was restricted to patients who self-reported severe head-ache, thereby excluding a large proportion of patients with less severe tension-type headaches.

## Frequency of ED Visits Among Patients with Cluster Headache

Cluster headache is a rare primary headache disorder. It appears to account for between 1.2 percent and 2.8 percent of all ED visits for headache [4,23,24]. Therefore, the proportion of cluster headache patients visiting the ED appears to be significant given its comparatively low prevalence in the general population at 0.07–0.4 percent [37]. Cluster headache patients use off-hours healthcare services, including the ED, much more frequently than the general population [38]. No data are available to show the relative propensity for cluster headache patients to use the ED as compared to patients with other primary headache disorders. However, it is possible that if one were to compare cluster headache to the other primary headaches, one would find that these patients have higher ED use, given the severity of the pain intensity and suffering associated with a cluster attack.

## Healthcare Costs and Resource Utilization Associated with ED Visits for Headache

### Use of Neuroimaging in Patients Visiting the ED for Headache

The overuse of neuroimaging among patients visiting the ED for headache has been extensively investigated. Inappropriate CT and MRI scans are costly to the healthcare system, and excessive CT use exposes patients to unnecessary risks due to ionizing radiation.

In the ED, the use of neuroimaging in the diagnostic evaluation of headache is increasing. Concurrently, the yield of neuroimaging in identifying cases with intracranial pathology appears to be decreasing. One study, carried out in the United States, reported that the proportion of ED headache patients undergoing neuroimaging increased from 12.5 percent to 31 percent over a ten-year period, whereas the proportion of neuroimaging studies uncovering pathology dropped from 10.1 percent to 3.5 percent over the same period [39]. Another US study examined the use of CT among adult patients presenting to the ED

with non-focal, atraumatic headaches without neurological symptoms, immunocompromised status, nor prior history of neurosurgery. In this group of patients, although 31.9 percent had abnormal CT findings, the vast majority were incidental and did not alter management, with only 1.02 percent resulting in management changes. The mean cost of each ED headache visit was $764 when accounting for the cost of CT. The authors compared this with the cost of an outpatient visit for headache of similar presentation, and found that the ED cost was triple the cost of an outpatient visit [40].

This trend has also been observed in pediatrics. In another US study, the proportion of children and adolescents undergoing CT head imaging for headache increased significantly from 1995 to 2008, with an initial rate of 11.6 percent and a final rate of 27.4 percent [41]. In a Canadian study that retrospectively assessed visits to a tertiary care pediatric neurology clinic for headache, 34 percent of the children and adolescents with normal neurologic exams had received CT scans of the head prior to referral. Of those patients, almost one-quarter had their CT scans ordered in the ED, suggesting a relatively high rate of unnecessary CTs in that setting [42].

Given the significant cost associated with neuroimaging, and given the risks associated with CT scans, it is concerning that a large proportion of patients presenting to the ED with headache are undergoing inappropriate neuroimaging. Advocating increased adherence to evidence-based neuroimaging guidelines could result in significant cost savings and reduced exposure to ionizing radiation in this patient population.

### Consultations for Patients Visiting the ED with Headache

Although the majority of patients presenting to the ED with headache are managed exclusively by ED physicians, the cost associated with consultations to specialists is substantial. Neurologists providing consultation services in the ED are very familiar with headache consultations. In a study carried out in Italy, headache was the second most common reason for neurological consultation in the ED, representing 22 percent of all ED consultations to neurology [43]. Migraine patients were seen by consultants 7.7 percent of the time in a US-based study, with neurology consultations accounting for the greatest proportion [44]. Therefore, apart from the cost of ED physician consultation, which represents one of the greatest overall costs associated with headache in the ED, consultant fees are also important to consider when calculating the economic burden of headache in this setting, though focusing exclusively on the immediate additional cost of involving a consultant could be misleading, as consultations may lead to cost savings in other forms (e.g., reduced use of neuroimaging and reduced return visits due to improved outpatient follow-up care).

## Disposition of Patients Visiting the ED for Headache

Although ED visits for headache are very common, they are less likely to result in admission than other types of ED visits. The vast majority of patients visiting the ED for headache are discharged home. In one US-based study, 82.3 percent of all patients visiting the ED were ultimately discharged. Among those with headache as the chief complaint, the ED visit resulted in discharge 97 percent of the time. Patients with migraine were more likely to be admitted than patients with other causes of headache: Whereas visits for headache of any cause resulted in admission in 2.4 percent of cases, visits for migraine lead to admission in 3.6 percent of cases. Women were 2.6 times more likely to be admitted for headache than men. Among patients admitted for headache, the proportion of women was higher and the mean age was lower compared to all inpatients [1]. These demographic characteristics reflect the epidemiology of migraine, given the high proportion of inpatient headache admissions due to migraine.

The cost of inpatient admissions for headache in the United States totaled $408 million in 2008. The average headache admission was shorter when compared to all admissions, with an average length of stay of 2.7 days, compared to 4.6 days for all admissions. Therefore, the total cost for headache admissions is less relative to other admissions. However, the cost per day appears to be equivalent, with headache admissions costing an average of $1900 per day and other admissions costing $2000 per day [1].

## Economic Burden of Primary Headaches in the ED

### Economics of Migraine in the ED

Migraine is prevalent in the ED and is associated with significant ED costs and resource utilization.

The annual cost of migraine care in the ED has been estimated at $520 million [45]. One relatively recent US study showed that the average cost of an ED visit for migraine totaled $1799 per patient, excluding the cost of transportation and radiologist fees [44]. Migraine patients in the general US population appear to have higher ED costs compared to controls without migraine [45,46]. However, in a US study carried out in 1998, the cost of individual ED visits was similar for migraine patients and patients visiting the ED for other reasons [47]. This may no longer be true, especially given the increasing use of neuroimaging, which could conceivably inflate the cost of an ED visit for migraine relative to other ED visits.

Use of the ED and ensuing costs vary considerably between migraine patients. In one study comparing the cost of healthcare utilization in an outpatient population of episodic and chronic migraine patients, the average cost of ED use in the past three months was $22 per chronic migraine patient and $29 per episodic migraine patient in the United States, and $78 per chronic migraine patient and $12 per episodic migraine patient in Canada [48]. Overall, patients with chronic migraine have higher total healthcare costs and also use more ED resources.

Although unnecessary in a sizable number of cases, a substantial proportion of migraine patients undergo neuroimaging in the ED. In one US study, 23 percent of migraine patients visiting the ED had a neuroimaging study, with 89 percent of those studies considered justified based on the indication documented in the chart. Patients who had imaging also had longer ED stays, with an average of two hours added to the length of stay among those who had imaging [44]. Therefore, although there are certainly several scenarios in which it is necessary to order neuroimaging in a migraine patient presenting to the ED, it is important that clinicians be judicious in ordering imaging studies in patients presenting to the ED with their typical migraine and the absence of red flags, given the associated cost and prolongation of length of stay.

### Economics of Other Primary Headache Disorders in the ED

Health resource utilization and cost of care are less well understood among primary headache disorders other than migraine. Migraine is associated with higher direct and indirect costs as compared to tension-type headache [49]. It is expected that ED costs for tension-type headache would also be significantly less both at the individual and societal level as compared to migraine, but this has not been well addressed in the literature. Conversely, healthcare costs associated with cluster headache are believed to be higher than those associated with migraine [50]. Because of the severity of cluster headache, its clinical features that mimic some severe secondary headaches and because of its relatively high prevalence in the ED as compared to its prevalence in the population, cluster headache is likely associated with higher ED costs and resource utilization for each patient as compared to migraine.

## Methods to Reduce the Costs and Resource Utilization Associated with Primary Headache in the ED

Severe modifiable factors related to outpatient management are associated with more frequent ED use among patients with primary headaches. These issues have been studied primarily among migraine patients, and the case of migraine is therefore the most illustrative. Patients with severe baseline migraine and those with chronic daily headache are most likely to use ED services [27]. Given that the appropriate outpatient management of migraine can result in reduced migraine severity and transition from chronic to episodic migraine, it is expected that it would also reduce the burden of migraine in the ED. Therefore, patients presenting to the ED with migraine require close follow-up and management in the community. Emergency department physicians should strongly consider referring primary headache patients to community care providers if they are not already being appropriately managed in the community.

It has also been shown that migraine patients using opioids have more frequent ED visits than opioid-naïve patients [32], a trend that is likely to be present across primary headache disorders. In addition, at least in the case of migraine, those receiving opioids appear to have worse short-term outcomes, with higher rates of return ED visits for headache within a week of discharge [51]. Community practitioners and ED physicians should therefore strive to avoid opioid use in patients with primary headache, especially given that opioids lack efficacy in this population and

can lead to short-term and long-term harm. Reducing opioid use among primary headache patients would very likely reduce the burden of headache not only in the ED but across the healthcare system.

Migraine patients using triptans [36] and preventive medications [35] on an outpatient basis are less likely to seek ED care for their migraines. It has been shown, in a retrospective database analysis, that the addition of preventive medications to the migraine treatment regimen can result in a significant decrease in the frequency of ED visits for migraine [35]. Therefore, community and ED providers should ensure that appropriate migraine-specific therapies are prescribed both for acute and preventive migraine management.

Psychiatric comorbidities are prevalent among patients with primary headache disorders. Patients with both migraine and psychiatric comorbidities are more likely to visit the ED compared to those with either migraine or psychiatric disorders alone [33]. Both community care providers and ED physicians have the opportunity to improve the management of psychiatric comorbidity in patients with primary headaches by screening for these disorders and ensuring appropriate management plans and referrals are in place. It is plausible that improved management of psychiatric comorbidities among patients with primary headaches could result in a lower headache burden in the ED and other areas of healthcare.

In addition to these strategies, improved access to patient health information is likely to reduce the cost of ED visits for headache. Health information exchange constitutes the sharing of patient health information across care providers within a geographic region. In one study, health information exchange resulted in better care and decreased resource utilization in a sample of patients presenting to the ED with primary headaches. Health information exchange use by ED providers resulted in fewer unwarranted imaging studies and improved adherence to evidence-based guidelines for the use of diagnostic neuroimaging in patients presenting to the ED with headache [52]. Therefore, several modifiable factors may help to prevent ED visits in migraine patients: optimal outpatient care; reduced reliance on opioids; improved outpatient migraine-specific acute and preventive management; management of psychiatric comorbidities; and improved information sharing between practitioners (Figure 2.4).

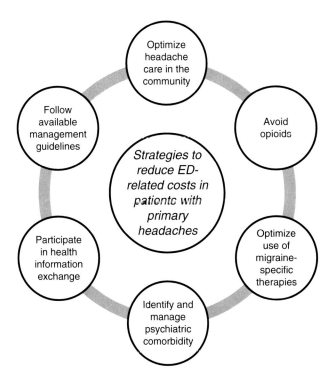

**Figure 2.4** Strategies to reduce ED resource utilization and costs in patients with primary headache.

## Summary

Headaches are among the most common chief complaints in the ED. Gender, socioeconomic status, age, and even environmental factors such as air pollution levels influence the likelihood of ED visits for headache. Although secondary headache etiologies must always be considered and are relatively common, primary headaches do account for a large proportion of ED visits due to headache. The cost associated with visiting the ED for headache is considerable, and appears to be increasing, at least in part due to increased use of neuroimaging in this setting. Although it is a common and expensive presentation, several strategies, primarily based on improved outpatient care, may help to reduce the burden of primary headache in the ED.

## References

1. Lucado J, Paez K, Elixhauser A. Headaches in US Hospitals and Emergency Departments, 2008: Statistical Brief #111. *Healthcare Cost and Utilization Project (HCUP) Statistical Briefs*. 2011;24:1–12.

2. Barton CW. Evaluation and treatment of headache patients in the emergency department: a survey. *Headache*. 1994;34(2):91–4.

3. Smitherman TA, Burch R, Sheikh H, Loder E. The prevalence, impact, and treatment of migraine and severe headaches in the United States: a review of statistics from national surveillance studies. *Headache*. 2013;53(3):427–36.

4. Dermitzakis EV, Georgiadis G, Rudolf J, et al. Headache patients in the emergency department of a Greek tertiary care hospital. *J Headache Pain*. 2010;11(2):123–8.

5. Fodden D, Peatfield R, Milsom P. Beware the patient with a headache in the accident and emergency department. *Emerg Med J*. 1989;6(1):7–12.

6. De Carli GF, Fabbri L, Cavazzuti L, et al. The epidemiology of migraine: a retrospective study in Italian emergency departments. *Headache*. 1998;38(9):697–704.

7. Cerbo R, Villani V, Bruti G, Di SF, Mostardini C. Primary headache in emergency department: prevalence, clinical features and therapeutical approach. *J Headache Pain*. 2005;6(4):287–9.

8. Bigal ME, Bordini CA, Speciali JG. Etiology and distribution of headaches in two Brazilian primary care units. *Headache*. 2000;40(3):241–7.

9. Maizels M. Health resource utilization of the emergency department headache "repeater." *Headache*. 2002;42(8):747–53.

10. Szyszkowicz M, Kaplan GG, Grafstein E, Rowe BH. Emergency department visits for migraine and headache: a multi-city study. *Int J Occup Med Environ Health*. 2009;22(3):235–42.

11. Szyszkowicz M, Rowe BH, Kaplan GG. Ambient sulphur dioxide exposure and emergency department visits for migraine in Vancouver, Canada. *Int J Occup Med Environ Health*. 2009;22(1):7–12.

12. Szyszkowicz M, Stieb DM, Rowe BH. Air pollution and daily ED visits for migraine and headache in Edmonton, Canada. *Am J Emerg Med*. 2009;27(4):391–6.

13. Szyszkowicz M. Ambient air pollution and daily emergency department visits for headache in Ottawa, Canada. *Headache*. 2008;48(7):1076–81.

14. Caperell K, Pitetti R. Seasonal variation of presentation for headache in a pediatric emergency department. *Pediatr Emerg Care*. 2014;30(3):174–6.

15. Kedia S, Ginde AA, Grubenhoff JA, et al. Monthly variation of United States pediatric headache emergency department visits. *Cephalalgia*. 2014;34(6):473–8.

16. Kan L, Nagelberg J, Maytal J. Headaches in a pediatric emergency department: etiology, imaging, and treatment. *Headache*. 2000;40(1):25–9.

17. Conicella E, Raucci U, Vanacore N, et al. The child with headache in a pediatric emergency department. *Headache*. 2008;48(7):1005–11.

18. Scagni P, Pagliero R. Headache in an Italian pediatric emergency department. *J Headache Pain*. 2008;9(2):83–7.

19. Hsiao HJ, Huang JL, Hsia SH, et al. Headache in the pediatric emergency service: a medical center experience. *Pediatr Neonatol*. 2014;55(3):208–12.

20. Burton LJ, Quinn B, Pratt-Cheney JL, Pourani M. Headache etiology in a pediatric emergency department. *Pediatr Emerg Care*. 1997;13(1):1–4.

21. Schobitz E, Qureshi F, Lewis D. Pediatric headaches in the emergency department. *Curr Pain Headache Rep*. 2006;10(5):391–6.

22. Leicht MJ. Non-traumatic headache in the emergency department. *Ann Emerg Med*. 1980;9(8):404–9.

23. Locker T. Headache management: are we doing enough? An observational study of patients presenting with headache to the emergency department. *Emerg Med J*. 2004;21(3):327–32.

24. Luda E, Comitangelo R, Sicuro L. The symptom of headache in emergency departments: the experience of a neurology emergency department. *Ital J Neurol Sci*. 1995;16(4):295–301.

25. McCarthy LH, Cowan RP. Comparison of parenteral treatments of acute primary headache in a large academic emergency department cohort. *Cephalalgia*. 2015;35(9):807–15.

26. Lafata JE, Moon C, Leotta C, et al. The medical care utilization and costs associated with migraine headache. *J Gen Intern Med*. 2004;19(10):1005–12.

27. Friedman BW, Serrano D, Reed M, Diamond M, Lipton RB. Use of the emergency department for severe headache: a population-based study. *Headache*. 2009;49(1):21–30.

28. Bloudek LM, Stokes M, Buse DC, et al. Cost of healthcare for patients with migraine in five European countries: results from the International Burden of Migraine Study (IBMS). *J Headache Pain*. 2012;13(5):361–78.

29. Sanderson JC, Devine EB, Lipton RB, et al. Headache-related health resource utilisation in chronic and episodic migraine across six countries. *J Neurol Neurosurg Psychiatry*. 2013;84(12):1309–17.

30. Gerth WC, Carides GW, Dasbach EJ, Visser WH, Santanello NC. The multinational impact of migraine symptoms on healthcare utilisation and work loss. *Pharmacoeconomics*. 2001;19(2):197–206.

31. Wilper A, Woolhandler S, Himmelstein D, Nardin R. Impact of insurance status on migraine care in the United States: a population-based study. *Neurology*. 2010;74(15):1178–83.

32. Buse DC, Pearlman SH, Reed ML, et al. Opioid use and dependence among persons with migraine: results of the AMPP study. *Headache*. 2012;52(1):18–36.

33. Minen MT, Tanev K. Influence of psychiatric comorbidities in migraineurs in the emergency department. *Gen Hosp Psychiatry*. 2014;36(5):533–8.

34. Lipton RB, Buse DC, Serrano D, Holland S, Reed ML. Examination of unmet treatment needs among persons with episodic migraine: results of the American Migraine Prevalence and Prevention (AMPP) Study. *Headache*. 2013;53(8):1300–11.

35. Silberstein SD, Winner PK, Chmiel JJ. Migraine preventive medication reduces resource utilization. *Headache*. 2003;43(3):171–8.

36. Lainez MJA. The effect of migraine prophylaxis on migraine-related resource use and productivity. *CNS Drugs*. 2009;23(9):727–38.

37. Russell M. Genetic epidemiology of migraine and cluster headache. *Cephalalgia*. 1997;17:683–701.

38. Jensen RM, Lyngberg A, Jensen RH. Burden of cluster headache. *Cephalalgia*. 2007;27(6):535–41.

39. Gilbert JW, Johnson KM, Larkin GL, Moore CL. Atraumatic headache in US emergency departments: recent trends in CT/MRI utilisation and factors associated with severe intracranial pathology. *Emerg Med J*. 2012;29(7):576–81.

40. Jordan YJ, Lightfoote JB, Jordan JE. Computed tomography imaging in the management of headache in the emergency department: cost efficacy and policy implications. *J Natl Med Assoc.* 2009;101(4):331–5.

41. Larson DB, Johnson LW, Schnell BM, et al. Rising use of CT in child visits to the emergency department in the United States, 1995–2008. *Radiology.* 2011;259(3):793–801.

42. Gandhi R, Lewis E, Evans J, Sell E. Investigating the necessity of computed tomographic scans in children with headaches: a retrospective review. *CJEM.* 2014;16:33–8.

43. de Falco FA, Sterzi R, Toso V, et al. The neurologist in the emergency department: an Italian nationwide epidemiological survey. *Neurol Sci.* 2008;29(2):67–75.

44. Friedman D, Feldon S, Holloway R, Fisher S. Utilization, diagnosis, treatment and cost of migraine treatment in the emergency department. *Headache.* 2009;49(8):1163–73.

45. Hawkins K, Wang S, Rupnow M. Direct cost burden among insured US employees with migraine. *Headache.* 2008;48(4):553–63.

46. Edmeads J, Mackell JA. The economic impact of migraine: an analysis of direct and indirect costs. *Headache.* 2002;42(6):501–9.

47. Joish VN, Cady PS, Shaw JW. Health care utilization by migraine patients: a 1998 Medicaid population study. *Clin Ther.* 2000;22(11):1346–56.

48. Stokes M, Becker WJ, Lipton RB, et al. Cost of health care among patients with chronic and episodic migraine in Canada and the USA: results from the International Burden of Migraine Study (IBMS). *Headache.* 2011;51(7):1058–77.

49. Linde M, Gustavsson A, Stovner LJ, et al. The cost of headache disorders in Europe: the Eurolight project. *Eur J Neurol.* 2012;19(5):703–11.

50. Gaul C, Finken J, Biermann J, et al. Treatment costs and indirect costs of cluster headache: a health economics analysis. *Cephalalgia.* 2011;31(16):1664–72.

51. Colman I, Rothney A, Wright S, Zilkalns B, Rowe BH. Use of narcotic analgesics in the emergency department treatment of migraine headache. *Neurology.* 2004;62(10):1695–700.

52. Bailey JE, Wan JY, Mabry LM, et al. Does health information exchange reduce unnecessary neuroimaging and improve quality of headache care in the emergency department? *J Gen Intern Med.* 2013;28(2):176–83.

# Approach to History Taking and the Physical Examination

Suzanne Christie
Garth Dickinson

## Abstract

The majority of patients presenting to the emergency department (ED) have non-life-threatening primary headaches such as migraine, tension-type, or cluster headache. It is important to differentiate this group from the smaller number of patients with a secondary headache disorder, which can be serious with potentially fatal outcomes.

A careful history and physical examination is the most important part of the evaluation of the patient presenting to the ED with headache. This helps to determine whether there is a significant risk for secondary headache and whether additional investigations are needed.

This chapter discusses how to approach adults who present to the ED with headache, with an emphasis on determining elements of the history indicative of an underlying secondary cause as well as important questions to ask patients presenting with a primary headache disorder. In addition, key elements of the general medical and neurological examination will be reviewed.

## Approach to the History

When it comes to headache patients, the history is the most important source of information for the physician. It is the history that allows a physician to determine risk for serious secondary headaches and to assign a primary headache diagnosis. Time spent up-front obtaining a meticulous headache history will ultimately save time and money by allowing the physician to avoid unnecessary testing. For patients with a typical exacerbation of a known headache disorder, a brief, focused history is sufficient. For patients with a new headache type, a complete history, detailed below, is more important. The detailed history will allow the physician to determine the need for diagnostic testing, point toward a specific

diagnosis, and form the basis for individualized management.

## General Outline of the History

To begin, the physician should determine why the patient has presented to the ED. Is it because he/she can no longer tolerate their usual headaches or is this a new headache? If it is a new headache, is it a first severe headache or is it sufficiently different from the usual headache that the patient is concerned enough to seek help [1]?

In addition to these initial questions, the elements of the history include the following, which will allow the physician to gauge risk of a serious secondary cause and help to render a specific diagnosis:

1. the age of the patient;
2. location of the pain;
3. quality of the pain (throbbing, pressure, severity);
4. onset of the pain (gradual vs. sudden);
5. associated symptoms (nausea, vomiting, photophobia, phonophobia, neck pain, fever);
6. associated neurological symptoms (visual change, numbness, tingling, focal paresis, vertigo, speech change, gait change, personality change, cognitive change, fluctuating level of consciousness or loss of consciousness);
7. current treatment;
8. previous treatment;
9. trigger (exercise, cough, strain, sex);
10. other present and past medical conditions;
11. family history;
12. social history including habits such as caffeine intake, alcohol, illicit drugs, and smoking;
13. review of systems (weight loss, night sweats, chills, myalgias, cough, shortness of breath, abdominal pain, change in bowel movements, urinary symptoms).

## Questions Pertaining to Suspected Primary Headaches

ED patients with recurrent headaches usually have a primary headache disorder. Most commonly, recurrent headaches will be migraine, tension-type headache, or cluster headache. The emergency physician should determine whether the headache description is consistent with the various primary headache diagnoses.

Migraine is a recurrent headache disorder lasting 4–72 hours. At least five attacks meeting pain and associated symptom criteria must have already occurred for the diagnosis to be made. The headache pain of migraine must include at least two of: unilateral location, throbbing quality, moderate to severe intensity, and aggravation by routine physical activity. In addition, patients must experience either nausea or vomiting or photophobia *and* phonophobia. It is important to remember that these features, while very sensitive for the presence of migraine, are very non-specific. Many sinister secondary causes of headache (e.g., arterial dissection, subarachnoid hemorrhage) may meet the headache and associated symptom criteria for migraine. Migraine can be either episodic (<15 days per month) or chronic (≥15 days per month, of which at least eight days meet the criteria for migraine or respond to a migraine-specific therapy, including triptans or ergotamine) [2].

Migraine occurs with or without aura. Aura consists of unilateral fully reversible visual, sensory, language, motor, or brainstem symptoms that generally develop gradually and are usually followed by headache and associated migraine symptoms. Each aura symptom onsets over at least five minutes and/or two or more symptoms occur in succession. Each aura symptom should last 5–60 minutes and the headache should follow within 60 minutes [2].

Visual aura is the most common type of aura, occurring in over 90 percent of patients. It often presents as a fortification spectrum: a zigzag figure near the point of fixation that may gradually spread right or left and assume a laterally convex shape with an angulated scintillating edge, leaving absolute or variable degrees of relative scotoma in its wake [2].

Next in frequency are sensory disturbances, in the form of pins and needles moving slowly from the point of origin and affecting a greater or smaller part of one side of the hand/arm, face, and/or tongue. Numbness may occur in its wake, but numbness may also be the only symptom [2].

Less frequent are speech disturbances; usually a form of aphasia occurs but it is often challenging to categorize [2].

Tension-type headaches last between 30 minutes and seven days. The features of tension-type headaches include at least two of: bilateral location, pressing or tightening (non-pulsating) quality, mild or moderate intensity, or not aggravated by routine physical activity. There is no associated nausea or vomiting and no more than one of photophobia or phonophobia. Tension-type headache can also be episodic (<15 days per month) or chronic (≥15 days per month) [2].

In the case of cluster headaches, attacks occur in series (daily or near-daily attacks) lasting for weeks or months (so called cluster periods), separated by remission periods usually lasting months or years. About 10–15 percent of patients have chronic cluster headache – at least one year of cluster headaches without a remission period lasting longer than one month [2]. Cluster headaches comprise attacks of severe, strictly unilateral pain which is orbital, supraorbital, temporal, or in any combination of these sites, lasting 15–180 minutes and occurring from once every other day to eight times per day. The pain is associated with ipsilateral conjunctival injection, lacrimation, nasal congestion, rhinorrhea, forehead and facial sweating, miosis, ptosis, and/or eyelid edema, and frequently accompanied by restlessness or agitation [2].

If there are any atypical features when taking a history from the patient who can no longer tolerate their usual headaches, it is imperative that the clinician considers a more serious underlying cause. Similarly, if it is a new headache or a headache that is sufficiently different from the usual headaches, it is also necessary to determine if this may be due to a serious underlying cause.

## Questions Pertaining to Suspected Secondary Headaches

The following are historical features of concern that should raise the clinician's suspicion for a secondary headache.

### The Presence of Systemic Symptoms, Illness, or Condition

The clinician should inquire about symptoms of infection that could potentially arise in the context of meningitis or of a cerebral abscess. Fever, night sweats, chills, malaise, lethargy, or rash are examples of symptoms that may indicate the presence of an underlying infection.

The use of medications such as anticoagulants, aspirin, or sympathomimetics could cause intracranial hemorrhage (ICH). Similarly, the use of illicit drugs such as cocaine and methamphetamine may also cause ICH or stroke [3,4].

Pregnancy can give rise to headaches as a result of pre-eclampsia/eclampsia, which can lead to hypertensive encephalopathy and/or posterior reversible encephalopathy syndrome (PRES) [5]. In addition, pregnancy and the puerperium carry an increased risk of cerebral venous sinus thrombosis (CVST) [6].

An active or history of malignancy and a new-onset headache or change in pattern from a preexisting headache disorder can arise from intracranial metastases with or without ICH, from ischemic stroke, or from CVST given the associated hypercoagulable state [7].

The use of immunosuppression drugs or diseases which compromise immune system function such as HIV may result in intracranial disease such as toxoplasmosis, stroke, brain abscess, meningitis, and malignancy of the central nervous system [8,9].

### The Presence of Neurological Symptoms

It is important to differentiate migraine aura from other neurological symptoms, as some medical conditions can produce symptoms that mimic migraine aura. These include stroke and transient ischemic attack (TIA), seizure disorders, tumors, CVST, arteriovenous malformation, and carotid artery dissection. Clinicians are commonly faced with the need to differentiate migraine aura from TIA. Migraine aura onsets gradually compared with TIAs, which are sudden in onset. Visual symptoms in aura are often positive, that is, characterized by shapes or structures that are not truly present and more often defined by loss of vision with TIA. Visual TIAs also generally do not gradually spread across the visual field. Sequential progression of aura symptoms is seen in migraine, as opposed to a simultaneous occurrence of symptoms in TIA. Headache is a more common occurrence in migraine but can occur in stroke [10] or transient ischemic attacks. Sensory disturbances associated with TIA do not involve the tongue, may involve the trunk, often involve all body parts (face, arm/hand, leg), do not involve sequential areas of the body (e.g., hand and then face), and do not evolve (sensory disturbances involve several body parts simultaneously) or spread (start in hand and spread up the arm).

A history of personality change, fluctuating level of consciousness, or seizures signals intracranial pathology [11,12] such as a CNS infection (e.g., herpes simplex encephalitis) or a space-occupying lesion.

### Sudden-Onset Severe Headache

Sudden-onset severe headaches are headaches that reach maximal intensity within seconds or minutes. All patients must be questioned about the time taken from onset to maximal intensity – asking the patient whether the onset was sudden is not discriminating enough. All sudden-onset severe headaches require a thorough investigation. An important consideration in the differential diagnosis of these types of headaches includes subarachnoid hemorrhage (SAH). Other etiologies could include reversible cerebral vasoconstriction syndrome, venous sinus thrombosis, pituitary apoplexy, carotid or vertebral artery dissection, hypertensive encephalopathy, colloid cyst of the third ventricle or acute angle-closure glaucoma [13].

### Onset Over Age 50

Although primary headaches including migraine, tension, and cluster headache can onset at any age, they typically do so before the age of 50 [14,15]. Onset of headaches after the age of 50 is still most likely to be a primary headache disorder, but advancing age increases the risk of secondary headaches. Examples of secondary headaches to consider in older patients include giant cell arteritis or intracranial space-occupying lesions [16].

### Progressive Worsening of Headache

Classically, clinicians have been taught to consider space-occupying lesions in patients with progressive headaches, which evolve subacutely and become continuous, with loss of headache-free intervals. However, this classic presentation of tumor-associated headaches may be less common. Intermittent headaches that appear similar to tension-type headache may be more common than constant headaches in patients with underlying tumors [17].

### Postural Component

Headaches worsened by being upright may be due to intracranial hypotension, which may onset spontaneously but may also be post-operative or post-traumatic (e.g., occurring after lumbar puncture) [18].

Conversely, headache worsened by recumbency may be due to increased intracranial pressure as a result of a space-occupying lesion, hydrocephalus, or idiopathic intracranial hypertension. Other symptoms associated with intracranial hypertension include pulsatile tinnitus, horizontal diplopia, and transient visual obscurations.

### Provocative Factors

Headaches precipitated by exertion should compel the clinician to consider the list of diagnoses associated with sudden-onset headache. For example, moderate to extreme physical exertion has been shown to almost triple the odds of subarachnoid hemorrhage within two hours of exercise [19]. In addition, the clinician should consider sinusitis or structural space-occupying lesions in this clinical scenario, such as Chiari malformation, which can cause headache triggered by coughing or straining [20].

### Other

Another important aspect to the history is the family history. For example, patients with a positive family history of SAH may be at increased risk for the development of aneurysms. This may be particularly true in the case of connective tissue disorders such as Ehlers–Danlos syndrome [21]. Polycystic kidney disease is also associated with intracerebral aneurysms [22].

Toxic exposure is also important to consider, particularly during the winter months when carbon monoxide poisoning can occur due to a faulty heating system [23].

Additionally, a history of new-onset headache in the context of head trauma may require additional investigation.

Box 3.1 provides a mnemonic for headache "red flags" [24].

## The Approach to the Physical Exam for Headache in the ED

The focus of the physical exam in the ED patient with headache will be guided by the presenting symptoms, the reason for seeking medical attention, and the overall alertness and mental status of the patient. A rapid assessment of mental status, signs of fever and meningismus, papilledema, and localizing or lateralizing abnormalities is necessary. Presence of these features or thunderclap headache suggesting a serious cause for the headache may require immediate intervention

---

**Box 3.1  Headache "Red Flags" – SNOOP**

**S**ystemic symptoms or illness
1. Fever
2. Anticoagulation
3. Pregnancy
4. Cancer
5. Immunosuppression (HIV infection)

**N**eurologic symptoms or signs
1. Papilledema
2. Asymmetric cranial nerve function
3. Asymmetric motor function
4. Abnormal cerebellar function

**O**nset recently or suddenly
**O**nset after age 50 years
**P**rior Headache History that is different or progressive
1. Progressive headache with loss of headache-free periods
2. Change in type of headache
3. Different location is less useful as predictor of serious cause
4. Pain response to standard headache therapy is not predictive of serious cause

**(Positional component)**
1. Increases when upright
2. Increases when recumbent

**(Provocative factors)**
1. Precipitated by coughing, exercise, sex

---

with therapeutic measures. In the stable patient, a more detailed neurological assessment can be performed while therapeutic and investigational plans are initiated.

The physical exam has two functions: (1) to help refine the differential diagnosis; and (2) to track disease progression. The physical exam should be perceived as a series of diagnostic tests. In stable patients, the history has already allowed the physician to form a differential diagnosis. If the physician is confident that the diagnosis is migraine, only substantial findings on the physical exam, such as persistent motor or speech deficits or papilledema, will alter the post-test probability of that diagnosis. If the physician is less confident in the diagnosis, findings on the physical exam such as sinus tenderness, muscular tightness, or reflex disparities may alter the physician's post-test diagnosis. For patients with malignant secondary causes of headache, physical exam features such as level of alertness and a motor exam will enable an assessment of disease progression.

# Approach to the General Medical Exam

The general medical exam can be used to confirm a clinician's impression of the diagnosis but should only rarely be used to change the clinician's diagnosis. For example, sinus tenderness supports a diagnosis of acute sinus headache, but not among patients in whom the clinician suspects migraine. Similarly, tenderness along the greater occipital nerve can support a diagnosis of occipital neuralgia, but not if the history is consistent with tension-type headache or migraine. At least two-thirds of patients with migraine experience cutaneous/mechanical allodynia, which results in tenderness/pain to palpation of pericranial muscles, sinuses, and nerves.

# Important Elements on the General Medical Exam

The physician instinctively performs a general assessment upon entering the patient's room. Is the pain unbearable? Is the patient avoiding light? A toxic appearance is suggestive of a CNS or systemic infection. The skin may be pale from anemia, cyanosed from hypoxemia, icteric from liver disease, cherry red from carbon monoxide poisoning, show petechiae from thrombocytopenia, telangiectasia from alcoholism, track marks from intravenous drug use, or a rash suggestive of a specific infection.

## Vital Signs

Vital signs are an important baseline assessment. Fever may be a reflection of meningitis, other CNS infections, sinusitis, or systemic viral or bacterial infections. Elevated blood pressure is frequently present in patients with headache and may be a simple reflection of acute pain in benign headaches. In the right setting, markedly elevated blood pressure may itself contribute to the headache etiology. A disparity in blood pressure between the left and right side may indicate arterial pathology.

## Head and Neck Exam

Among patients who experienced head trauma, scalp contusions and hematomas or open wounds may cause pain. Signs of basal skull fracture, including hemotympanum, periorbital ecchymosis (raccoon eyes), retroauricular ecchymosis (Battle's sign), and CSF rhinorrhea or otorrhea, may be delayed. The presence of any of these physical signs of basal skull fracture is an indication for computed tomography of the head [25].

Meningismus is frequently present with meningitis and may be seen with SAH or cervical muscle spasm. The three classical signs of meningeal irritation are nuchal rigidity (pain, resistance, or inability to passively flex the neck so that the chin touches the chest), Kernig's sign (pain or resistance to knee extension when one hip is flexed to 90 degrees in the supine patient), and Brudzinski's sign (flexion of the hips with neck flexion while supine). All three signs may be absent in early meningitis. Nuchal rigidity appears to be the most sensitive of the traditional signs of meningeal irritation [26]. Jolt accentuation of headache (worsening of headache with the rapid rotation of the neck) has been reported to be a more sensitive sign of meningitis in alert patients [27,28]. However, the absence of any or all of these signs of meningismus is not sufficient to obviate the need for spinal fluid analysis in a patient with suspected meningitis.

Sinusitis may be a cause of headache. The three cardinal features of acute rhinosinusitis are purulent nasal discharge accompanied by nasal obstruction with symptoms of facial pain, pressure, fullness, or both [29]. Accentuation of pain by leaning forward or by percussion of the sinuses may be supportive of the diagnosis.

Examination of the mouth may show evidence of dental caries, which may be the source of headache, or of a bitten tongue, which may indicate a recent seizure. Headache due to temporomandibular joint disorder is supported by findings of irregular or limited jaw opening and tenderness over the temporomandibular joint [30]. Temporomandibular joint disorders should not be suspected without these physical findings.

In patients over 50 with an unexplained headache, enlargement of the temporal artery, absence of pulsations or tenderness of the artery are suggestive of giant cell arteritis [31] and necessitate further investigations to establish or refute the diagnosis.

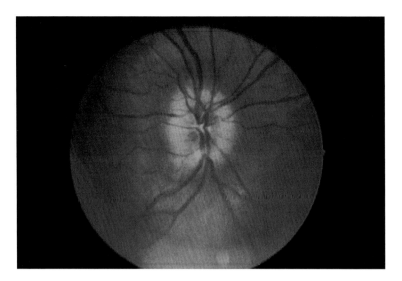

**Figure 3.1** Papilledema (photo Dr. M.L. Reardon, reproduced with permission).

Carotid bruits are the result of turbulent blood flow and may occur in headache patients with suspected cerebrovascular events such as stroke or carotid artery dissection.

### Ophthalmologic Exam

Among patients who report unilateral ocular or peri-orbital pain, examination of the eyes may suggest a cause of the headache. With cluster headache, severe orbital, supraorbital, or temporal pain in a restless individual may be accompanied by conjunctival injection, lacrimation, eyelid edema, nasal congestion, rhinorrhea, sweating or flushing of the forehead and face, a sensation of aural fullness, ptosis, and miosis [2].

Severe eye pain accompanied by headache, visual loss, and frequently nausea and vomiting should compel an urgent eye examination. Findings of conjunctival injection, reduced visual acuity, a fixed or sluggish mid-point pupil, corneal edema on slit lamp exam, and elevated intraocular pressure with tonometry are indicative of acute angle-closure glaucoma, which requires immediate treatment to lower intraocular pressure and emergency ophthalmology consultation [32].

On initial examination, the overall appearance of the eyes should be assessed for symmetry. Headache patients with new-onset unilateral ptosis may have Horner syndrome or a third nerve palsy. Horner syndrome (ptosis, miosis, anhydrosis) results from disruption of the sympathetic tract, either centrally (brainstem) or peripherally. An acute Horner syndrome with neck or face pain requires investigation for carotid artery dissection [33].

In the patient with headache, examination for papilledema (swollen optic disk) is essential (Figure 3.1). Papilledema is the result of increased intracranial pressure from intracranial mass lesions, cerebral edema, or obstruction of cerebral venous outflow. The visualization of spontaneous retinal venous pulsations excludes elevated intracranial pressure; however, they are often difficult to observe with an ophthalmoscope at the bedside and they are absent in some normal individuals [34]. Papilledema is usually bilateral. Unilateral papilledema usually results from local interference of the optic nerve or its vasculature. Ischemic optic neuropathy, which appears as a pale, swollen optic disc with blurred margins, is associated with giant cell arteritis. Fundoscopy may also reveal retinal hemorrhages, a pale ischemic retina from central retinal artery occlusion (Figure 3.2), a congested, hemorrhagic, edematous fundus (blood and thunder fundus) from central retinal vein occlusion, or signs of hypertensive or diabetic retinopathy.

## Approach to the Neurologic Exam

Any new neurologic finding in a patient presenting to the ED with headache is a strong predictor for serious underlying intracranial pathology and requires further urgent investigation [35]. Focal findings may be obvious, as in hemiparesis with stroke, or subtle, as with a mild pronator drift resulting from a slow-growing tumor. Similarly, non-focal findings range

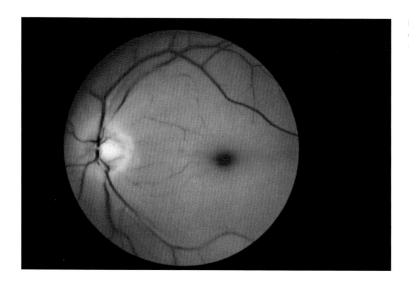

**Figure 3.2** Central retinal artery occlusion (photo Dr. M.L. Reardon, reproduced with permission).

from unconsciousness to subtle confusion or behavioral change. In migraine with aura, neurologic findings may transiently accompany migraine headache in a recurrent, predictable pattern. Any new or atypical focal neurologic deficit should not be attributed to migraine until other causes have been reasonably excluded.

For patients with a typical exacerbation of a well-defined recurrent headache disorder, a focused neurological exam focusing on mental status, speech, and gait is sufficient.

## Mental Status Examination

A patient with headache and any abnormality in level of consciousness requires urgent investigation for malignant pathology, including space-occupying intracranial lesions, CNS infection, or toxic/metabolic processes such as carbon monoxide poisoning.

The level of consciousness is usually immediately apparent on initial patient contact. An alert patient without cognitive impairment is able to give a detailed and coherent history and does not require further specific testing. If headache is accompanied by new cognitive impairment, a diagnostic work-up is indicated. The Standardized Mini-Mental State Examination [36] can be used to measure cognition. Inattention, confusion, or lethargy suggests impairment and may alter the approach to history taking and the physical examination. A standardized scale to describe level of consciousness is helpful in communicating with others and following changes in clinical condition.

**Table 3.1** Glasgow Coma Scale

| | | |
|---|---|---|
| Eye opening response | Spontaneous | 4 |
| | To speech | 3 |
| | To pain | 2 |
| | No response | 1 |
| Best verbal response | Normal | 5 |
| | Confused | 4 |
| | Inappropriate words | 3 |
| | Incomprehensible sounds | 2 |
| | No response | 1 |
| Best motor response | Obeys commands | 6 |
| | Localizes pain | 5 |
| | Withdraws from pain | 4 |
| | Flexion (decorticate) response | 3 |
| | Extension (decerebrate) response | 2 |
| | No response | 1 |
| Total score | | 15 |

The Glasgow Coma Scale (Table 3.1) is most commonly used to describe level of consciousness in the emergency department and prehospital setting. It consists of a 15-point scale on which normal is defined as a score of 15 and lower scores indicate a progressive deterioration in consciousness. It is divided into three parts, with a score of 1 to 4 for eye opening, a score of 1 to 5 for best verbal response, and a score of 1 to 6 for best motor response. It is useful for describing the degree of impaired consciousness and changes over time [37].

## Cranial Nerve Examination

### Olfactory Nerve (CN I)

The olfactory nerve is rarely assessed. However, it is the most commonly injured cranial nerve following head trauma [38].

### Optic Nerve (CN II)

A complete optic nerve exam involves assessment of the pupils, visual acuity, color vision, visual fields, and fundoscopy. A screening exam should involve, at minimum, examination of the pupils, a rapid screen of visual acuity and visual fields, and fundoscopy.

Anisocoria in a patient with headache may be long-standing and physiologic. In this case, the pupillary asymmetry will be similar in a dark or light environment. In one study, 19 percent of healthy participants had physiologic anisocoria, defined as pupillary asymmetry of 0.4 mm or greater [39]. Ordinarily, the difference in pupillary size in physiologic anisocoria is less than 1 mm. New-onset anisocoria in the patient with headache suggests a serious etiology. If anisocoria is more prominent in the dark, the small pupil is abnormal. If the miosis is accompanied by a mild ptosis, it is indicative of a partial Horner syndrome and the possibility of a carotid dissection. Pupillary asymmetry more prominent in bright light indicates an abnormality on the side of the large pupil and may be seen in traumatic mydriasis or third nerve palsy.

An afferent pupillary defect (Marcus Gunn pupil) is demonstrated by pupillary dilatation when a bright light is shone from a normal eye to the affected eye (swinging light test) and can indicate an optic nerve lesion. In a patient with eye pain, reduced vision, and often a history of multiple sclerosis, this defect suggests optic neuritis and mandates an ophthalmology consultation [40].

For a screening assessment, visual fields are tested in each eye by confrontation (comparison to one's own visual fields). A bitemporal hemianopia in a patient with headache suggests a lesion in the optic chiasma, such as a pituitary tumor. A homonymous hemianopia results from a lesion in the visual pathways from behind the chiasma to the visual (occipital) cortex.

Fundoscopy, which is integral to the examination of the optic nerve, was reviewed above.

### Eye Movements (CN III, IV, VI)

The oculomotor, trochlear, and abducens nerves are examined together during assessment of eye movements.

Diplopia and abnormal eye movements in association with headache requires further investigation. A patient with headache and diplopia due to a new third nerve palsy may have SAH from a posterior communicating artery aneurysm, infarction, tumor, or pituitary apoplexy. In a complete third nerve palsy, examination will demonstrate a dilated pupil, ptosis, and dysconjugate gaze with the affected eye directed inferiorly and laterally ("down and out"), though even in cases of definite posterior communicating artery aneurysms, the palsy may be incomplete [41]. Headache and sixth nerve palsy with horizontal diplopia may co-occur in patients with increased intracranial pressure or cavernous sinus thrombosis. Tolosa Hunt syndrome (THS) is a painful ophthalmoplegia usually presenting with horizontal or vertical diplopia and unilateral severe retroorbital or periorbital pain of acute onset. Tolosa Hunt syndrome is caused by inflammation of the cavernous sinus or superior orbital fissure. If the inflammation extends to involve the orbit, patients may report visual loss due to involvement of the optic nerve. Since the first division of the trigeminal nerve may be involved along with cranial nerves III, IV, and VI in the cavernous sinus, the patient may also report paresthesias or sensory loss along the forehead.

### Trigeminal Nerve (CN V)

Assessment of the trigeminal nerve involves examining facial sensation in the V1, V2, and V3 distributions, and assessment of the muscles of mastication: the medial and lateral pterygoids, masseters, and temporalis. This can be done rapidly by assessing sensation in the face and by asking the patient to clench their jaw. A loss of sensation in any division of the trigeminal nerve may suggest either inflammation or compression of the trigeminal nerve anywhere along its course from the brainstem to its course and exit from the skull base. Central brainstem lesions may also affect trigeminal sensation, though other brainstem findings are usually present.

Trigeminal neuralgia is a syndrome of severe intensity, unilateral, recurring, brief (a fraction of a second to two minutes) paroxysmal attacks of electric shock-like pain in the trigeminal nerve distribution without neurologic deficits.

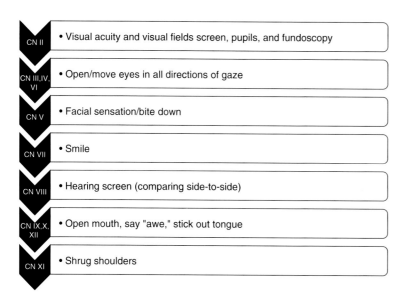

**Figure 3.3** Rapid cranial nerve (CN) exam.

### Facial Nerve (CN VII)

Strength and symmetry of facial movements must be assessed as part of a screening neurologic exam. This can be done rapidly by observing the patient's face during a relaxed state, then asking the patient to forcefully close their eyes, raise their eyebrows, smile, and puff out their cheeks.

Patients with facial weakness present to the ED because of the obvious abnormality in facial expression and concern about the possibility of a stroke. Bell's palsy is an acute peripheral facial nerve palsy, with a differential diagnosis that includes viral infection, Lyme disease, and demyelinating disease. Symptoms of facial weakness develop progressively over a day or two. Headache is not a common symptom. The finding of the absence of forehead weakness suggests a central lesion, rather than a Bell's palsy, and should prompt further investigation.

### Vestibulocochlear Nerve (CN VIII)

Cranial nerve VIII is assessed by comparing hearing side-to-side. During a screening exam, the clinician can rub their fingers together and ask if the patient is able to hear the rubbing equally in each ear.

### Glossopharyngeal and Vagus Nerves (CN IX and X)

In a conscious patient, symmetrical elevation of the palate and uvula indicates intact glossopharyngeal and vagus nerves. In an obtunded patient, a gag reflex can assess the function of these nerves.

### Accessory Nerve (CN XI)

In examining the accessory nerve, the clinician should ask the patient to elevate the shoulders in order to assess the strength of the trapezius muscles, and to rotate the head in order to assess the strength of the sternocleidomastoid muscles.

### Hypoglossal Nerve (CN XII)

When assessing the hypoglossal nerve, the clinician should look for deviation of the tongue and weakness of the tongue, which can be brought out by asking the patient to rapidly move their tongue side-to-side.

### Motor Exam

New asymmetry of motor strength in the major muscle groups is a red flag for nervous system pathology and warrants further investigation. Pronator drift is a simple method of testing for upper motor neuron pattern weakness in the upper extremity. It is assessed by having the patient hold the arms outstretched with palms facing upward and maintaining the position with the eyes closed. Drifting of an arm downward with the palm turning toward the floor is a sign of a subtle upper motor neuron disorder [41]. The forearm roll test is also a very sensitive test for detecting upper motor neuron weakness. Patients are asked to rotate one arm over the other and repeat the test in reverse. Asymmetry in speed, fluidity, and/or dexterity becomes obvious on the affected side. Tendon stretch reflexes should be assessed bilaterally for symmetry.

An extensor plantar reflex (Babinski sign) is an important sign of an upper motor neuron lesion.

### Sensory Exam

A screening sensory exam involves assessment of light touch and one modality from each of the major sensory systems in the face and limbs: pain or temperature for the spinothalamic tract and proprioception or vibration for the dorsal-column medial lemniscus tract.

The Romberg test, whereby the patient is asked to stand with their feet together with eyes first open then closed, helps to differentiate a sensory ataxia, where the unsteadiness will be worse with the eyes closed, from a cerebellar ataxia, where the unsteadiness will be present even with the eyes open.

### Coordination and Gait Exam

Coordination can be assessed with a variety of tests. Typically, a basic coordination exam involves testing rapid alternating movements, finger–nose testing, heel–shin testing, and tandem gait.

A gait exam provides the clinician with valuable information and should always be carried out in the mobile headache patient.

# Conclusion

Headache is a common reason for patients to present to the ED. Most will have a non-life-threatening cause for their headache and require therapeutic intervention to reduce their pain, and words of assurance to relieve their concerns. A careful history and focused physical examination is essential to identify those few patients who may have more serious and potentially fatal underlying causes for headache. Identifying any red flags in the clinical assessment of an ED patient with headache necessitates further diagnostic investigation to guide therapeutic interventions and optimize outcomes.

# References

1. Edmeads J. Challenges in the diagnosis of acute headache. *Headache*. 1990;30:537–40.

2. Headache Classification Committee of the International Headache Society (IHS). The International Classification of Headache Disorders, 3rd edition (beta version). *Cephalalgia*. 2013;33(9):629–808.

3. Pozzi M, Roccatagliata D, Sterzi R. Drug abuse and intracranial hemorrhage. *Neurol Sci*. 2008;29(Suppl. 2):S269–70.

4. McGee SM, McGee DN, McGee MB. Spontaneous intracranial hemorrhage related to methamphetamine abuse: autopsy findings and clinical correlation. *Am J Forensic Med Pathol*. 2004;25(4):334–7.

5. Cozzolino M, Bianchi C, Mariani G, et al. Therapy and differential diagnosis of posterior reversible encephalopathy syndrome (PRES) during pregnancy and postpartum. *Arch Gynecol Obstet*. 2015;292(6):1217–23.

6. Coutinho JM. Cerebral venous sinus thrombosis in women. *Stroke*. 2009;40(7):2356–61.

7. Rogers LR. Cerebrovascular complications in cancer patients. *Neurol Clin*. 2003;21(1):167–92.

8. Berger JR. Pearls: neurologic complications of HIV/AIDS. *Semin Neurol*. 2010;30(1):66–70.

9. Sheikh HU, Cho TA Clinical aspects of headache in HIV. *Headache* 2014;54(5):939–45.

10. Dodick D. Diagnosing headache: clinical clues and clinical rules. *Adv Stud Med*. 2003;3(2):87–92.

11. Sobri M, Lamont AC, Alias NA, Win MN. Red flags in patients presenting with headache: clinical indications for neuroimaging. *Br J Radiol*. 2003; 76(908):532–5.

12. Dodick D. Headache as a symptom of ominous disease: what are the warning signals? *Postgrad Med*. 1997;101(5):46–50.

13. Ward TN, Levin M, Phillips JM. Evaluation and management of headache in the emergency department. *Med Clin North Am*. 2001;85:971.

14. Stewart WF, Wood C, Reed ML, et al. Cumulative lifetime migraine incidence in women and men. *Cephalalgia*. 2008;28:1170–8.

15. Swanson JW, Yanagihara T, Stang PE, et al. Incidence of cluster headaches: a population-based study in Olmstead County, Minnesota. *Neurology*. 1994;44:433–7.

16. Bravo, TP. Headaches of the elderly. *Curr Neurol Neurosci Rep*. 2015;15(30):1–9.

17. Kahn K, Finkel A. It is a tumor: current review of headache and brain tumor. *Curr Pain Headache Rep*. 2014;18(6):421.

18. Schievink WI, Deline CR. Headache secondary to intracranial hypotension. *Curr Pain Headache Rep*. 2014;18:457.

19. Anderson C, Mhurchu N, Scott D, et al. Triggers of subarachnoid hemorrhage: role of physical exertion, smoking, and alcohol in the Australasian Cooperative Reseach on Subarachnoid Hemorrhage Study (ACROSS). *Stroke*. 2003;34(7):1771–6.

20. Alvarez R, Ramón C, Pascual J. Clues in the differential diagnosis of primary vs secondary cough, exercise, and sexual headaches. *Headache*. 2014;54(9):1560–2.

21. Debette S, Germain DP. Neurologic manifestations of inherited disorders of connective tissue. *Handb Clin Neurol.* 2014;119:565–76.

22. Ring T, Spiegelhalter D. Risk of intracranial aneurysm bleeding in autosomal-dominant polycystic kidney disease. *Kidney Int.* 2007;72(11):1400–2.

23. Zorbalar N, Yesilaras M, Aksay E. Carbon monoxide poisoning in patients presenting to the emergency department with a headache in winter months. *Emerg Med J.* 2014;31(1):66–70.

24. Adapted from Dodick D. Diagnosing headache: clinical clues and clinical rules. *Adv Stud Med.* 2003;3(2):87–92.

25. Stiell IG, Wells GA, Vandemheen K, et al. The Canadian CT head rule for patients with minor head injury. *Lancet.* 2001;357(9266):1391–6.

26. Thomas KE, Hasbun R, Jekel J, Quagliarello VJ. The diagnostic accuracy of Kernig's sign, Brudzinski's sign, and nuchal rigidity in adults with suspected meningitis. *Clin Infect Dis.* 2002;35:46–52.

27. Uchihara T, Tsukagoshi H. Jolt accentuation of headache: the most sensitive sign of CSF pleocytosis. *Headache.* 1991;31(3):167–71.

28. Nakao JH, Jafri FN, Shah K, Newman DH. Jolt accentuation of headache and other clinical signs: poor predictors of meningitis in adults. *Am J Emerg Med.* 2014;32(1):24–8.

29. Rosenfeld RM, Piccirillo JF, Chandrasekhar SS, et al. Clinical practice guideline (update): adult sinusitis. *Otolaryngol Head Neck Surg.* 2015;152(Suppl. 2): S1–39.

30. Graff-Radford SB. Dental causes of headache. Available from: www.americanheadachesociety.org/assets/1/7/Steven_Graff_Radford_-_Dental_Causes_for_Migraine.pdf.

31. Smetana GW, Shmerling RH. Does this patient have temporal arteritis? *JAMA.* 2002;287(1):92–101.

32. Lama DSC, Thama CCY, Laia JSM, Leung DYL. Current approaches to the management of acute primary angle closure. *Curr Opin Ophthalmol.* 2007;18:146–51.

33. Lyrer PA, Brandt T, Metso TM, et al. Clinical import of Horner syndrome in internal carotid and vertebral artery dissection. *Neurology.* 2014;82:1653–9.

34. Jacks AS, Miller NR. Spontaneous retinal venous pulsation: aetiology and significance. *J Neurol Neurosurg Psychiatry.* 2003;74:7–9.

35. Detsky ME, McDonald DR, Baerlocher MO, et al. Does this patient with headache have a migraine or need neuroimaging? *JAMA.* 2006;296:1274–83.

36. Vertesi A, Lever JA, Molloy DW, et al. Standardized mini-mental state examination: use and interpretation. *Can Fam Physician.* 2001;47:2018–23.

37. Teasdale G, Jennett B. Assessment of coma and impaired consciousness: a practical approach. *Lancet.* 1974;304(7872):81–4.

38. Coello AF, Canals AG, Gonzalez JM, Martín JJA. Cranial nerve injury after minor head trauma. *J Neurosurg.* 2010;113(3):547–55.

39. Lam BL, Thompson HS, Corbett JJ. The prevalence of simple anisocoria. *Am J Ophthalmol.* 1987;104(1):69–73.

40. Optic Neuritis Study Group. The clinical profile of optic neuritis: experience of the optic neuritis treatment trial. *Arch Ophthalmol.* 1991;109:1673–8.

41. Darcy P, Moughty AM. Pronator drift. *N Engl J Med.* 2013;369(16):e20.

**Chapter 4**

# Approach to Investigations

Meir H. Scheinfeld

Benjamin W. Friedman

## Abstract

A variety of testing modalities are available in the emergency department (ED) to enable diagnosis of headache. For an emergency care provider, the goal is to order those tests that will facilitate diagnosis in a timely manner, without burdening the patient and healthcare system with unnecessary tests, particularly those tests that are time-consuming, uncomfortable, or expensive. Available diagnostic tests include analyses of blood, urine, and cerebrospinal fluid (CSF), as well as a variety of neuroimaging modalities. In this chapter, we discuss the utility, indication, and best practice with regard to the many tests commonly available in an ED.

## Introduction to Laboratory Testing

Laboratory testing is unlikely to be useful for most patients who present to an ED with headache. With the exception of CSF analysis and serum biomarkers of infection, which may indicate a specific headache diagnosis, currently available laboratory testing is not pathognomonic for specific headache disorders. In general, both sensitivity and specificity of specific laboratory tests for specific headaches is poor. Laboratory tests may help alert the clinician to the presence of a secondary cause of headache. However, relying on laboratory testing to differentiate primary from secondary headaches may lead the clinician astray. Specific instances in which laboratory testing may be useful are discussed below.

## Urine

**Pregnancy Testing.** Though the later stages of pregnancy and parturition are associated with malignant secondary causes of headache, including venous sinus thrombosis and pituitary apoplexy, the first trimester of pregnancy, when the diagnosis of pregnancy may not be apparent, is not considered a high-risk period for secondary headaches. However, primary headache disorders, especially migraine, may worsen during the first trimester and awareness of early pregnancy is important because choice of acute medication may depend on pregnancy status. Medications such as dihydroergotamine and valproic acid have unfavorable pregnancy ratings and should be avoided. Pregnancy should be excluded prior to treatment with medications with unfavorable pregnancy ratings.

**Specific Gravity.** Migraine patients may present to the ED dehydrated because of the nausea, vomiting, and anorexia that often accompany acute migraine attacks. An elevated specific gravity may reinforce a clinical impression of dehydration and allow the patient to be treated with intravenous fluids.

**Ketones.** As with specific gravity, ketonuria may indicate dehydration requiring treatment with intravenous fluids.

## Blood

Routine blood tests including a complete blood count and chemistry panel are unlikely to provide useful information with regard to diagnosis of an acute headache. Nausea, vomiting, and anorexia associated with acute migraine may cause electrolyte abnormalities. A serum chemistry panel should be ordered for those patients with a physical exam consistent with marked dehydration.

**Markers of Inflammation.** Two markers of systemic inflammation, the erythrocyte sedimentation rate (ESR) and C-reactive protein (CRP) have been assessed for their ability to exclude giant cell arteritis from the differential diagnosis. The sensitivity of ESR for giant cell arteritis, when adjusted for age, is as low as 76 percent [1]. The sensitivity of CRP has been reported as low as 87 percent [2]. The combination of the two tests has been reported to have near-perfect sensitivity and thus should be considered in elderly patients with a new headache type [1,2]. An elevated ESR is included in the American College of Rheumatology's diagnostic criteria for giant cell arteritis, though an ESR <50 mm/hr does not exclude the disease [3].

**Markers of Thrombophilia.** The d-dimer, a serum marker of thrombus formation, may be elevated in patients with venous sinus thrombosis. However, this test is imperfect. In a meta-analysis of 1134 patients, the sensitivity was 94 percent [4]. Thus, as with other thromboembolic diseases such as pulmonary embolism or deep vein thrombosis, this test is best reserved to rule out the diagnosis in patients with low pre-test probability of disease. However, unlike pulmonary embolism and deep vein thrombosis, a low-risk population has not been well defined – clinicians are therefore left to use their own judgment to determine if venous sinus thrombosis is likely enough that further testing should be pursued in the setting of a normal d-dimer.

**Markers of Infection.** In North America, a serum antibody assay is sufficient to rule out Lyme neuroborreliosis. In Europe, because of heterogeneity in strains of *B. burgdorferi*, it is more difficult to rule out Lyme neuroborreliosis with blood tests, though in Europe Lyme is less likely to present as an isolated headache [5]. Among patients with cryptococcal meningitis, the sensitivity of assays for serum cryptococcal antigen depends on the specific assay used, and ranges from 83 to 100 percent [6].

## Cerebrospinal Fluid

Analysis of CSF allows for the exclusion of two important secondary headaches from the differential diagnosis: meningitis and subarachnoid hemorrhage (SAH). Meningitis, which is defined by markers of inflammation within the CSF, can be caused by a variety of infectious agents, inflammatory diseases, or medications. An absence of white blood cells in the CSF excludes meningitis as the diagnosis, with the exception of cryptococcal meningitis among patients with AIDS and T-cell counts less than 100, who may present with an acellular CSF [7]. Cerebrospinal fluid cryptococcal antigen should be ordered when meningitis is suspected in these patients. An elevated opening pressure is consistent with cryptococcal meningitis, though the differential diagnosis for elevated opening pressure includes infection, space-occupying lesion, venous sinus thrombosis, and idiopathic intracranial hypertension.

In the right clinical setting, the presence of xanthochromia or red blood cells in the CSF raises concern for SAH. The absence of both of these findings excludes the diagnosis [8]. Unfortunately, both of these tests are imperfect. The sensitivity of xanthochromia is time-dependent. If fewer than six hours have elapsed since the headache began, xanthochromia is frequently not present and one must rely on the presence of red blood cells to exclude disease [9]. However, relying on presence of red blood cells results in false positive rates as high as one in three [10]. Spectrophotometric analysis for xanthochromia may increase sensitivity at the cost of specificity [8], but inspecting the CSF for visual rather than spectrophotometric xanthochromia is standard in clinical laboratories across the United States [11]. There are reports of patients who were ultimately diagnosed with aneurysmal SAH with clear CSF and as few as 100 red cells in tube 4 [12].

## Introduction to Neuroimaging

Neuroimaging for headache is extremely common in the emergency setting as it is a reliable and accurate method of diagnosing intracranial pathology. Headache is the second most common reason for obtaining ED head CTs (head trauma is the most common indication) [13]. When normal, appropriate neuroimaging offers reassurance that the patient can be discharged safely. Imaging has a clear role in the diagnostic evaluation of headache patients as ED physicians cannot rule out a space-occupying lesion, SAH, or other vascular causes of headache based on clinical considerations alone [14]. The need to image is not always obvious – in one Canadian study, 5.4 percent of patients with SAH were missed in their initial ED encounter despite availability of a CT scanner [15]. Additionally, the limitations of neuroimaging must be recognized – neuroimaging will not identify all patients with intracranial pathology, particularly if the wrong imaging study is ordered. Nevertheless, during the last 15 years the frequency of head neuroimaging has increased markedly with a concurrent decline in discovery of intracranial pathology, indicating that factors contributing to neuroimaging have evolved [16]. In addition to costs, imaging may entail the risk of radiation (for CT), contrast material (for

CT angiography [CTA] and contrast-enhanced magnetic resonance angiography [MRA]), and detection of incidental findings leading to unnecessary work-up and invasive procedures.

The goals of the remainder of this chapter are to define when neuroimaging is indicated and the preferred imaging pathway for certain conditions. When available, we will discuss society recommendations. At the time of this writing, there were no Cochrane Reviews on the topic of neuroimaging for headache. There are, however, the following society guidelines or recommendations: American College of Emergency Physicians (ACEP) clinical policy for ED headache management [14]; American College of Radiology (ACR) appropriateness criteria for headache [17]; American Academy of Neurology practice parameter for migraine headache [18]; and the US Headache Consortium evidence-based guidelines for neuroimaging in patients with non-acute headache [19]. Common among these guidelines is the discretion granted to treating physicians to image even when not fully supported by the data, in situations where there is considerable concern for underlying intracranial pathology or the need to conclusively rule out pathology.

Headaches lasting longer than four weeks are considered non-acute and are best evaluated in the outpatient setting. However, patients may present to the ED with this complaint. Often the emergency physician cannot be sure of adequate outpatient follow-up. Therefore, the need for neuroimaging in these patients will be relevant for the ED clinician. Regardless of headache duration, the ultimate goals of neuroimaging for the patient presenting with headache to the ED are to exclude secondary causes of headache, to offer reassurance for safe discharge, and as a preamble for performing lumbar puncture (LP).

## What Neuroimaging Tests are Available?

CT and MRI are the two commonly used neuroimaging techniques used to image the brain parenchyma. Each has advantages and disadvantages. CT is typically the first-line technique used to evaluate the brain for intracranial pathology due to its relatively low cost, brief exam time, and compatibility with implanted electronic or ferromagnetic devices. It has the disadvantage of delivering a dose of ionizing radiation to the head, which has been associated with a statistically

significant but small increased risk of brain tumors in children and adolescents [20]. MRI lacks ionizing radiation, has superior soft-tissue resolution, and eliminates streak artifacts from the calvarial bone, which is of particular concern in the posterior fossa. Its disadvantages are a longer exam time, fewer hours of availability in some EDs, requirement of special MR-safe monitoring equipment, increased cost, and non-compatibility with certain implantable devices such as most pacemakers. Either pre-contrast and post-contrast CT (iodine-based) or MRI (gadolinium-based) should generally be performed when there is concern for an intracranial infection, mass, or a vascular lesion.

There are three types of neurovascular imaging techniques: CTA, MRA, and digital subtraction angiography. CTA has excellent spatial resolution (as low as 0.5 mm) but requires intravenous contrast, may be degraded by bone or metal artifacts, and delivers a dose of ionizing radiation to the head. MRA may be performed with or without contrast and does not use ionizing radiation but is susceptible to MRI-specific flow-type artifacts and metal artifacts. Contrast-enhanced MRA with gadolinium is contraindicated in patients with low GFR, including dialysis patients and pregnant patients. Digital subtraction angiography is considered the gold standard for diagnostic neurovascular imaging. Also, angiography allows for interventions to be performed concurrent with diagnosis. However, because it is an invasive procedure, it is not considered a first-line modality

## What is the Role of Imaging in Headache Differential Diagnosis?

Since SAH is the most common cause of malignant secondary headache in the ED [14], and administration of contrast may interfere with detection of SAH, once the clinician decides to obtain imaging in a patient suspected of having an SAH, a non-contrast head CT is the best initial imaging test. Based on the results of this initial CT and clues from the history and physical exam, the clinician can then decide to pursue other tests. Many secondary headaches can be diagnosed with the assistance of specific imaging modalities and protocols, and these should be considered when there are specific diagnoses on the differential diagnosis (Table 4.1; Figures 4.1 and 4.2). Other conditions such as primary headache syndromes do not have typical imaging findings, and in these patients

**Table 4.1** Neurological conditions associated with headache and typical imaging findings using CT and MRI

| Condition | Imaging findings | Comments |
| --- | --- | --- |
| Carbon monoxide poisoning | NC CT – characteristic appearance is low attenuation in the medial aspects of the globi pallidi<br>NC MRI* – medial aspects of the globi pallidi have high T2-weighted signal, low T1-weighted signal, and elevated signal on diffusion-weighted imaging | People may present with carbon monoxide poisoning with headache and flu-like symptoms especially during the winter months. Symptoms commonly effect co-habitants [21] |
| Cavernous sinus thrombosis | NC CT – high density within the cavernous sinuses with the sinuses bulging outward. There are also distended superior ophthalmic veins<br>CE CT, CE MRI* – non-enhancement of the cavernous sinuses | May have associated dural sinus thrombosis. |
| Colloid cyst with acute hydrocephalus | NC CT* – high-density rounded mass in the anterior third ventricle which obstructs the foramina of Monro causing acute hydrocephalus | Low density in the periventricular white matter is indicative of trans-ependymal CSF flow and acute hydrocephalus |
| Dissection of cervical artery | CTA of the neck* – cutoff of the contrast column in the carotid or vertebral artery<br>MRI/MRA of the neck* – lack of flow-related enhancement within the dissected vessel. On T2-weighted images or T1-weighted fat-suppressed images there is a crescent of high signal within the vessel due to hemorrhage into the vessel wall | If there is a brain infarct due to the dissection, there may also be evidence of infarct on non-contrast CT |
| Dural sinus thrombosis (Figure 4.1) | NC CT – high density along the course of a dural sinus, but this finding has a low sensitivity<br>CE CT/CTV, CE MRI* – non-enhancement of a dural sinus, or a tubular filling defect within the contrast-enhanced lumen of a dural sinus<br>NC MRV – lack of flow-related enhancement within a dural sinus | CE MRI is preferred. In pregnant patients and patients with renal insufficiency/failure who cannot receive gadolinium, non-contrast MRV is an alternative but is prone to artifacts. CE CT will also yield a diagnosis but entails radiation and should not be performed in patients with renal insufficiency. If accompanied by venous infarct there is the imaging appearance of stroke in a non-arterial territory distribution ± hemorrhagic conversion |
| Encephalitis (herpes) | High T2-weighted signal and restricted diffusion in the areas of involvement, most commonly within the temporal lobes | Headache is generally not the only presenting symptom |
| Idiopathic intracranial hypertension (pseudotumor cerebri) [22] | NC MRI*, NC CT – flattening of the posterior sclera, partially empty sella (best seen on sagittal images), tortuosity of optic nerves, prominent subarachnoid space about the optic nerves<br>CE MRI – optic nerve prelaminar enhancement (i.e., enhancement within the posterior globe at the optic nerve insertion site)<br>CTV/MRV – bilateral stenoses within the transverse sinuses without evidence of prior or current thrombosis | Despite the possibility of identifying findings that are commonly seen in idiopathic intracranial hypertension, the primary purpose of performing neuroimaging is to exclude serious conditions including brain tumor and hydrocephalus |
| Intracranial hypotension | CT or MRI – there is descent of midline structures, high dural T2-weighted signal, and subdural collections<br>CE MRI – dural enhancement | These headaches are generally postural, becoming symptomatic when the head is erect |
| Intraparenchymal hemorrhage | NC CT* – high density within the substance of the brain<br>NC MRI – signal on T1- and T2-weighted images varies with the age of the hemorrhage [23] | On MRI, in amyloid angiopathy, there are multiple foci of cortical susceptibility (low signal on gradient-echo or SWI images) |
| Leptomeningitis | NC CT – usually normal. Source of meningitis such as sinusitis or mastoiditis may be revealed<br>CE MRI* – high subarachnoid signal on FLAIR images as well as leptomeningeal enhancement | MRA may demonstrate areas of vessel narrowing |

*(Continued)*

**Table 4.1** (*cont.*)

| Condition | Imaging findings | Comments |
|---|---|---|
| Migraine and tension-type headache | NC MRI – there may be white matter foci of high T2-weighted signal [24] | MRI findings in primary headaches are usually normal |
| Pituitary apoplexy | NC CT – expanded high-density pituitary, best seen on sagittal images<br>NC MRI* – pituitary mass with high T1-weighted signal due to blood. Fluid–fluid levels are also characteristic | Caused by acute hemorrhagic infarction of a pituitary adenoma or the pituitary itself causing rapid expansion [25]<br>MRI can be used to determine effects of adjacent structures, most importantly the optic chiasm [26] |
| Posterior reversible encephalopathy syndrome (PRES) | NC CT – low density within the posterior cerebral (predominantly) white matter without mass effect<br>NC MRI* – high signal within posterior cerebral (predominantly) white matter without mass effect. DWI is usually normal | Despite its name, edema may involve gray matter as well as anterior portions of the brain |
| Reversible cerebrovascular syndrome (RCVS) | MRA/CTA – multifocal narrowing of cerebral vessels with a "string of beads" configuration. In uncomplicated cases there is no SAH, but in complicated cases there may be small areas of cerebral cortical SAH | The angiographic appearance must resolve within three months to be considered "reversible" |
| Acute sinusitis | NC CT of the sinuses* – findings are generally not specific and there is no standard diagnostic criteria. A frothy air–fluid level is the best imaging signs of acute sinusitis. Additional non-specific imaging signs include mucosal thickening greater than 4 mm and an air–fluid level | In chronic sinusitis there is commonly thickening of the bony walls around the sinus consistent with a chronic sinus obstructive process. Circumferential mucosal thickening may be seen in acute or chronic sinusitis |
| Stroke [27,28] | NC CT – early findings in stroke are loss of gray matter/white matter differentiation and gyral edema<br>NC MRI* – high signal on diffusion-weighted imaging and reciprocal low signal on the apparent diffusion coefficient (ADC) map | Stroke, whether ischemic or hemorrhagic, may be accompanied with headache or even a thunderclap headache. Association is strongest in younger patients, patients with migraines, and with cerebellar stroke |
| Subarachnoid hemorrhage (Figure 4.2) | NC CT* – high density within the subarachnoid space<br>NC MRI – high signal within the subarachnoid space on FLAIR images and low signal in the subarachnoid space on gradient-echo or susceptibility-weighted images | The differential diagnosis for high subarachnoid signal on MRI FLAIR images includes: SAH, hyperoxygenation, meningitis, leptomeningeal carcinomatosis, and recent gadolinium administration. For CT there may be "pseudo-subarachnoid hemorrhage" in intracranial hypotension, meningitis such as *Cryptococcus*, contrast in the CSF from prior contrast-enhanced study, diffuse cerebral edema, or obstructive hydrocephalus |
| Temporal or giant cell arteritis | US – focused on the temporal artery, where there is thickening of the artery and a surrounding dark halo. Still, interpretation of imaging findings is highly influenced by pre-test probability for temporal arteritis [29]<br>CTA – may demonstrate vascular stenoses or aneurysms<br>CE MRI – may demonstrate wall thickening and enhancement [30] | Diagnosis is usually clinical and with biopsy |

CE, contrast-enhanced; CTA, CT angiography; CTV, CT venography; DWI, diffusion-weighted imaging; MRA, MR angiography; MRV, magnetic resonance venography; NC, non-contrast; SWI, susceptibility-weighted imaging; US, ultrasound. * indicates the test which is best used to demonstrate the pathology.

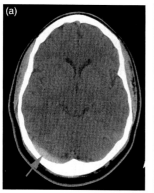
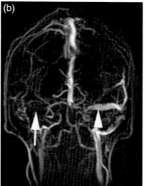
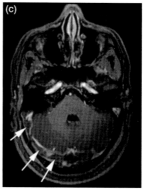

**Figure 4.1** Dural sinus thrombosis in a 16-year-old male. (a) Axial CT image of the head demonstrating high density in the right transverse sinus (arrow), consistent with presence of thrombus. (b) Coronal maximum intensity projection (MIP) image from phase-contrast (i.e., no gadolinium contrast) magnetic resonance venography (MRV) demonstrating flow in the left transverse sinus (arrowhead), but lack of flow-related enhancement in the right transverse sinus, consistent with thrombosis (arrow). (c) Axial image from contrast-enhanced MRI demonstrating filling defect (low signal irregular material) in the right transverse sinus (arrows), consistent with presence of thrombus.

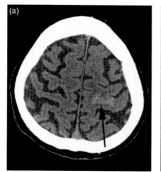
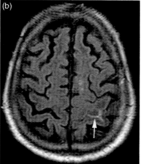
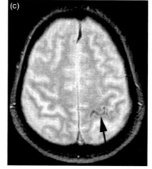

**Figure 4.2** Subarachnoid hemorrhage in a 75-year-old male. (a) Axial CT image demonstrating high-density SAH (arrow) within the left central sulcus. (b) Axial FLAIR image demonstrating high signal within the left central sulcus (arrow), consistent with hemorrhage. (c) Axial gradient-echo image demonstrating low signal within the left central sulcus (arrow), consistent with hemorrhage.

the only role of imaging is to rule out secondary headache etiologies.

## Is There a Clinical Decision Rule to Predict Who Does and Does Not Need a CT for Headache?

In an attempt to determine clinical predictors of positive and negative imaging exams and to decrease the number of CTs performed on patients with headache, Perry et al. initially described three rules with sensitivity of 100 percent and specificities ranging between 28.4 percent and 38.8 percent [31]. When using each of these rules, the presence of any one element of the rule is an indication for imaging. The three rules are: (1) age ≥40 years, neck pain or stiffness, witnessed loss of consciousness, onset during exertion; (2) age ≥45 years, arrival by ambulance, vomiting, diastolic BP >100 mmHg; and (3) age 45–55 years, neck pain or stiffness, arrival by ambulance, systolic BP >160 mmHg. Because of inadequate sensitivity in a validation sample, the first rule above was combined with thunderclap headache and limited neck flexion on examination to constitute the Ottawa SAH rule [32] (i.e., age ≥40 years, neck pain or stiffness, witnessed loss of consciousness, onset during exertion, thunderclap headache, limited neck flexion on examination), which was shown to have a sensitivity of 100 percent and specificity of 15.3 percent [31]. It is important to realize the limitations of this rule, which are as follows: applies only to patients older than 15 years old with a new non-traumatic headache, without new neurologic deficit, without previous aneurysm, without previous SAH, without brain tumor, and without a history of recurrent headaches (defined as more than three episodes over the course of six or more months). Pending validation in an independent sample of patients, this rule may be used to exclude SAH without any diagnostic testing.

## What are the "Red Flags" That Would Indicate the Need for Neuroimaging?

Other than the high-risk predictors identified in the Ottawa SAH rule, the published literature has identified a multitude of factors termed "red flags," which are proposed triggers for neuroimaging. Some of these red flags are evidence-based or components of the decision rules above; however, others are based on more tenuous evidence, being derived from a single study or dogma (Box 4.1) [18,31–34]. It is important to realize that despite the extensive list of red flags, the absence of a red flag does not completely rule out a serious intracranial abnormality [35]. In children, a guideline from the American Academy of Neurology states that neuroimaging is indicated for headache patients only for an abnormal neurologic exam, the presence of seizure activity, or headaches of recent onset or a change in the headache characteristics [36].

Many of the red flag items are discussed elsewhere in this chapter, but we will provide a few notes on others which are not. Headache associated with cough or Valsalva may be due to a Chiari 1 malformation or other posterior fossa abnormality, where there is intermittent obstruction to the flow of CSF at the level of the foramen magnum [37]. This may be investigated with CT (with sagittal images best for visualizing this pathology) or preferably with MRI, where CSF flow may also be assessed using special phase-contrast CSF flow MRI sequences. Exertional headache or headache associated with sexual activity may represent a primary headache syndrome, but reversible cerebral vasoconstriction may account for a significant proportion of these cases. Sudden severe headache also raises concern for SAH, arterial dissection, or space-occupying lesion. Headache in patients who are in the latter half of pregnancy or the postpartum period may be due to dural puncture headache, pituitary apoplexy, or cortical vein, or dural or cavernous sinus thrombosis. Stroke, metastatic or primary brain tumor, or

**Box 4.1 Clinical "Red Flags" for Which Neuro-imaging Should be Obtained or Considered in Patients Presenting with Headache**

Age greater than 40/45/50 with new onset (CSDR, CP class C, OSAHR)

Altered mental status or decreased level of consciousness (CP class B)

Ambulance as mode of arrival (CSDR)

Abnormal or focal neurological exam (EBGPC, CP class B)

Atypical features for a primary headache syndrome (EBGPC)

Cancer history

Changed headaches (increased frequency or increased severity)

Coagulopathy or anticoagulation

Exertion or sexual activity as trigger (CSDR, OSAHR)

Family history of intracranial aneurysm or polycystic kidney disease

First or first of a certain headache type

Hypertension (diastolic greater than 100 mmHg or systolic greater than 160 mmHg) (CSDR)

Immunodeficiency or immunosuppression (CP class B)

Lack of coordination

Loss of consciousness (CSDR, OSAHR)

Meningeal symptoms (e.g., fever, stiff neck) (CSDR, OSAHR)

Neck pain (OSAHR)

Occipital location of pain

Papilledema

Positional headache

Pregnancy or postpartum

Seizure accompanying headache

Sensory symptoms including numbness, tingling, or visual symptoms

Syncope at the time of onset

Systemic symptoms (e.g., fever, weight loss)

Temporal headache (i.e., pain over temporal arteries)

Thunderclap (CP class B, OSAHR)

Transient ischemic attack

Trauma

Valsalva maneuver or cough triggering the headache

VP shunt

Vomiting (CSDR)

Waking from sleep due to the headache

Worst headache of life

Red flags from the following sources are indicted in parenthesis.

EBGPC = Evidence-based guidelines for non-acute headache in primary care; CP = ACEP clinical policy; CSDR = components of Canadian subarachnoid decision rule; OSAHR = Ottawa SAH rule temporal arteritis should be considered in patients who present with headache in older age. Papilledema raises concern for meningitis or raised intracranial pressure from a space-occupying mass or decreased venous outflow.

## What is the Role of CT in the Diagnosis of Subarachnoid and Other Intracranial Hemorrhage?

In patients presenting with abrupt onset headache, the role of CT is to diagnose or rule out SAH. Subarachnoid hemorrhage may be found in 11 percent of patients with a true thunderclap headache [38]. Among patients with SAH, ruptured aneurysm causes 80–85 percent of cases, arteriovenous malformations (AVM) account for 10 percent, and the remainder are due to other causes such as mycotic aneurysm, trauma, vasculitis, or perimesencephalic hemorrhage. The differential diagnosis for isolated SAH along the cortical convexities includes pial AVM, dural arteriovenous fistula (AVF), arterial dissection, dural or cortical venous thrombosis, vasculitis, reversible cerebral vasoconstriction syndrome (RCVS), posterior reversible encephalopathy syndrome (PRES), cerebral amyloid, coagulopathy, trauma, septic aneurysm, cavernoma, or brain tumor [39]. Intraparenchymal hemorrhage may be due to hypertension (typically in the central gray and white matter), amyloid angiopathy (typically cortical and in older patients), hemorrhagic metastases, vascular malformation, or coagulopathy (e.g., hemorrhagic venous infarction).

Anticoagulant use is a risk factor for intracranial hemorrhage. Even with minor head trauma, anticoagulated patients should be imaged prior to continuing anticoagulation [40]. Warfarin (Coumadin®) and, to a lesser extent, dabigatran (Pradaxa®) increase the risk of intracranial hemorrhage [41]. Aspirin (acetylsalicylic acid) increases the risk of intracranial hemorrhage by 0.2 events per 1000 patient years [42]. In one study, clopidogrel and ticlopidine demonstrated risk for SAH that was marginally higher than aspirin [43]. Coagulopathies such as hemophilia may also be a risk factor for intracranial hemorrhage. As an incidental note, anticoagulated patients with intracranial hemorrhage on CT may have characteristic "fluid–fluid levels" due to red blood cells settling out of the serum of the non-clotted blood.

## What are the Sensitivities of Different Neurovascular Imaging Modalities for Aneurysm?

Sensitivity of the neurovascular imaging modalities (CTA, MRA, and angiography) for aneurysm varies by aneurysm size. Using angiography as the gold standard, for aneurysms ≥5 mm, CTA has a sensitivity of 95–100 percent, while for aneurysms <5 mm, sensitivity ranges between 64 and 83 percent [44]. For non-contrast time-of-flight MRA, sensitivity for aneurysms ≥5 mm is 85–100 percent, while for aneurysms <5 mm sensitivity is 56 percent [44]. In one study, among patients with diagnosed SAH, contrast-enhanced MRA was more sensitive for aneurysm than time-of-flight MRA (95 percent versus 86 percent) with equal specificity (80 percent) [45]. In a study from 2007, also using angiography as the gold standard, Romijn et al. found subtraction CTA (where pre-contrast images were used for bone subtraction of the post-contrast images) with a four-slice CT scanner to be 99 percent sensitive for aneurysms greater than 3 mm, but only 38 percent for aneurysms of less than 3 mm [46]. Luo et al., using a state-of-the art 320-slice multiple detector CT scanner, found subtraction CTA to be 100 percent sensitive and specific for all aneurysms compared to angiography, even those less than 3 mm in diameter (11 in the study) [47]. Despite angiography being considered the gold standard, there is one study in which 4 of 43 patients with negative angiography had an aneurysm on CTA, and 1 of 43 had an aneurysm using MRA [48]. This illustrates how continued development of imaging technology may lead to shifts in what is considered the gold standard.

## Does a Negative Non-Contrast CT of the Head Rule Out SAH?

Many studies have reported on sensitivity of CT or MR for the detection of SAH. It should be noted that the generalizability of many of these studies is limited because the studies were performed at referral centers where imaging equipment is the most modern and radiology staff have greater expertise or subspecialization in neuroradiology. Furthermore, when reading the literature from the 1990s and early 2000s, one must pay attention to the type of CT scanner used, as CT technology has evolved considerably during this time period.

Time plays a crucial role in the ability to diagnose SAH using CT. Within 12 hours of symptom onset, and even more so within six hours, sensitivity for detection of SAH is very high. In the first 12 hours after SAH, CT has a sensitivity for SAH of 98–100 percent [44]. By 24 hours it drops to 93 percent, and by six days it is as low as 57 percent [44]. In an older study in which patients with known SAH were scanned serially with CT, the sensitivity for SAH decreased to 85 percent by five days and 50 percent by one week [19]. In another study, in patients presenting within six hours of symptom onset, sensitivity of non-contrast CT was 98.5 percent, whereas with greater than six hours the sensitivity was 90 percent [50].

In one study, CT had a sensitivity of 95 percent for detection of SAH among patients presenting within 12 hours when modern 16- or 64-slice CT scanners were used [51]. In more recent studies, a 100 percent sensitivity was found using modern CT equipment (4- to 320-slice CT scanners) when the patient was scanned within six hours of headache onset [52]. Based on the results of two prospective studies, some have recommended no further evaluation after negative head CT performed within six hours of symptom onset when two caveats are met: the patient presents with headache (rather than with, for example, neck pain) and the CT scans are being read by experienced neuroradiologists [53]. However, in one case-control study performed in 21 emergency departments over a 12-year period, there were only seven cases of missed vascular lesions (six aneurysms and one AVM) on head CT performed within six hours; this would amount to a miniscule risk for an individual practitioner or patient [54]. In a patient with pre-test probability of SAH of 1 in 14 (the risk of SAH among patients with a headache that peaks in intensity within one hour), a negative head CT yields a post-test probability of about 1 in 700 if imaging was performed within 12 hours, whereas the post-test probability is 1 in 80 if negative imaging was performed greater than 24 hours after headache onset [55].

According to the ACEP clinical policy (Level B recommendation), LP is indicated for patients who present with an abrupt onset of headache and who have a normal non-contrast head CT because of the limitations in CT, which include artifacts from bone (particularly in the posterior fossa), decreased sensitivity in the context of anemia, decreased sensitivity with time, and decreased sensitivity with small amounts of subarachnoid blood [14].

## Can MRI be Used as the First Imaging Test When SAH is Suspected?

Many studies have compared the sensitivity of MRI versus CT for SAH, some of which are summarized in Table 4.2. Four of these studies were performed with human subjects [56–59], while the study by Woodcock et al. [60] was performed using a rabbit animal model in which blood was injected into the subarachnoid

**Table 4.2** Sensitivity of CT and MR sequences for SAH in selected studies

| Author | Symptom onset until MR | Gap between CT and MR | Gold standard test used for initial diagnosis | CT | FLAIR | GE/T2* | SWI | DIR | FLAIR + SWI |
|---|---|---|---|---|---|---|---|---|---|
| Woodcock [60] | 2–5 h | CT performed "immediately after MR imaging" | Rabbit model- blood injected ("high volume" data) | 56% | 100% | | | | |
| Wiesmann [56] | 2–12 h | NA | CT | Gold standard | 100% | | | | |
| Verma [59] | 2.25 d (mean) | 48 h (mean) | CT or MR | 75% | 87% | | 88% | | 100% |
| Yuan [57] | ≤5 d | <12 h | LP or surgery | 91% | 100% | 91% | | | |
| Yuan [57] | 6–30 d | <12 h | LP or surgery | 46% | 33% | 100% | | | |
| Hodel [58] | 14–16 d | 2–5 h | Initial CT | 28% | 60% | 56% | 60% | 100% | |

FLAIR, fluid attenuation inversion recovery; GE, gradient-echo; SWI, susceptibility-weighted imaging; DIR, double inversion recovery; NA, not available.

space and then CT and MR imaging was performed. In summary, MRI performs equivalent to or better than CT when appropriate MRI sequences are performed and interpreted. Despite this, CT is still generally performed as the first-line test due to its availability, rapidity, and lower cost.

## What Should be the First Neuroimaging Test Obtained in Patients Presenting with Headache?

Non-contrast CT of the head should be obtained first to rule out life-threatening conditions such as acute intracranial hemorrhage, herniation, or acute hydrocephalus, as it is a rapid test that is nearly universally available in North American EDs. Following this, other more specialized and more time-consuming tests such as CTA or MRI may be obtained.

If acute headache is unilateral and there is suspicion for carotid or vertebral artery dissection, CTA of the head and neck or MRA of the head and neck (including T1 fat-saturated images) are the most appropriate diagnostic studies, as per the ACR appropriateness criteria [17]. For trigeminal neuralgia pain, temporomandibular joint pain, suspicion for temporal arteritis, or headache in immunosuppressed/immunocompromised patients, MRI of the head without and with contrast is the most appropriate test following the non-contrast head CT [17]. The skull base, orbital, or periorbital areas are best evaluated with MRI of the head and orbits without and with contrast [17]. Orthostatic headache without prior dural puncture can be investigated with CT or MRI of the entire spine with the goal of demonstration of an extraspinal/juxtaspinal fluid collection presumably caused by a CSF leak [17]. If this is negative, diagnosis can be made with demonstration of brain MRI findings of intracranial hypotension associated with either low opening pressure on LP, a meningeal diverticulum, or resolution with a blood patch [61].

## What is the First Study to Perform in a Pregnant Patient with Headache?

Approximately one-quarter of pregnant patients with headache who are imaged will have a cause found on neuroimaging [62]. According to the ACR appropriateness criteria, non-contrast MRI and CT are categorized as usually appropriate, with MR preferred due to lack of ionizing radiation [17]. Despite the fetal dose from maternal head CT possibly being as low as zero [63], it would seem prudent to use MRI when equivalent information may be obtained. Iodinated contrast may be used if necessary in pregnant patients, but gadolinium contrast is contraindicated. Aside from SAH, the differential diagnosis of headache in a pregnant patient includes posterior reversible encephalopathy syndrome (PRES), cortical vein or dural or cavernous sinus thrombosis, and intracranial tumors such as meningioma, which may grow in response to the altered hormonal milieu of pregnancy. During the postpartum period, Sheehan's syndrome and postdural puncture headache should also be considered.

## If CT Head is Negative, What is the Second Test to Obtain?

If non-contrast CT of the head is negative, the current standard of care and ACEP recommendation for the work-up of potential SAH is LP [14,44]. If CT and LP are both negative there is no need for catheter angiography according to the ACEP clinical policy (Level B recommendation) [14]. In a prospective study of nearly 600 patients, the combination of CT followed by LP was found to have a sensitivity of 100 percent and a negative likelihood ratio of 0 for SAH, validating the current practice [64].

LP has the advantage of allowing for opening pressure measurements to diagnose intracranial hypotension or hypertension, collection of CSF to diagnose meningitis, and allowing for the detection of xanthochromia in the context of SAH, which may be detected for as long as two weeks after the hemorrhage. Because of decreasing attenuation of SAH on CT with time, the LP becomes more important (as discussed above). For example, in one study evaluating 30 patients with negative CT but positive xanthochromia on LP, aneurysms were found in 0 of 2 patients presenting within 3 days, 8 in 18 (44 percent) patients presenting within 4–7 days, and in 5 of 10 (50 percent) presenting within 8–14 days [65]. This would suggest that the CT false negative rate increases with time in patients with confirmed xanthochromia.

There are some challenges with LP though. The test is invasive and commonly time-consuming. With abnormal coagulation tests or infection overlying the puncture zone, LP cannot be safely performed. Accurate needle placement may be hampered by patient body habitus, and patients may refuse the procedure for a variety of reasons. Even once the procedure is performed, there may be the complication of postdural puncture headache [66]. For these reasons, imaging-based modalities have appeal as the next test to perform. These include MRI, CTA, and MRA. The role of MRI in diagnosing SAH has been discussed above, particularly regarding MRI's superior ability to diagnose SAH after a longer duration of symptoms. MRI has other advantages over CT and LP, such as diagnosis of dural or cavernous sinus thrombosis, and pituitary apoplexy [67].

The role of CTA/MRA in the work-up of headache is to diagnose an aneurysm or AVM, which could be possible sources of SAH, rather than to diagnose hemorrhage itself. Regarding cost, a mathematical model has shown that there was no "overwhelming" cost-effectiveness difference between CT followed by LP versus CT followed by CTA or MR/MRA for the diagnosis of aneurysm-related SAH [68]. Unruptured aneurysms may cause symptoms; however, these are most commonly ischemia due to downstream emboli or mass effect from the aneurysm itself, rather than an isolated headache [69]. If there is indeed a headache related to an unruptured aneurysm, it may improve after open or endovascular treatment [70].

Reasoning that a clinical trial would require enrolling over 3000 patients, a decision analysis concluded that a CT/CTA pathway would be an acceptable method to rule out aneurysmal or AVM-related SAH with a greater than 99 percent post-test probability [66].

Other than time, expense, radiation risk, and risk of contrast reaction, an additional drawback of performing CTA or MRA is the uncertainty associated with identifying an asymptomatic, incidentally discovered aneurysm, which autopsy studies reveal are present in 2 percent of the general population [71].

Increased use of vascular imaging (prior to diagnosis of SAH using CT or LP) poses the risk of discovering incidental non-culprit aneurysms that would lead to increased downstream imaging and interventions (as there is currently no way of prospectively excluding an aneurysm from eventual rupture) with potential complications from these interventions [69]. Also, these additional diagnoses may lead to patient anxiety [69].

In patients with thunderclap headache who have no evidence of hemorrhage on CT or in CSF, vascular imaging is indicated to exclude other serious vascular causes which are often or always undetectable on CT/CSF [72]. These include RCVS, which has emerged as one of the most common causes of thunderclap headache [73]. Since RCVS may be associated with intracranial hemorrhage within the first week or ischemic stroke within the second week after onset, prompt diagnosis is urgent. It is important to remember that even in patients with documented RCVS, the initial non-invasive vascular imaging is normal in up to 20 percent of patients. It is therefore important to ensure that these patients have outpatient follow-up and imaging if indicated within 7–10 days. In addition, non-invasive vascular imaging (CTA/MRA) may identify carotid or vertebral artery dissection or cerebral venous sinus thrombosis. Each of these disorders may present with thunderclap headache in isolation and easily go undetected on CT or CSF analysis.

## Must CT of the Head be Performed Prior to Lumbar Puncture?

There is a level C recommendation in the ACEP clinical policy guideline that in adults with signs of increased intracranial pressure (papilledema, absent venous pulsation on fundoscopic exam, altered mental status, focal neurological deficit or meningismus) should have a CT prior to LP. Otherwise, LP can be performed without neuroimaging [14].

## When and What Imaging Should be Performed in Headache Following Trauma?

Acute post-traumatic headache most commonly presents as a migraine [74]. Headache may occur as part of the post-concussion syndrome, which may include psychological and cognitive changes [75]. Although advanced MRI imaging can be used to image subtle white matter changes and axonal damage, in the acute phase, CT is most appropriate to exclude hemorrhage and skull fracture [17]. Intracranial hemorrhage in trauma is classically multi-compartmental, involving multiple spaces of the following: subdural, epidural, subarachnoid, intraparenchymal, and intraventricular. Hemorrhagic contusion of the brain parenchyma commonly involves the inferior frontal lobes and anterior temporal lobes. Vascular injuries are also possible. Even minor trauma may cause cervical artery dissection, especially in patients with underlying vascular abnormalities (such as Ehlers–Danlos type 4).

**Table 4.3** ACEP recommendations to obtain or to consider obtaining non-contrast CT of the head following minor trauma

| Level A ACEP Recommendation **to obtain** non-contrast head CT for mild head trauma: | Level B ACEP Recommendation **to consider** non-contrast head CT for mild head trauma: |
|---|---|
| Loss of consciousness **OR** post-traumatic amnesia, AND one or more of the following: | **NO** loss of consciousness **AND NO** post-traumatic amnesia, AND one or more of the following: |
| • Headache<br>• Vomiting<br>• Age older than 60 years<br>• Intoxication (drug or alcohol)<br>• Short-term memory deficits<br>• Evidence of trauma above the clavicle<br>• Post-traumatic seizure<br>• GCS score less than 15<br>• Focal neurologic deficit<br>• Coagulopathy | • Focal neurologic deficit<br>• Vomiting<br>• Severe headache<br>• Age 65 years or greater<br>• Signs of a basilar skull fracture<br>• GCS score less than 15<br>• Coagulopathy<br>• Dangerous mechanism of injury (including ejection from a motor vehicle, struck pedestrian, and a fall from a height of more than 3 feet or 5 stairs) |

According to the ACR appropriateness criteria, when there is mild closed head trauma with a GCS of 13 or greater and no neurological deficit or risk factors, head CT is at the lower end of "usually appropriate." For moderate or severe closed head trauma or for mild trauma if there is a neurological deficit and risk factors for hemorrhage, then a head CT is at the upper end of "usually appropriate" [76]. If there is additional concern for carotid or vertebral dissection, CTA or MRA (with T1 fat-saturated images) of the neck is usually appropriate [64]. ACEP recommendations to obtain or to consider obtaining a non-contrast CT of the head following minor trauma are summarized in Table 4.3 [77].

## For Chronic Headache with a Normal Neurologic Exam, is Imaging Indicated?

A practice parameter from the US Headache Consortium states that neuroimaging is not usually warranted for a patient with a migraine headache and a normal neurological exam [18]. A meta-analysis indicates that the prevalence of brain abnormality in patients with migraine headache is 0.2 percent, with an upper 95 percent confidence interval of 0.6 percent. This is less than the prevalence of 0.8 percent of AVM and 2 percent of saccular aneurysm in the general population [19,78,79]. In their Choosing Wisely campaign, one of the items specified by the American Headache Society pertains to not imaging stable migraine headaches. This is also an item on the American College of Radiology's Choosing Wisely

list, although the ACR item is broader and includes all stable headaches, while the American Headache Society mentions only migraine [80].

If the patient or family is "disabled by their fear of serious pathology" or the provider is suspicious of an abnormality, CT or MRI may be considered even though there would be no true indication for imaging [18,19]. In one study, patients randomized to receive an MRI scan for chronic headache had less anxiety in the short term (three months) and lower overall costs in the long term (one year) [81]. Additionally, in the evidence-based guidelines for neuroimaging in patients with non-acute headache released by the US Headache Consortium in 2000, it acknowledges that there may be a role for imaging if the doctor is concerned with medicolegal liability for an incidental finding unrelated to the headache (applies to all headache types) despite belief that risk is equal to the general population or if the patient or family particularly requests an imaging exam [17,82].

Regarding other (non-migraine) types of chronic headache, in a retrospective study on 402 adult patients with chronic headache, multivariate analysis showed abnormalities such as glioma, meningioma, pituitary macroadenoma, and hydrocephalus in 14.1 percent of patients with "atypical headaches" [83]. In an older study, 89 patients received a CT scan for chronic isolated headache; none of the scans yielded "important new information" (95 percent CI, 0–3 percent) [84]. Furthermore, in a sample of 40 patients with malignant brain tumors and patients requiring craniotomy for other reasons, none of the patients had isolated headache at the time of diagnosis, and only 5 percent sought medical attention for headache alone [84]. According to the ACR appropriateness criteria, when there is chronic headache with no new features and no neurological exam abnormalities, MRI of the head is classified on the lower end of appropriateness in the "may be appropriate" category. Otherwise, other imaging would be classified as "usually not appropriate." For non-migraine headaches, aside from the ACR Choosing Wisely list, which does not recommend imaging for any "uncomplicated headache," there are no specific recommendations.

The greatest reason to image only when indicated is that there is a greater likelihood of identifying an incidental finding rather than a true cause for the headache in the situation in which an indication for imaging is lacking [85]. In this context, imaging may lead to greater harm as incidental findings may compel work-up, which will lead to treatments and interventions that may unnecessarily harm the patient.

When the decision has been made to image a patient with chronic headache, MRI is more sensitive for pathology; however, the additional sensitivity may only detect insignificant abnormalities rather than elucidating the cause of the headache [19]. There are currently no comparative effectiveness studies with an endpoint of clinical relevance to inform whether CT or MR should be performed. According to the ACR appropriateness criteria, for chronic headache with new features or neurological deficit, MRI is rated slightly higher for appropriateness as compared to CT [17]. Of the primary headaches, cluster headaches may raise the most concern for a secondary etiology given that they commonly cause referred headache to the orbit, retroorbital region, and/or the temporal region. A Horner syndrome may also be present, further suggesting a secondary cause. In these situations, MRI of the brain and orbit with and without contrast would be appropriate to determine if there is an underlying abnormality [17,86] and MRA of the neck would be appropriate to exclude the possibility of carotid dissection.

## For Headache in a Patient with a Known Primary Neoplasm, What Imaging Test Should be Performed?

Patients with a primary malignancy and a new or changed headache may have intracranial metastatic disease. Brain metastases occur in 15–40 percent of patients with cancer; often these are asymptomatic [87]. Metastases may occur within the substance of the brain or within the surrounding skull, pachymeninges, or leptomeninges. Classically, metastases to the brain parenchyma localize to the gray–white matter junction [87]. When brain metastases are the primary concern, head CT should be obtained to rule out cerebral metastases, obstructive hydrocephalus, or herniation (transtentorial, subfalcine). Head CT is especially indicated in patients with abrupt neurological deterioration or impaired levels of consciousness. A gadolinium enhanced MRI should be performed in all cases, whether the head CT is positive or negative, to rule out parenchymal, leptomeningeal, and dural metastatic lesions and to determine the number and location of the metastatic lesions [88]. MRI is significantly more sensitive than CT for the detection of cerebral metastatic disease.

## If There is Suspected Sinus Headache, When and What Type of Imaging is Indicated?

The diagnosis of a headache secondary to sinus pathology may be made clinically and treated empirically [89], although migraine and other primary headache disorders are frequently misdiagnosed (by both patient and physician) as sinus headache. When there is a need for imaging confirmation, sinus radiographs have moderate sensitivity to detect a sinus air–fluid level or opacification, which are typical radiographic findings in acute sinusitis [90]. However, expertise in interpreting these radiographs is commonly limited, particularly now that the primary focus is placed on cross-sectional imaging such as CT. CT can be performed using a low radiation dose technique, although no study has been performed to assess its sensitivity and specificity relative to the gold standard of sinus puncture [90]. It is believed that CT has a high sensitivity and relatively low specificity as sinus fluid or mucosal thickening may have many causes, including allergy, upper respiratory infection, dental infection, trauma, or recent sinus lavage. A sinus CT may also be indicated to look for anatomic abnormalities that increase the risk for sinusitis [17]. If there is suspicion of intracranial or intraorbital complications of sinusitis, MRI of the brain and orbits without and with contrast is considered "usually appropriate" by the ACR appropriateness criteria [17,89]. The Infectious Diseases Society of America favors CT over MRI in such situations [91]. Non-contrast CT or MRI of the head is considered "maybe appropriate" [17]. Brain or orbital imaging may be particularly necessary in immunocompromised patients, as they are at higher risk of intraorbital and intracranial extension.

## Summary

A large variety of testing modalities are available for patients who present to an ED with headache. Though many diagnostic tests are now ordered routinely for headache patients, careful consideration of the appropriate test to order will increase efficiency and decrease cost.

## References

1. Parikh M, Miller NR, Lee AG, et al. Prevalence of a normal C-reactive protein with an elevated erythrocyte sedimentation rate in biopsy-proven giant cell arteritis. *Ophthalmology*. 2006;113(10):1842–5.

2. Kermani TA, Schmidt J, Crowson CS, et al. Utility of erythrocyte sedimentation rate and C-reactive protein for the diagnosis of giant cell arteritis. *Semin Arthritis Rheum*. 2012;41(6):866–71.

3. Murchison AP, Gilbert ME, Bilyk JR, et al. Validity of the American College of Rheumatology criteria for the diagnosis of giant cell arteritis. *Am J Ophthalmol*. 2012;154(4):722–9.

4. Dentali F, Squizzato A, Marchesi C, et al. D-dimer testing in the diagnosis of cerebral vein thrombosis: a systematic review and a meta-analysis of the literature. *J Thromb Haemost*. 2012;10(4):582–9.

5. Pachner AR, Steiner I. Lyme neuroborreliosis: infection, immunity, and inflammation. *Lancet Neurol*. 2007;6(6):544–52.

6. Makadzange AT, McHugh G. New approaches to the diagnosis and treatment of cryptococcal meningitis. *Semin Neurol*. 2014;34(1):47–60.

7. Bahr NC, Boulware DR. Methods of rapid diagnosis for the etiology of meningitis in adults. *Biomark Med*. 2014;8(9):1085–103.

8. Chu K, Hann A, Greenslade J, Williams J, Brown A. Spectrophotometry or visual inspection to most reliably detect xanthochromia in subarachnoid hemorrhage: systematic review. *Ann Emerg Med*. 2014;64(3):256–64.

9. Edlow JA. Diagnosis of subarachnoid hemorrhage. *Neurocrit Care*. 2005;2(2):99–109.

10. Perry JJ, Alyahya B, Sivilotti ML, et al. Differentiation between traumatic tap and aneurysmal subarachnoid hemorrhage: prospective cohort study. *BMJ*. 2015;350:h568.

11. Edlow JA, Bruner KS, Horowitz GL. Xanthochromia. *Arch Pathol Lab Med*. 2002;126(4):413–15.

12. Heasley DC, Mohamed MA, Yousem DM. Clearing of red blood cells in lumbar puncture does not rule out ruptured aneurysm in patients with suspected subarachnoid hemorrhage but negative head CT findings. *AJNR Am J Neuroradiol*. 2005;26(4):820–4.

13. Raja AS, Andruchow J, Zane R, Khorasani R, Schuur JD. Use of neuroimaging in US emergency departments. *Arch Intern Med*. 2011;171(3):260–2.

14. Edlow JA, Panagos PD, Godwin SA, et al. Clinical policy: critical issues in the evaluation and management of adult patients presenting to the emergency department with acute headache. *Ann Emerg Med*. 2008;52(4):407–36.

15. Vermeulen MJ, Schull MJ. Missed diagnosis of subarachnoid hemorrhage in the emergency department. *Stroke*. 2007;38(4):1216–21.

16. Gilbert JW, Johnson KM, Larkin GL, Moore CL. Atraumatic headache in US emergency departments: recent trends in CT/MRI utilisation and factors associated with severe intracranial pathology. *Emerg Med J*. 2012;29(7):576–81.

17. Douglas AC, Wippold FJ 2nd, Broderick DF, et al. ACR appropriateness criteria headache. *J Am Coll Radiol*. 2014;11(7):657–67.

18. Silberstein SD. Practice parameter: evidence-based guidelines for migraine headache (an evidence-based review): report of the Quality Standards Subcommittee of the American Academy of Neurology. *Neurology*. 2000;55(6):754–62.

19. Frishberg B, Rosenberg JH, Matchar DB, Pietrzak MP, Rozen TD. Evidence-based guidelines in the primary care setting: neuroimaging in patients with nonacute headache. 2000 Available from the American Academy of Neurology. Available at: http://tools.aan.com/professionals/practice/pdfs/gl0088.pdf.

20. Pearce MS, Salotti JA, Little MP, et al. Radiation exposure from CT scans in childhood and subsequent risk of leukaemia and brain tumours: a retrospective cohort study. *Lancet*. 2012;380(9840):499–505.

21. Zorbalar N, Yesilaras M, Aksay E. Carbon monoxide poisoning in patients presenting to the emergency department with a headache in winter months. *Emerg Med J*. 2014;31(e1):e66–70.

22. Brodsky MC, Vaphiades M. Magnetic resonance imaging in pseudotumor cerebri. *Ophthalmology*. 1998;105(9):1686–93.

23. Bradley WG Jr. MR appearance of hemorrhage in the brain. *Radiology*. 1993;189(1):15–26.

24. De Benedittis G, Lorenzetti A, Sina C, Bernasconi V. Magnetic resonance imaging in migraine and tension-type headache. *Headache*. 1995;35(5):264–8.

25. Randeva HS, Schoebel J, Byrne J, et al. Classical pituitary apoplexy: clinical features, management and outcome. *Clin Endocrinol (Oxf)*. 1999;51(2):181–8.

26. Boellis A, di Napoli A, Romano A, Bozzao A. Pituitary apoplexy: an update on clinical and imaging features. *Insights Imaging*. 2014;5(6):753–62.

27. Tentschert S, Wimmer R, Greisenegger S, Lang W, Lalouschek W. Headache at stroke onset in 2196 patients with ischemic stroke or transient ischemic attack. *Stroke*. 2005;36(2):e1–3.

28. Schwedt TJ, Dodick DW. Thunderclap stroke: embolic cerebellar infarcts presenting as thunderclap headache. *Headache*. 2006;46(3):520–2.

29. Karassa FB, Matsagas MI, Schmidt WA, Ioannidis JP. Meta-analysis: test performance of ultrasonography for giant-cell arteritis. *Ann Intern Med*. 2005;142(5):359–69.

30. Bley TA, Uhl M, Carew J, et al. Diagnostic value of high-resolution MR imaging in giant cell arteritis. *AJNR Am J Neuroradiol*. 2007;28(9):1722–7.

31. Perry JJ, Stiell IG, Sivilotti ML, et al. High risk clinical characteristics for subarachnoid haemorrhage in patients with acute headache: prospective cohort study. *BMJ*. 2010;341:c5204.

32. Perry JJ, Stiell IG, Sivilotti ML, et al. Clinical decision rules to rule out subarachnoid hemorrhage for acute headache. *JAMA*. 2013;310(12):1248–55.

33. Grimaldi D, Nonino F, Cevoli S, et al. Risk stratification of non-traumatic headache in the emergency department. *J Neurol*. 2009;256(1):51–7.

34. De Luca GC, Bartleson JD. When and how to investigate the patient with headache. *Semin Neurol*. 2010;30(2):131–44.

35. Sempere AP, Porta-Etessam J, Medrano V, et al. Neuroimaging in the evaluation of patients with non-acute headache. *Cephalalgia*. 2005;25(1):30–5.

36. Lewis DW, Ashwal S, Dahl G, et al. Practice parameter: evaluation of children and adolescents with recurrent headaches – report of the Quality Standards Subcommittee of the American Academy of Neurology and the Practice Committee of the Child Neurology Society. *Neurology*. 2002;59(4):490–8.

37. Pascual J, González-Mandly A, Martín R, Oterino A. Headaches precipitated by cough, prolonged exercise or sexual activity: a prospective etiological and clinical study. *J Headache Pain*. 2008;9(5):259–66.

38. Landtblom AM, Fridriksson S, Boivie J, et al. Sudden onset headache: a prospective study of features, incidence and causes. *Cephalalgia*. 2002;22(5):354–60.

39. Cuvinciuc V, Viguier A, Calviere L, et al. Isolated acute nontraumatic cortical subarachnoid hemorrhage. *AJNR Am J Neuroradiol*. 2010;31(8):1355–62.

40. Nishijima DK, Offerman SR, Ballard DW, et al. Risk of traumatic intracranial hemorrhage in patients with head injury and preinjury warfarin or clopidogrel use. *Acad Emerg Med*. 2013;20(2):140–5.

41. Hart RG, Diener HC, Yang S, et al. Intracranial hemorrhage in atrial fibrillation patients during anticoagulation with warfarin or dabigatran: the RE-LY trial. *Stroke*. 2012;43(6):1511–17.

42. Gorelick PB, Weisman SM. Risk of hemorrhagic stroke with aspirin use: an update. *Stroke*. 2005;36(8):1801–7.

43. Garbe E, Kreisel SH, Behr S. Risk of subarachnoid hemorrhage and early case fatality associated with outpatient antithrombotic drug use. *Stroke*. 2013;44(9):2422–6.

44. Bederson JB, Connolly ES Jr, Batjer HH, et al. Guidelines for the management of aneurysmal subarachnoid hemorrhage: a statement for healthcare professionals from a special writing group of the Stroke Council, American Heart Association. *Stroke*. 2009;40(3):994–1025.

45. Pierot L, Portefaix C, Rodriguez-Régent C, et al. Role of MRA in the detection of intracranial aneurysm in the acute phase of subarachnoid hemorrhage. *J Neuroradiol*. 2013;40(3):204–10.

46. Romijn M, Gratama van Andel HA, van Walderveen MA, et al. Diagnostic accuracy of CT angiography with matched mask bone elimination for detection of intracranial aneurysms: comparison with digital subtraction angiography and 3D rotational angiography. *AJNR Am J Neuroradiol*. 2008;29(1):134–9.

47. Luo Z, Wang D, Sun X, et al. Comparison of the accuracy of subtraction CT angiography performed on 320-detector row volume CT with conventional CT angiography for diagnosis of intracranial aneurysms. *Eur J Radiol*. 2012;81(1):118–22.

48. Delgado Almandoz JE, Jagadeesan BD, Refai D, et al. Diagnostic yield of computed tomography angiography and magnetic resonance angiography in patients with catheter angiography-negative subarachnoid hemorrhage. *J Neurosurg*. 2012;117(2):309–15.

49. van Gijn J, van Dongen KJ. The time course of aneurysmal haemorrhage on computed tomograms. *Neuroradiology*. 1982;23(3):153–6.

50. Backes D, Rinkel GJ, Kemperman H, Linn FH, Vergouwen MD. Time-dependent test characteristics of head computed tomography in patients suspected

of nontraumatic subarachnoid hemorrhage. *Stroke.* 2012;43(8):2115–19.

51. Stewart H, Reuben A, McDonald J. LP or not LP, that is the question: gold standard or unnecessary procedure in subarachnoid haemorrhage? *Emerg Med J.* 2014;31(9):720–3.

52. Perry JJ, Stiell IG, Sivilotti ML, et al. Sensitivity of computed tomography performed within six hours of onset of headache for diagnosis of subarachnoid haemorrhage: prospective cohort study. *BMJ.* 2011;343:d4277.

53. Edlow JA, Fisher J. Diagnosis of subarachnoid hemorrhage: time to change the guidelines? *Stroke.* 2012;43(8):2031–2.

54. Mark DG, Hung YY, Offerman SR, et al. Nontraumatic subarachnoid hemorrhage in the setting of negative cranial computed tomography results: external validation of a clinical and imaging prediction rule. *Ann Emerg Med.* 2013;62(1):1–10.

55. Fine B, Singh N, Aviv R, Macdonald RL. Decisions: does a patient with a thunderclap headache need a lumbar puncture? *CMAJ.* 2012;184(5):555–6.

56. Wiesmann M, Mayer TE, Yousry I, et al. Detection of hyperacute subarachnoid hemorrhage of the brain by using magnetic resonance imaging. *J Neurosurg.* 2002;96(4):684–9.

57. Yuan MK, Lai PH, Chen JY, et al. Detection of subarachnoid hemorrhage at acute and subacute/chronic stages: comparison of four magnetic resonance imaging pulse sequences and computed tomography. *J Chin Med Assoc.* 2005;68(3):131–7.

58. Hodel J, Aboukais R, Dutouquet B, et al. Double inversion recovery MR sequence for the detection of subacute subarachnoid hemorrhage. *AJNR Am J Neuroradiol.* 2014;36(2):251–8.

59. Verma RK, Kottke R, Andereggen L, et al. Detecting subarachnoid hemorrhage: comparison of combined FLAIR/SWI versus CT. *Eur J Radiol.* 2013;82(9):1539–45.

60. Woodcock RJ Jr, Short J, Do HM, Jensen ME, Kallmes DF. Imaging of acute subarachnoid hemorrhage with a fluid-attenuated inversion recovery sequence in an animal model: comparison with non-contrast-enhanced CT. *AJNR Am J Neuroradiol.* 2001;22(9):1698–703.

61. Schievink WI, Maya MM, Louy C, Moser FG, Tourje J. Diagnostic criteria for spontaneous spinal CSF leaks and intracranial hypotension. *AJNR Am J Neuroradiol.* 2008;29(5):853–6.

62. Ramchandren S, Cross BJ, Liebeskind DS. Emergent headaches during pregnancy: correlation between neurologic examination and neuroimaging. *AJNR Am J Neuroradiol.* 2007;28(6):1085–7.

63. McCollough CH, Schueler BA, Atwell TD, et al. Radiation exposure and pregnancy: when should we be concerned? *Radiographics.* 2007;27(4):909–17.

64. Perry JJ, Spacek A, Forbes M, et al. Is the combination of negative computed tomography result and negative lumbar puncture result sufficient to rule out subarachnoid hemorrhage? *Ann Emerg Med.* 2008;51(6):707–13.

65. Horstman P, Linn FH, Voorbij HA, Rinkel GJ. Chance of aneurysm in patients suspected of SAH who have a "negative" CT scan but a "positive" lumbar puncture. *J Neurol.* 2012;259(4):649–52.

66. McCormack RF, Hutson A. Can computed tomography angiography of the brain replace lumbar puncture in the evaluation of acute-onset headache after a negative noncontrast cranial computed tomography scan? *Acad Emerg Med.* 2010;17(4):444–51.

67. Swadron SP. Pitfalls in the management of headache in the emergency department. *Emerg Med Clin North Am.* 2010;28(1):127–47.

68. Ward MJ, Bonomo JB, Adeoye O, Raja AS, Pines JM. Cost-effectiveness of diagnostic strategies for evaluation of suspected subarachnoid hemorrhage in the emergency department. *Acad Emerg Med.* 2012;19(10):1134–44.

69. Edlow JA. What are the unintended consequences of changing the diagnostic paradigm for subarachnoid hemorrhage after brain computed tomography to computed tomographic angiography in place of lumbar puncture? *Acad Emerg Med.* 2010;17(9):991–5.

70. Kong DS, Hong SC, Jung YJ, Kim JS. Improvement of chronic headache after treatment of unruptured intracranial aneurysms. *Headache.* 2007;47(5):693–7.

71. Rinkel GJ, Djibuti M, Algra A, van Gijn J. Prevalence and risk of rupture of intracranial aneurysms: a systematic review. *Stroke.* 1998;29(1):251–6.

72. Devenney E, Neale, H, Forbes R, Raeburn B. A systematic review of causes of sudden and severe headache (thunderclap headache): should lists be evidence based? *J Head Pain.* 2014;15:49.

73. Ducros A, Hajj-Ali RA, Singhal AB, Wang SJ. Reversible cerebral vasoconstriction syndrome. *JAMA Neurology.* 2014;71:368.

74. Lucas S, Hoffman JM, Bell KR, Dikmen S. A prospective study of prevalence and characterization of headache following mild traumatic brain injury. *Cephalalgia.* 2014;34:93–102.

75. Ryan LM, Warden DL. Post concussion syndrome. *Int Rev Psychiatry.* 2003;15(4):310–16.

76. https://acsearch.org/docs/69481/Narrative.

77. Jagoda AS, Bazarian JJ, Bruns JJ Jr, et al. Clinical policy: neuroimaging and decision making in adult

mild traumatic brain injury in the acute setting. *Ann Emerg Med.* 2008;52(6):714–48.

78. Neff MJ. Evidence based guidelines for neuroimaging in patients with nonacute headache. *Am Fam Physician.* 2005;71(6):1219–22.

79. Rinkel GJ, Djibuti M, Algra A, van Gijn J. Prevalence and risk of rupture of intracranial aneurysms: a systematic review. *Stroke.* 1998;29(1):251–6.

80. Loder E, Weizenbaum E, Frishberg B, Silberstein S; American Headache Society Choosing Wisely Task Force. Choosing wisely in headache medicine: the American Headache Society's list of five things physicians and patients should question. *Headache.* 2013;53(10):1651–9.

81. Howard L, Wessely S, Leese M, et al. Are investigations anxiolytic or anxiogenic? A randomised controlled trial of neuroimaging to provide reassurance in chronic daily headache. *J Neurol Neurosurg Psychiatry.* 2005;76(11):1558–64.

82. Evans RW. Medico-legal headaches: trials and tribulations. In *Advanced Therapy of Headache*, 2nd ed. Edited by Purdy RA, Rapoport A, Sheftell F, Tepper S. Hamilton, ON: BC Decker; 2005, 229–38.

83. Wang HZ, Simonson TM, Greco WR, Yuh WT. Brain MR imaging in the evaluation of chronic headache in patients without other neurologic symptoms. *Acad Radiol.* 2001;8(5):405–8.

84. Weingarten S, Kleinman M, Elperin L, Larson EB. The effectiveness of cerebral imaging in the diagnosis of chronic headache. *Arch Intern Med.* 1992;152(12):2457–62.

85. Sudlow C. US guidelines on neuroimaging in patients with non-acute headache: a commentary. *J Neurol Neurosurg Psychiatry.* 2002;72(Suppl. 2):ii16–18.

86. Waldman CW, Waldman SD, Waldman RA. Pain of ocular and periocular origin. *Med Clin North Am.* 2013;97(2):293–307.

87. Fink KR, Fink JR. Imaging of brain metastases. *Surg Neurol Int.* 2013;4(Suppl. 4):S209–19.

88. Expert Panel on Radiation Oncology-Brain Metastases, Lo SS, Gore EM, et al. ACR Appropriateness Criteria® pre-irradiation evaluation and management of brain metastases. *J Palliat Med.* 2014;17(8):880–6.

89. Cornelius RS, Martin J, Wippold FJ 2nd, et al. ACR appropriateness criteria sinonasal disease. *J Am Coll Radiol.* 2013;10(4):241–6.

90. Anzai Y. Evaluation of sinusitis: evidence-based neuroimaging. In *Evidence-Based Neuroimaging Diagnosis and Treatment*. Edited by Medina LS, Sanelli PC, Jarvik JG. New York: Springer; 2013, 581–97.

91. Chow AW, Benninger MS, Brook I, et al. IDSA clinical practice guideline for acute bacterial rhinosinusitis in children and adults. *Clin Infect Dis.* 2012;54(8):e72–112.

# Thunderclap Headache in the Emergency Department

James Ducharme

*Put simply, the sun should not set on an undiagnosed thunderclap headache.*

*JF Rothrock*

## Abstract

A person presenting with a thunderclap headache is at high risk of a life-threatening condition – 4–5 times greater risk than those who are in the "rule-out MI" or "rule-out pulmonary embolism" category. Of those who do have a high-risk condition, 30–50 percent will not have a subarachnoid hemorrhage (SAH). Many emergency physicians discharge people with thunderclap headaches after a computed tomography (CT) and a lumbar puncture (LP) have ruled out an SAH, but this strategy needs to change and encompass consultation and additional imaging if that first series of investigations is negative. There are many other conditions that can present with a thunderclap headache. This chapter will review the differential diagnosis, and the signs and symptoms of each; it will conclude with recommendations on a comprehensive approach in the emergency department (ED) for someone presenting with a thunderclap headache.

## Introduction

A thunderclap headache is normally defined as severe in character and reaching maximum severity within seconds to minutes of onset. An even more restrictive definition states that it must be of instantaneous onset, reaching maximum intensity within one minute. The term "thunderclap headache" is listed as one of the critical red flags used to identify patients with headache who are at risk for life-threatening pathology. Every emergency physician is wary of the patient who presents with such a clinical presentation as they have linked that presentation with the possibility of an SAH. Emergency physicians have perhaps associated too strongly the clinical presentation of "thunderclap

headache" with "rule-out SAH": a patient who has a negative diagnostic work-up is often felt to be safe to be sent home, having had the possibility of SAH ruled out. At times, these patients need a more extensive work-up.

It is important to recognize from the start of this chapter that thunderclap headaches are neither sensitive nor specific for the diagnosis of SAH – about 50 percent of patients with SAH present with a thunderclap headache, while SAH is the identified cause in only 11–21 percent of patients who present with thunderclap headache [1]. The location of the headache, while retrospectively helpful for cohort pattern descriptions, cannot accurately guide the clinician to a diagnosis prior to work-up: headaches related to dissection, for example, *usually* are focal (occipital or unilateral in the neck) but do not seem to be *consistently* focal enough to rely on that localization to rule in or rule out dissection. Many life-threatening conditions other than SAH can present with a thunderclap headache, some of which will not be identified with a "CT and LP" approach (Table 5.1). Overall, in this author's experience, approximately 25 to 30 percent of patients presenting to an emergency department with a thunderclap headache will be suffering from a life-threatening condition, making this one of the most high-risk symptoms emergency physicians encounter. *A significant proportion of these life-threatening conditions will not be an SAH.*

Taking the *next* diagnostic step after a negative CT and LP in patients with thunderclap headache has remained inconsistent – whereas in most EDs patients are discharged without further work-up, in some departments none are discharged without an MRI/MRA. The American College of Emergency Physicians (ACEP) 2008 policy on acute headache states as a level B recommendation: "Patients with a sudden-onset, severe headache who have negative findings on a head CT, normal opening pressure, and

**Table 5.1** Differential diagnosis of thunderclap headache

| Identifiable with CT | Identifiable with LP | Normal CT and LP |
| --- | --- | --- |
| Subarachnoid hemorrhage | Subarachnoid hemorrhage | Arterial dissection extracranial -Carotid -Vertebral Intracranial |
| Intracerebral hemorrhage | Meningitis -bacterial -viral | Symptomatic aneurysm with mass effect |
| Intraventricular hemorrhage | | Reversible cerebral vasoconstriction syndrome |
| Acute subdural hemorrhage | | Posterior reversible encephalopathy syndrome |
| Ischemic stroke | | Cerebral venous sinus thrombosis |
| Tumor (third ventricle colloid cyst, posterior fossa tumor) | | Pituitary apoplexy |
| Hydrocephalus (aqueductal stenosis, Chiari type 1 malformation) | | Intracranial hypotension (usually unidentified CSF leak) |
| | | Ischemic stroke in first three hours |
| | | Temporal arteritis |
| | | Myocardial ischemia |
| | | Aortic dissection |

negative findings in CSF analysis do not need emergent angiography and can be discharged from the ED with follow-up recommended" [2]. When looking at the differential diagnosis, one cannot help but notice that most conditions are vascular in origin – abrupt onset severe pain anywhere is almost always vascular or ischemic in nature, be it a ruptured ectopic pregnancy, testicular torsion, or an SAH. It is understandable, therefore, why it is felt by many that vascular imaging is mandatory for a patient presenting with a thunderclap headache. There is an over-diagnosis risk, especially with regards to discovering an incidental aneurysm, as prospective autopsy studies have identified that approximately 3.6 percent of the population have an intracranial aneurysm at the time of death, but unrelated to their cause of death [3]. The time, money, and patient risk inherent with over-diagnosis

has to be considered therefore in any discussion about investigating a patient with a thunderclap headache.

In this chapter we identify conditions the emergency physician needs to diagnose at the first visit, and review the value of certain clinical symptoms in distinguishing one disease from another. We follow that with a review of the investigative approach, discuss the value of testing, and attempt to recommend a coherent diagnostic strategy that ensures the clinician does not miss a critical illness.

## Diagnostic Possibilities

### "Can't Miss" Conditions

**Intracranial Bleeding**. The first hemorrhagic condition to consider is SAH, since it represents a large subset of the life-threatening conditions associated with thunderclap headaches. Warning, or sentinel leaks associated with aneurysmal expansion, may precede major, clinically devastating SAH in up to half of cases. Typically the thunderclap headache is the only symptom in such sentinel events, and can resolve within hours to days. It is important to recognize that a thunderclap headache related to a sentinel bleed may have resolved by the time the patient is seen in the ED – such patients must not be ignored despite their normal appearance and absence of headache at the time of their evaluation. Other patients with SAH may present with headache or neck pain/rigidity, with a less obvious "thunderclap" presentation. Associated symptoms can include loss of consciousness, nausea, and emesis.

Arteriovenous malformations (AVMs) or hemorrhagic tumors/metastasis may also present with a thunderclap headache. Decreased mental status or focal findings are more typical in intraparenchymal bleeding compared to hemorrhage that is confined to the subarachnoid space; in all cases, decreased mental status is associated with worse outcomes [4]. Patients with cerebellar hemorrhages must be seen emergently by neurosurgery as they may deteriorate rapidly after onset. If a patient presents with symptoms typical of a cerebellar hemorrhage, but has a normal CT, an urgent MRI is required to exclude a cerebellar ischemic stroke.

**Arterial Dissection**. Neck pain is the most prevalent symptom for vertebral or carotid artery dissection (CAD). It may be the presenting symptom in 50–60 percent of patients with vertebral artery dissection

(VAD), and can precede any other symptom by up to two weeks [5]. Thunderclap headache as the initial symptom occurs about 20 percent of the time [2]. The headache is classically occipital and may be bilateral in those with unilateral VAD. In those with CAD, the pain may involve the neck, jaw, face, and periorbital and/or temporal region on the ipsilateral side, and is invariably unilateral. Diagnosis must be rapid: the mean time from headache onset to the occurrence of ischemic stroke may be as short as 15 hours [6]. Carotid artery dissection often occurs after seemingly trivial trauma – hyperextension of the neck, rapidly shaking the head, even massage and manipulation. Acute headache accompanies CAD in at least 60 percent of cases [7]. Isolated head or neck pain is the only symptom of cervical artery dissection in 8 percent of cases [5]. Patients with *aortic* dissection will have no history of trauma; one must consider this possibility in the young person (Marfan's syndrome) or in the over-50 person with hypertension, obesity, or atherosclerotic heart disease. Unless complicated by hemorrhagic or ischemic stroke, cervical arterial dissection will not result in abnormal findings on either non-contrast head CT or LP.

**Cerebral Venous Sinus Thrombosis.** The headache may be thunderclap in approximately 15 percent of cases; headache of some form will be present in up to 90 percent of cases and may be the sole manifestation of the condition in as many as 10 percent [6]. Initial early CT (with or without contrast) may be normal. Non-invasive venography (CT or MR) is often diagnostic. It is felt that the obstruction of venous return leads to a rapid rise in intracranial pressure and thus an abrupt onset headache. Symptoms can be non-specific, with headache lasting months or years. In most, however, the clinical course is fulminant, with rapid clinical deterioration involving focal neurological deficits and seizures [8].

**Posterior Reversible Encephalopathy Syndrome (PRES).** This almost always occurs in relationship to a hypertensive crisis (eclampsia or hypertension emergency), though other provoking factors have been identified, such as certain immunosuppressive medications. Rapid neurological deterioration may follow the thunderclap headache – seizures, decreased mental status, and visual symptoms. There may be segmented vasoconstriction identified on MRA. Posterior reversible encephalopathy syndrome can also occur in normotensive people who develop acute hypertension from illicit drug

use (cocaine), other types of sympathomimetics (nasal decongestants containing pseudoephedrine), reversible cerebral vasoconstriction syndrome, or pheochromocytoma [8].

## Non-Life-Threatening Conditions

**Reversible Cerebral Vasoconstriction Syndrome (RCVS).** Until roughly ten years ago, 70 percent or more of patients with thunderclap headache were felt to have a benign headache of unknown origin. They were often felt to occur in patients already suffering from tension-type headache or migraine [1]. At that time there were isolated case reports of diffuse multifocal segmental cerebrovascular vasospasm, without focal neurological signs or symptoms. In 2012, a systematic review by Ducros highlighted that reversible cerebral vasoconstriction is more common than previously thought [9]. Reversible cerebral vasoconstriction syndrome presents as isolated headaches in about 75 percent of cases [8]. While Ducros et al. feel that RCVS accounts for most cases of thunderclap headache previously identified as "benign thunderclap headache" [9], others have found it to represent less than 10 percent of these patients [10].

Many patients with this disorder may have several thunderclap headaches over several weeks. As would be expected, CT and cerebrospinal fluid (CSF) are normal in most, although roughly 20 percent have been found to have a small sulcal subarachnoid hemorrhage [9]. Diagnosis requires non-invasive vascular imaging (CTA/MRA) demonstrating diffuse, segmental, multifocal vasoconstriction [11]. This diagnosis is often missed initially – hence the previous belief of thunderclap headache to be of unknown origin – as the vasoconstriction may take 1–2 weeks to appear after the first headache and usually peaks at week three. RCVS-associated vasoconstriction normally reverses within 12 weeks of onset.

**Intracranial Hypotension.** While most cases of intracranial hypotension occur after dural puncture, spontaneous intracranial hypotension from CSF leak is well-recognized [12,13]. Thunderclap headache may be the presenting feature in approximately 15 percent of people with this disorder [13]. After the abrupt onset, the symptoms resemble a postdural puncture leak with a positional headache that occurs or worsens while sitting or standing and is relieved by recumbency. The diagnosis suspected on the basis of the history of a postural headache, and supported by typical findings on gadolinium-enhanced MRI of the brain, including pachymeningeal thickening and enhancement, cerebellar tonsillar descent, flattening of the tectum and anterior pons, enlarged dural venous sinuses, and pituitary enlargement with diffuse homogeneous enhancement. The etiology is usually a CSF leak in the low cervical or upper thoracic region and extra-arachnoid or extra-dural CSF can be demonstrated with an unenhanced MRI spine [14].

## The Cause of Thunderclap Headache Cannot be Made Based on Clinical Symptoms Alone

There are no pathognomonic signs or symptoms associated with thunderclap headache with sufficient sensitivity or specificity to narrow the differential diagnosis with certainty. The sentinel symptom alone engenders a standardized work-up. If the first phase of investigations (CT, LP) do not disclose a diagnosis, associated symptoms may guide subsequent diagnostic evaluation. Table 5.2 lists symptoms normally associated with different pathologies that may present with thunderclap headache and illustrates the considerable overlap of associated symptoms.

## Investigation of a Thunderclap Headache

### First Step of Investigation: Head CT

It is well-recognized, as outlined in the previous chapter, that the sensitivity of head CT for identifying an SAH decreases with the passage of time. With ever-improving technology, the question has been raised of whether CT can be sensitive enough to stand alone as a means to diagnose SAH in the first few hours [15]. In a 2011 study, Perry et al. showed that overall CT sensitivity was unacceptably low, at 92 percent. Restricting assessment of sensitivity to an a-priori established six-hour cutoff after headache onset yielded CT sensitivity of 100 percent for SAH. There were some concerns about the generalizability of the conclusions. Scanners were not standard in the 11 sites, varying from 4- to 320-slice machines, and nine of the sites had neuroradiological and neurosurgical teams where expertise was high. Since there were only 121 patients with SAH in the study window of six hours, the confidence

**Table 5.2** Symptoms associated with diagnoses presenting with thunderclap headache

| Diagnosis | Associated symptoms |
|---|---|
| Carotid artery dissection | Ipsilateral neck pain of gradual onset, up to two weeks prior to headache or neurological symptoms. Onset with minor neck trauma |
| Vertebral artery dissection | Occipitonuchal pain of gradual onset, vertigo, posterior circulation neurological findings. Onset with minor neck trauma |
| Aortic dissection | Chest pain |
| RCVS | Recurrent abrupt headaches over 2–3 weeks |
| Intracerebral hemorrhage | Vomiting, decreased level of consciousness, focal neurological findings. "Focal findings trump headache" [6] |
| Cerebral sinus thrombosis | Diplopia, blurred vision, focal headache, seizures, decreased mental status |
| SAH | Nausea, vomiting, syncope, photophobia, nuchal rigidity. "Headache trumps focal findings" [6] |
| PRES | Seizures, decreased mental status, visual symptoms |
| Intracranial hypotension | Orthostatic symptoms, recent dural puncture |
| Temporal arteritis (vasculitis) | Polymyalgia rheumatica, xerostomia, masseter claudication, abrupt loss of vision from one eye, non-contiguous focal deficits |
| Hydrocephalus | Nausea, vomiting, decreased mental status |

interval for sensitivity was as low as 97 percent. While this initial study by Perry et al. showed that the chance of a missed SAH in a person presenting to one of these study centers with a thunderclap headache within the first six hours and having a normal CT would be very low (less than 0.1 percent), these findings must be replicated before this approach can be accepted broadly. In a more recent study in non-academic centers, Blok et al. attempted to provide external validation of this six-hour cutoff [16]. In that study, 52 patients had an SAH, with one being missed (98 percent sensitivity, with a lower confidence interval of 92 percent); this study therefore failed to confirm this approach. Mark et al. also failed to validate the six-hour rule: In their study, 20 percent of patients with SAH were missed using the Perry criteria [17]. Teleradiology is now widely available, but it is uncommon for a neuroradiologist to be available during off-hours. It is acknowledged that a CT *after* six hours from onset can only rule in SAH; further testing is required to rule it out. However, as seen from Table 5.1, there are many conditions presenting with a thunderclap headache that will not be identified by CT.

## Lumbar Puncture

It has been argued that, in a patient presenting with an acute onset headache, a head CT is not required prior to LP [18]. In his theoretical model, Schull argues that up to 80 percent of CTs could be eliminated with such an approach. If we accept Perry's model that states that CT after six hours is not sensitive enough, it could be argued that, in a patient with a thunderclap headache and normal mentation presenting after six hours, LP should be the first investigation as it would carry a greater chance of identifying the SAH. Any patient with a negative CT will have to have an LP, so it would seem reasonable to start with the LP in this subset. If the LP was positive, the next imaging would be a vascular study, and not a routine CT. While LP would also identify all infectious and some inflammatory causes of thunderclap headache, such an approach would fail to diagnose many conditions listed in Table 5.1 that would be identified on CT.

Another weakness of the LP-first approach is that xanthochromia may take up to 12 hours to become evident. It is xanthochromia that is diagnostic of an SAH, not the presence of red blood cells, for the latter may be present from a traumatic tap. There is still debate as to whether "clearing" of red cells between the first tube and the fourth tube collected can establish the difference between a traumatic tap and an SAH [19]. In this 2015 study, the authors concluded that – no matter when the LP was performed in relation to headache onset – the absence of xanthochromia *and* less than $2000 \times 10^6$/L red blood cells safely ruled out SAH, even though the low range of the sensitivity confidence interval was 74.7 percent. The traditional (and conservative) approach has been (and remains) to rule-out SAH only if there is no xanthochromia after 12 hours or if there are (almost) no red blood cells on the initial tap.

## Both CT and LP are Negative: Now What?

Almost all life-threatening conditions are vascular in origin. When a patient gives a clear history of thunderclap headache, the emergency physician should have the expectation that further imaging will be required. Inherent to the process should be the understanding that – with both CT- and LP-negative thunderclap headache – any aneurysm identified is *not* the source of the headache, unless no other cause is identified and the aneurysm is abnormally large. This line of thinking is important, for MRA or CTA will usually be the next step in investigation – and inferring causality from an identified aneurysm *that is not the actual cause* will lead to increased morbidity from both missing the true diagnosis and the steps taken as a result of over-diagnosis.

In a patient with a documented SAH, CTA or MRA will identify if the bleeding is aneurysmal in origin. If not, treatment is conservative and does not require further intervention, unless the location and size of the aneurysm warrants intervention even if the finding is *incidental* to the thunderclap headache. In a patient where dissection is suspected, or where an AVM is a possibility, then vascular imaging is required – CTA or MRA are equally sensitive. It is important when SAH is no longer in the differential diagnosis that the arterial imaging be for the head *and* neck, as dissection may be extracranial and not identified with imaging only of the head. This discussion should take place with the neurologist or radiologist prior to imaging. MRA will also demonstrate the segmental vasospasm of RCVS.

For other conditions, arterial imaging will not be of value. When considering cerebral venous sinus thrombosis, CT or MR venography are often required but the choice should be made in consultation with radiology/neuroradiology. Clinicians should not be dissuaded from this critical decision-making discussion because they do not have magnetic resonance capacity in-house or available at night.

## Cut to the Chase: What is the Best Approach?

Of all patients presenting to an ED with a thunderclap headache, approximately 30 percent will have a life-threatening etiology of one kind or another. Let's place that in context: In most centers the rule-in rate for myocardial infarction clinical presentations can be less than 5–7 percent [20]. The risk of sepsis in a patient presenting with febrile neutropenia after chemotherapy is around 14 percent [21]. Extensive work-ups are performed for all of these conditions, with many staying for 24 hours or more to complete the work-up. Despite the higher risk to the patient presenting with a thunderclap headache and despite the data showing that at least 30–40 percent of these conditions will not be identified with a CT + LP approach, that approach is often the only one taken, and is currently the approach endorsed by ACEP.

If we return to the quote by Rothrock at the start of this chapter, when a patient presents with a thunderclap headache, the CT + LP process can be but the first step in our investigation. If either suggests the presence of an SAH, then a CT/MRI or catheter angiogram of the head is required to identify if an aneurysm is the cause.

If the CT + LP are negative, the job is not done: Consultation with a neurologist or radiologist should be the next step, in order to discuss which form of cervicocephalgic vascular imaging should be performed. The range of imaging options is extensive and the local expertise variable enough that the emergency physician should discuss options with a consultant, factoring in as much as possible the associated symptoms, no matter how (un)reliable they are for narrowing the differential diagnosis.

## Conclusion

In this chapter we have provided a review of the differential diagnosis of thunderclap headache with an emphasis on conditions that are imperative to diagnose in the ED setting. We then reviewed the breadth of investigations for thunderclap headache. Finally, we proposed a strategy for the diagnostic evaluation of patients with thunderclap headache in the ED.

## References

1. Landtblom AM, Fridriksson S, Boivie J, et al. Sudden onset headache: a prospective study of features, incidence and causes. *Cephalalgia* 2002;22:354–60.

2. Edlow JA, Panagos PD, Godwin SA, Thomas TL, Decker WW. Clinical policy: critical issues in the evaluation and management of adult patients presenting to the emergency department with acute headache. *Ann Emerg Med*. 2008;52(4):407–36.

3. Rinkel GJ, Djibuti M, Algra A, van Gijn J. Prevalence and risk of rupture of intracranial aneurysms: a systematic review. *Stroke*. 1998;29:251–6.

4. Chotai S, Ahn SY, Moon HJ, et al. Prediction of outcomes in young adults with aneurysmal subarachnoid hemorrhage. *Neurol Med Chir*. 2013;53(3):157–62.

5. Hsu YC, Sung SF. Spontaneous vertebral artery dissection with thunderclap headache: a case report and review of the literature. *Acta Neurol Taiwan*. 2014;23:24–8.

6. Silbert PL, Mokri B, Schievink WI. Headache and neck pain in spontaneous internal carotid and vertebral artery dissections. *Neurology*. 1995;45:1517–22.

7. Fisher CM, Ojemann RG, Roberson GH. Spontaneous dissection of cervicocerebral arteries. *Can J Neurol Sci*. 1978;5:9–19.

8. Stam J. Thrombosis of the cerebral veins and sinuses. *N Engl J Med*. 2005;352:1791–8

9. Ducros A. Reversible cerebral vasoconstriction syndrome. *Lancet Neurol*. 2012;11:906–17.

10. Grooters GS, Sluzewski M, Tijssen CC. How often is thunderclap headache caused by the reversible cerebral vasoconstriction syndrome? *Headache*. 2014;54:732–5.

11. Rothrock JF. Headache caused by vascular disorders. *Neurol Clin*. 2014;32:305–19.

12. Ducros A, Bousser MG. Thunderclap headache. *BMJ*. 2012;345:e8557.

13. Schievink WI, Wijdicks EF, Meyer FB, Sonntag VK. Spontaneous intracranial hypotension mimicking aneurysmal subarachnoid hemorrhage. *Neurosurgery* 2001;48:513–16.

14. Mokri B. Spontaneous low pressure, low CSF volume headaches: spontaneous CSF leaks. *Headache*. 2013;53:1034–53.

15. Perry JJ, Stiell IG, Sivilotti ML, et al. Sensitivity of computed tomography performed within six hours of onset of headache for diagnosis of subarachnoid haemorrhage: prospective cohort study. *BMJ*. 2011;343:d4277.

16. Blok KM, Rinkel GJE, Majoie CBLM, et al. CT within 6 hours of headache onset to rule out subarachnoid hemorrhage in nonacademic hospitals. *Neurology* 2015;84:1927–32.

17. Mark DG, Hung YY, Offerman SR, et al. Nontraumatic subarachnoid hemorrhage in the setting of negative cranial computed tomography results: external validation of a clinical and imaging prediction rule. *Ann Emerg Med*. 2013;62:1–10.e1.

18. Schull M. Lumbar puncture first: an alternative model for the investigation of lone acute sudden headache. *Acad Emerg Med*. 1999;6:131–6.

19. Perry JJ, Alyahya B, Sivilotti ML, et al. Differentiation between traumatic tap and aneurysmal subarachnoid hemorrhage: prospective cohort study. *BMJ*. 2015;350:h568. doi: 10.1136/bmj.h568.

20. Gaspoz JM, Lee TH, Weinstein MC, et al. Cost-effectiveness of a new short-stay unit to "rule out" acute myocardial infarction in low risk patients. *J Am Coll Cardiol.* 1994;24:1249–59.

21. Freifeld AG, Bow EJ, Sepkowitz KA, et al. Clinical practice guideline for the use of antimicrobial agents in neutropenic patients with cancer: 2010 update by the Infectious Diseases Society of America. *Clin Infect Dis.* 2011;52:e56–93.

# Other Secondary Headaches in the Emergency Department

Michael J. Marmura

Benjamin W. Friedman

## Abstract

A wide range of diseases can present to the ED with headache as the major or only symptom. Infectious diseases, inflammatory diseases, autoimmune diseases, and malignancy can cause headache. Processes that raise or lower intracranial pressure can also result in headache. In this chapter, we discuss the epidemiology, pathophysiology, diagnosis, and treatment of other secondary headaches including brain tumor headache, post-traumatic headache, high- and low-pressure headache, cervicogenic headache, trigeminal neuralgia, and headaches attributed to infection, Chiari malformation, arteritis, disorders of the eye, substances or withdrawal headache, and autonomic dysreflexia. In this chapter we also discuss primary (idiopathic) stabbing headache.

## Introduction

Diseases that affect pain-sensitive intracranial tissues that can generate pain, including the dura mater and cervicocephalic arteries and veins, can result in headache. In addition, diseases that can refer pain to the head, ranging from cervical musculoskeletal disorders to angina and aortic dissection, may present with headache as the predominant or only symptom. This chapter will review the range of disorders that may present to the emergency department (ED) with headache as a predominant symptom.

## Brain Tumor Headache

Although headache occurs in many patients with brain tumors, there is no specific headache quality that suggests the diagnosis [1]. Over half of patients with intracranial tumors experience headache, which is often similar in quality to tension-type headache [2]. Brain tumor headache is usually progressive and more common in persons with infratentorial and intraventricular tumors or cerebral edema [3]. Large tumors are not more likely to cause headache,

however, and brain tumor headache may not lateralize to the side of the neoplasm. An exception may be infratentorial tumor-related headaches, which are more common in children and usually localize to the occiput [4]. There is some evidence that morning headache suggests brain tumor in children [5], but a significant minority worsen during Valsalva maneuvers [6]. Although headache is one of the most common initial symptoms of brain tumor, the vast majority of persons have abnormal signs and symptoms suggestive of serious neurologic disease at the time of presentation to medical attention, especially children [7]. Young and middle-aged patients without focal neurological findings have an extremely low risk of tumor [8].

The treatment of brain tumors may also produce headache. Temozolomide, a chemotherapeutic agent often used as the initial treatment for malignant CNS tumors, commonly causes headache [9]. Corticosteroids may be an effective treatment for this complication. Brain radiation may lead to acute headache and encephalopathy, or can present many months later as cerebral radiation necrosis with headache and focal symptoms corresponding to the areas involved [10]. Post-craniotomy pain after surgery occasionally leads to emergency evaluation. Suboccipital craniotomies, such as in those with acoustic neuroma, are more likely to cause chronic headache [11].

A new headache type or the onset of new headache in any patient with a history of a known systemic cancer requires urgent evaluation. Brain metastases may present with headache, seizure, gait instability, delirium, or other cognitive difficulties (Figure 6.1) [12]. Lung (especially small-cell) cancer and melanoma are among the most likely primary cancers to metastasize to the brain, followed by breast and renal cell cancers [13]. Acute symptoms due to brain metastases frequently result from hemorrhage into the area, especially in patients with systemic melanoma

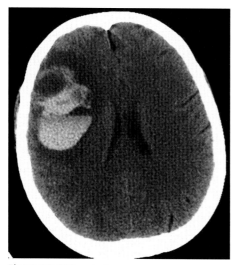

**Figure 6.1** Brain metastases.

or germ cell tumors, such as choriocarcinoma [14]. Patients with a history of brain or systemic cancer should receive prompt attention and neuroimaging for a new-onset headache, especially when accompanied by other symptoms such as malaise or delirium. MRI with gadolinium is the procedure of choice as it is far more sensitive to parenchymal brain lesions than CT. Leptomeningeal metastases may also produce severe headache, often with meningismus, cranial nerve exam abnormalities, or radicular pain. Breast, lung, melanoma, leukemia, and lymphoma are the most common tumors associated with carcinomatous meningitis. Diagnostic lumbar puncture can confirm the diagnosis [15].

Although headache associated with intracranial neoplasm is usually non-specific, there are a few specific headache syndromes known to be associated with cancer:

- Orbital apex or Jacod syndrome: severe eye pain with cranial nerve deficits including proptosis, diplopia, and ophthalmoplegia. Etiologies may include either neoplasm or inflammatory disorders such as neurosarcoidosis, Wegener's granulomatosis, or systemic lupus erythematosus.
- Parasellar syndrome: unilateral frontal headache, diplopia, ocular paresis, and facial pain may occur. Associated with diseases of the cavernous sinuses such as meningioma, internal carotid artery aneurysms, and inflammatory disorders such as Tolosa Hunt syndrome [16].

- Occipital condyle syndrome: severe, unilateral occipital pain and unilateral twelfth nerve palsy. Usually associated with skull-based metastasis [17].

## Pituitary Neoplasms and Headache

Pituitary tumors account for about 9 percent of all intracranial neoplasms, but are more likely than most to cause headache [18]. Pituitary tumor-associated headache can present with migraine or tension-type features, but also may mimic unusual headache syndromes such as short-lasting unilateral neuralgiform headache attacks with conjunctival injection and tearing (SUNCT), cluster headache, and primary stabbing headache [18]. When cavernous sinus invasion occurs, the patient may present with a more severe phenotype, but severe headaches such as cluster can occur without invasion of the cavernous sinus [19]. Besides headache, pituitary tumors may lead to vision loss, most commonly bitemporal hemianopia from compression of the optic chiasm (Figure 6.2). Less common clinical manifestations include autonomic symptoms, fatigue, or diabetes insipidus due to hypothalamic invasion or obstructive hydrocephalus and third ventricle obstruction [20]. The endocrinologic manifestations of pituitary tumors may be subtle and are not usually evaluated in the ED. MRI is superior for the evaluation of pituitary tumors, but CT scans can usually identify emergency situations such as acute hemorrhage or cavernous sinus invasion.

Pituitary apoplexy is a neurologic emergency in patients with pituitary tumors caused by hemorrhagic infarction of the tumor or the pituitary gland itself (Figure 6.3). Chronic hemorrhage into the pituitary gland or gradual infarction may occur without symptoms. Sudden hemorrhage or infarction is a medical emergency. Signs and symptoms include severe headache, diplopia, blurred vision, visual loss or visual field defects, extraocular motor palsies, and delirium that may progress to coma. Fever is common and may result from subarachnoid bleeding, acute hypoadrenalism, or hypothalamic compression [21]. Early recognition is essential as treatment with surgical decompression can improve visual outcomes [22].

## Post-Traumatic Headache

Post-traumatic headache is characterized not by the description of the headache or the underlying pathology, but by the temporal relationship between the

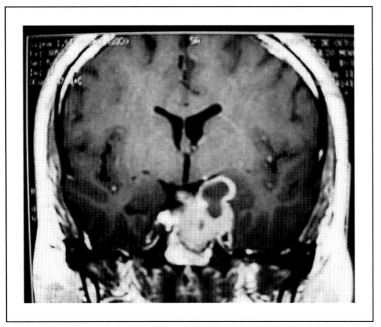

**Figure 6.2** Pituitary tumor.

headache and the antecedent events, a feature that distinguishes post-traumatic headache from other common headache diagnoses. Post-traumatic headache cannot be distinguished clinically from primary headaches such as migraine and tension-type headache because post-traumatic headache often takes the form of one of these. International classification relies on proximity of headache onset to the traumatic event to make the diagnosis [24]. Headache onset within seven days of trauma is required for the diagnosis of post-traumatic headache, though the vast majority of headaches that occur as a result of trauma occur at the onset or within 24 hours of the head trauma. The most recent version of the International Classification of Headache Disorders recognizes two broad categories of post-traumatic headache: *Acute* headache attributed to traumatic injury to the head and *Persistent* headache attributed to traumatic injury to the head, with a three-month headache period used as the defining cutoff point [24]. When a patient presents to the ED complaining of headache in the setting of trauma, the emergency physician must exclude a life-threatening cause of headache, reassure the patient who may have concerns about the underlying headache etiology, treat the acute headache, and provide guidance as to the expected course. The immediate focus is excluding headache etiologies that require specific

treatment, such as an intracranial hematoma or a skull or vertebral fracture. Superficial musculoskeletal injuries such as scalp hematomas or contusions, or muscle strains, may also cause headache in this context. Once these have been excluded, post-traumatic headache becomes the default diagnosis. The term post-concussive headache is often used interchangeably with post-traumatic headache but relies on the diagnosis of concussion, which in some cases may not be applied reliably.

Traumatic brain injury causes nearly 2.5 million visits to US EDs annually, during which the vast majority of patients are treated and released [25]. The prevalence of persistent or recurrent headache after traumatic brain injury has varied substantially in published reports, with a weighted average of more than 50 percent [26]. Headache was less likely among military personnel injured in combat and among those with more severe brain injury. In fact, for reasons that are unclear, an inverse relationship has been described between the severity of the initial trauma and the risk of post-concussion syndrome at three months post-injury [27]. The design of many studies makes it difficult to determine how often headache develops de novo after the traumatic injury versus how often it is a continuation or exacerbation of an underlying primary headache disorder. Post-traumatic headaches take the form of migraine or

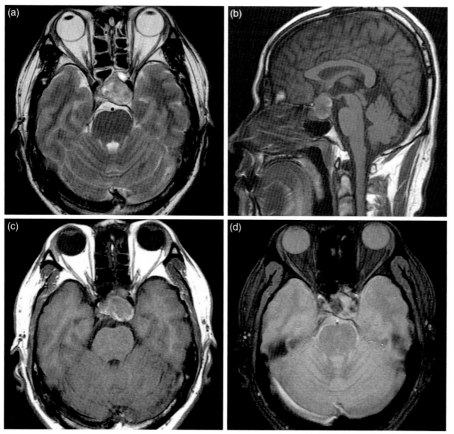

**Figure 6.3** Pituitary apoplexy: (a) T1-weighted axial MRI image demonstrating pituitary mass with mixed signal intensity; (b) and (c) T1-weighted sagittal and axial images demonstrating pituitary mass with peripheral high signal intensity; (d) Multiple areas of low signal intensity within pituitary mass shown on gradient-echo T2-weighted axial image suggesting intralesional hemorrhage. Source: [23].

probable migraine in about half of all patients [28,29]. An Italian study of patients hospitalized for traumatic brain injury excluded patients with a history of headache prior to the trauma. These investigators reported headache in 54 percent of patients one year later and in 30 percent of patients two years later [30].

The pathophysiology of post-traumatic headache is multifactorial. Patients can develop subtle white matter abnormalities in the setting of relatively minor head trauma [31]. It is likely that many patients with post-traumatic headache have pathological findings that are finer than the resolution of common imaging modalities. In fact, a large body of evidence using advanced neuroimaging techniques has demonstrated that subjects with concussion have microstructural alterations in white matter integrity that

are not visualized on CT or routine MRI brain scans [32–34].

Other physical symptoms that may accompany post-traumatic headache and that are commonly seen in subjects with concussion include nausea, photophobia and phonophobia, dizziness, and unsteadiness. Difficulties concentrating, sleepiness, insomnia, and psychiatric symptoms including depression, anxiety, and irritability may occur as well.

Emergency physicians can use published clinical decision rules to stratify head trauma patients with headache into high- and low-risk strata (Box 6.1) [35]. High-risk patients require head imaging or observation. Low-risk patients are candidates for outpatient observation. Only 1.5 percent of all patients with mild TBI require neurosurgical intervention. The

**Box 6.1 Published Decision Rules of Clinical Characteristics to Exclude Clinically Significant Injuries in Patients with Minor Head Trauma**

The absence of all of these features is required if head CT is to be avoided.

**New Orleans Criteria [37]**

- Headache
- Vomiting
- Seizure
- Intoxication
- Short-term memory deficit
- Age > 60 years
- Injury above the clavicles

**Canadian CT Head Rule [38]**

- Failure to reach GCS 15 within two hours
- Suspected open skull fracture
- Sign of basilar skull fracture
- Vomiting > 2 episodes
- Age > 65 years
- Amnesia before impact > 30 minutes
- Dangerous mechanism of injury

**Test Characteristics for Clinically Important Findings in an Independent Sample [39]**

- NOC: sensitivity 97.7 percent (95 percent CI: 92.1, 99.4 percent), specificity 5.5 percent (95 percent CI: 2.6, 8.7 percent)
- CCHR: sensitivity 87.2 percent (82.5, 90.9 percent), specificity 39.3 percent (36.6, 42.0 percent)

frequency of neurosurgical intervention is even less among those who present to an ED with GCS of 15 – in these patients, fewer than 1 in 200 required intervention, though as many as 8 percent have abnormal findings on head CT [35]. A non-contrast head CT is the current standard diagnostic modality for patients who have experienced head trauma. One normal head CT excludes intracranial hematoma in the vast majority of patients. This test does not need to be repeated, even among those using anticoagulants, if symptoms do not progress [36].

Primarily because of a significant lack of evidence on how to manage post-traumatic headaches, treatment is generally no different from the headache type it resembles. Once intracranial injury has been excluded, nonsteroidal anti-inflammatory drugs, dopamine antagonists, and triptans may be used to treat post-traumatic headaches that resemble migraine. Nonsteroidal anti-inflammatory drugs and dopamine antagonists may have efficacy for acute post-traumatic headaches that phenotypically resemble tension-type headache. Nausea and dizziness can be treated symptomatically. Patients may be counseled to engage in cognitive and physical rest for 24–48 hours followed by symptom-limited physical and cognitive activity. All patients with headache in the setting of trauma should be referred to a healthcare provider with expertise in the management of post-traumatic headache. On subsequent visits to the ED, patients with a history of head injury should be treated no differently than those with primary headache disorders without such a history.

Upon discharge from the ED, patients should be counseled as to their risk of persistent headache and other symptomatology. Persistence of symptoms is variable and difficult to predict. Broad risk factors for persistent symptoms include female sex [40] and mild rather than moderate or severe TBI [26].

# Headache Attributed to Infection

In patients presenting to an ED with headache and fever, altered mental status, or neck rigidity, CNS infection must be considered. While many of these patients merely require symptomatic relief including anti-pyretics and analgesics, a subset requires aggressive early management with antibiotics and corticosteroids. It can be challenging to differentiate aseptic meningitis from bacterial meningitis and meningitis itself from systemic febrile illness. In addition to bacterial and viral meningitis, headache can be caused by a variety of CNS infections including Lyme neuroborreliosis and herpetic encephalitis. Brain abscess and non-herpetic viral encephalitis may also present with headache and fever. Cryptococcal meningitis and other fungal infections, as well as mycobacterial infection, should be considered in immunocompromised patients.

Among immunocompetent adults with a normal mental status, bacterial meningitis is uncommon. In one case series conducted in an urban ED in the United States, among 230 patients with normal mental status who underwent a lumbar puncture to evaluate for meningitis, only three were culture-positive with causative organisms, including one patient with *Neisseria meningitidis*, one with *Cryptococcus neoformans*, and one with *Enterovirus* [41]. The infrequent presentation of bacterial meningitis can largely be attributed to vaccines against *Pneumococcus*, *Meningococcus*, and *Haemophilus influenzae*, which have decreased the incidence of bacterial meningitis to a fraction of what it was 50 years ago [42].

Common infections among immunocompetent adults include viruses, most commonly enteroviruses and herpes viruses. Common CNS bacterial pathogens include *Neisseria*, *Pneumococcus*, and *Listeria*. *Haemophilus influenzae* has become an uncommon pathogen. *Lyme neuroborreliosis* may occur in endemic areas. *Tuberculous meningitis* is an uncommon CNS infection in the developed world. *Staphylococcus aureus* is a common cause of brain abscess.

The classic triad of fever, mental status changes, and neck stiffness occurs in just 46 percent of patients with meningitis, though any two of these occur in 95 percent of patients with meningitis [43]. Bacterial meningitis is a progressive disease. These patients typically do not demonstrate sustained improvement after treatment with just intravenous fluid and antipyretics. Classic findings on physical exam including Kernig and Brudzinski signs, and jolt accentuation, are inadequately sensitive for CSF pleocytosis, with sensitivities of less than 25 percent [41,44]. Among North American patients with Lyme neuroborreliosis, most will remember the classic erythema migrans rash [45].

When evaluating patients with fever and headache, it is often difficult to determine who requires lumbar puncture to exclude a malignant infection. Immunocompetent patients with a normal neurological exam are unlikely to have bacterial meningitis or herpetic encephalitis. In well-appearing patients with a normal neurological exam, it is reasonable to observe the patient's response to intravenous fluids and anti-pyretics. Substantial improvement in symptomatology means that antibiotics are unlikely to be needed emergently.

For patients in whom meningitis is suspected, an analysis of CSF is required to confirm the diagnosis of meningitis. Prior to performing a lumbar puncture, brain imaging is often performed to exclude a space-occupying lesion. Neuroimaging, however, is not required prior to lumbar puncture among patients younger than 50 with headache and fever if they have no comorbidities, have a normal neurologic exam, and have no papilledema [46]. In addition to excluding a space-occupying lesion for safety purposes, neuroimaging will also identify brain abscesses.

Patients with bacterial meningitis require prompt antibiotic therapy, tailored to the age and medical history of the patient. Similarly, patients in whom herpetic encephalitis is suspected should be treated promptly with parenteral antiviral agents. The bulk of published data support the use of corticosteroids in patients with bacterial meningitis [47]. Similarly, fungal causes of meningitis need prompt treatment with antifungals. Viral meningitis should be treated supportively with fluids, nonsteroidal anti-inflammatory drugs, and acetaminophen, as needed.

The prognosis of patients with bacterial meningitis is variable and depends on prompt recognition of disease and initiation of antibiotics. Viral meningitis almost always has a benign course and good prognosis.

# High- and Low-Pressure Headache

Low-pressure headaches are characterized by their orthostatic features – low-pressure headaches worsen when assuming an upright position and improve or resolve with recumbency. Low-pressure headaches are most commonly iatrogenic in origin. Patients will frequently present with low-pressure headache in the days following a diagnostic lumbar puncture or an epidural anesthesia procedure. Spontaneous intracranial hypotension is increasingly recognized with the widespread use of advanced neuroimaging. High CSF pressure can be caused by a variety of intracranial processes including space-occupying lesions and processes that obstruct CSF or venous blood. *Idiopathic intracranial hypertension*, a syndrome characterized by transient visual obscurations, pulsatile tinnitus, progressive visual fields deficits and headache, is a diagnosis of exclusion once specific causes of intracranial hypertension have been excluded. The terms "pseudotumor cerebri" and "benign intracranial hypertension" have fallen out of favor with increased understanding of the disease and its natural history.

## Idiopathic Intracranial Hypertension

Idiopathic intracranial hypertension is a rare disease in the population as a whole, with a higher prevalence in young, obese, women [48]. Cases in the ED are uncommon though the diagnosis is subtle and may be missed [49]. The mechanism underlying this disease is unknown. It is thought that increased intracranial pressure may relate to inadequate resorption of CSF.

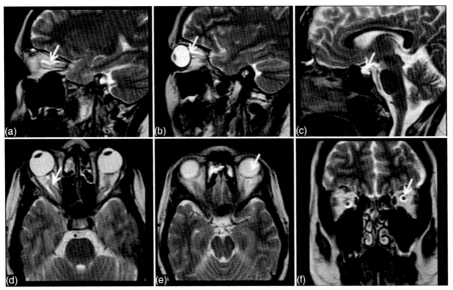

**Figure 6.4** MRI findings in idiopathic intracranial hypertension. T2-weighted MRI brain showing: tortuosity of the optic nerve (a,d), flattening of the globe and prominence of the optic nerve head (b,e), partially empty sella turcica (c), and prominent perioptic nerve sheath (d,f).
Source: [53].

Headache is often pulsatile and associated with nausea and vomiting [50]. The headache phenotype resembles migraine. A substantial number of these patients have comorbid migraine, which is not surprising given the overlapping epidemiological profiles [51]. In addition to headache, transient visual obscurations, pulse synchronous tinnitus, and back pain are common among patients with established disease [51]. Papilledema is common though not universal [52]. Afferent pupillary defects and cranial nerve palsies are uncommon [51]. Visual loss, in the form of enlarged blind spots and visual field deficits, is present in the majority of cases in which formal visual field testing is performed [50].

While idiopathic intracranial hypertension may be suggested by the constellation of symptoms reported above, diagnosis is contingent on demonstrating an opening pressure of at least 25 cm H$_2$O in the CSF [23]. Specific causes of elevated intracranial pressure including venous sinus thrombosis, primary angiitis of the central nervous system and cryptococcal meningitis should be considered. MRI is often normal, but evidence of elevated intracranial pressure may be suggested by an empty or partially empty sella turcica, tortuosity of the optic nerves, prominence of the perioptic nerve sheath and optic nerve head, and/or flattening of the posterior sclera of the globes (Figure 6.4).

Removal of CSF may relieve symptoms of patients with elevated intracranial hypertension [52]. Lack of relief after removal of enough CSF to lower the intracranial pressure can occur with idiopathic intracranial hypertension but should also cause the clinicians to consider alternate diagnoses.

Modest weight loss appears to improve the long-term prognosis. Acetazolamide, using doses titrated up to 4 g daily and combined with dietary advice, improves visual field deficits and overall quality of life but does not improve headaches more than dietary advice alone [54].

Idiopathic intracranial hypertension is a chronic illness requiring ongoing care. These patients should be referred to neurology and ophthalmology. Many patients experience remission of headaches with ongoing medical care, though chronic headache is common [55]. Cognitive dysfunction has been reported [55].

## 6.6.2 Low-Pressure Headaches

*Postdural puncture headache* is a common complication of spinal anesthesia and diagnostic lumbar puncture. It can occur in up to 40 percent of spinal

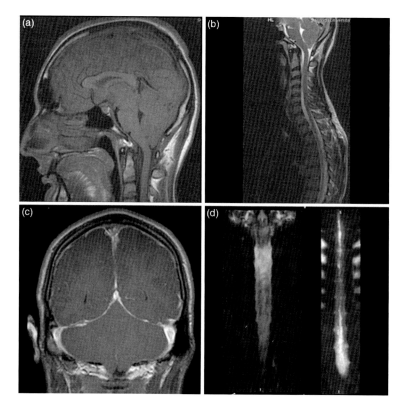

**Figure 6.5** MRI findings of intracranial hypotension. (a) Sagittal T1-weighted brain MRI demonstrating brainstem descent with mild herniation of the cerebellar tonsils, flattening of the pons, dilated sagittal sinus, and enlarged pituitary gland. (b) Sagittal T2-weighted MRI of the spine showing subdural fluid collection anterior to the spinal cord at the levels of C5–T1 causing posterior displacement of the cord and symmetrically dilated vascular structures with venous engorgement anterior to the spinal cord from the atlanto-occipital junction to C4. (c) Coronal T1-weighted brain MRI demonstrating diffuse pachymeningeal enhancement. (d) MR myelogram which was unremarkable in this case (no evidence of dural tear). Source: [60].

procedures [56]. Techniques to decrease the incidence of postdural puncture headache have been described and include positioning the bevel of the needle in parallel with dural fibers (oriented toward the patient's hip), using a smaller gauge needle, removing smaller volumes of fluid, and using non-traumatic blunt-tip needles.

*Spontaneous intracranial hypotension headache* is uncommon and often unrecognized. One ED-based cohort identified 11 new patients during a four-year period [57]. Connective tissue disorders and recent trauma are associated with this disorder [58].

Low-pressure headaches are characteristically orthostatic. The headache generally occurs within 30 seconds of assuming an upright posture, though may lag for minutes or rarely even hours [59]. Nausea, tinnitus, and dizziness are common [59]. By definition, postdural puncture develops within five days of the procedure [23].

Without a recent procedure, diagnosis of CSF hypotension is difficult because of the rarity of presentation. Lumbar puncture may reveal an opening pressure of <60 mm CSF but may be normal in up to 40 percent of patients and is often not necessary in making the diagnosis [23]. MRI of the brain and spinal cord has high sensitivity for documenting brain sag and evidence of a spinal fluid leak, often at the cervical and/or thoracic spinal level. MRI brain with gadolinium may reveal diffuse, smooth, pachymeningeal enhancement and thickening, dural venous sinus engorgement, pituitary enlargement and enhancement, cerebellar tonsillar herniation, flattening of the anterior portion of the pons, and midbrain/tectal compression (Figure 6.5). Subdural collections including hygromas and hematomas may also be present [58].

Pharmacological treatment with caffeine, theophylline, gabapentin, and hydrocortisone may improve outcomes for patients with low-pressure headache [61]. It is unclear if intravenous fluids improve symptoms. An autologous epidural blood patch, repeated up to three times, may be necessary for resolution of symptoms. When patients do not respond to these measures, myelography may be required to document the precise site of a leak [62]. Autologous blood patches directed toward the site

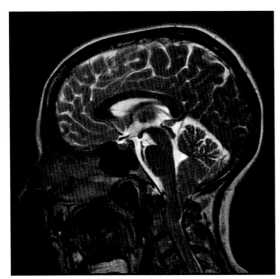

**Figure 6.6** Chiari type 1 malformation. T2-weighted sagittal brain MRI sequence showing a Chiari 1 malformation with tonsillar descent to the level of C1 and a slight increase in signal in the upper cervical spinal cord.
Source: [65].

of the leak, fibrin glue injections, or surgical repair may be necessary for patients with spontaneous CSF leaks and persistent symptoms despite conservative treatment.

## Headache Attributed to Chiari Malformations

Chiari malformations are a collection of cerebellar structural defects in which brain tissue descends into the spinal canal. A type 1 Chiari malformation requires a 5 mm caudal descent of the cerebellar tonsils or 3 mm descent with crowding of the subarachnoid space at the craniocervical junction on MRI (Figure 6.6). Chiari-related headache is short-lasting (<5 minutes), usually occipital, and triggered by coughing or Valsalva maneuvers [23]. Some patients with Chiari 1 malformations are asymptomatic until adulthood. Headaches are a more common symptom than seizure or developmental delay [63]. Chiari disorders may also be associated with either a cervical cord syrinx, causing central cord syndrome and upper extremity symptoms, or brainstem or cerebellar dysfunction. It is important to distinguish intracranial hypotension-related tonsillar descent from Chiari malformations. Orthostatic headache and radiological findings such

as pachymeningeal enhancement are suggestive of low-pressure headache, and a *secondary* Chiari malformation. In many cases, Chiari malformations are incidental findings in persons with migraine. Surgical decompression may worsen headache and a very careful presurgical evaluation is required by a headache specialist and neurosurgeon [64].

## Headache Attributed to Arteritis

Systemic vasculitis is an important cause of secondary headache. Giant cell arteritis is as common as migraine among elderly patients with new-onset headache [66]. Temporal or giant cell arteritis should be considered in any patient older than 60 years with unexplained headache of recent onset. Systemic symptoms such as fatigue, weight loss, jaw claudication, and polymyalgia rheumatica raises the level of concern. Elevations of either the Westergren erythrocyte sedimentation rate (ESR) or C-reactive protein (CRP) level are very common. C-reactive protein generally rises before the ESR, and the sensitivity and specificity of CRP is high (98.6 percent and 75.7 percent, respectively). A complete blood count will often reveal a normocytic normochromic anemia and thrombocytosis. Alpha2 globulin, interleukin-6, liver transaminases, and fibrinogen may also be elevated. While neither an ESR nor a CRP can exclude the disease from consideration, the combination of these two tests is very sensitive (99 percent) and can exclude the need for biopsy among patients who do not have a high pre-test probability of disease [67]. Biopsy-proven giant cell arteritis has occurred in patients with either normal ESR or normal CRP levels [68]. Complications of temporal arteritis include blindness due to anterior ischemic optic neuropathy, central retinal artery occlusion, stroke, or aortic aneurysm. If giant cell arteritis is considered likely because of markedly elevated ESR and typical symptoms, corticosteroid treatment should be initiated. Prednisone is typically dosed at no less than 40 mg/day. For those patients with visual or neurological symptoms, high-dose oral prednisone 80–100 mg or three days of high-dose intravenous methylprednisolone (250–1000 mg) is indicated. These patients should be referred for a long segment temporal artery biopsy [69], optimally within one week of starting steroids.

Headache can be the initial symptom in other types of systemic vasculitis [70]. Granulomatosis with polyangiitis, or Wegener granulomatosis, typically presents with respiratory tract disease, sinusitis, serous otitis media, sensorineural hearing loss, cranial neuropathies, and headache [71]. Headache is also a common symptom of systemic autoimmune disease such as Sjögren syndrome and systemic lupus erythematosus. Behcet disease may cause headache, eye disturbances, and oral or genital ulcers. Neurosarcoidosis can cause severe headache, cranial neuropathies, enhancing mass lesions, and pachymeningeal enhancement on MRI. Children are more likely to experience seizures due to space-occupying lesions [72].

Primary angiitis of the CNS without systemic involvement is relatively uncommon. Progressively worsening headache, rather than thunderclap headache, is more typical for primary CNS vasculitis [73]. Angiographic features may mimic reversible cerebral vasoconstriction syndromes with beading and/or segmental narrowing of intracranial arteries. Neuroimaging can also reveal multifocal white matter hyperintense lesions and cortical and subcortical infarctions in multiple vascular territories. Atypical "multiple sclerosis-like lesions" or larger mass lesions [74] may also be seen. Brain biopsy is almost always needed to confirm the diagnosis of angiitis.

## Headache Attributed to Disorders of the Eye

Many primary headache disorders present with eye pain and visual symptoms, such as migraine and cluster headache. Serious ocular disease, however, is relatively unusual as a cause of severe headache, especially when the sclerae are normal-appearing, pupils are equal and reactive, and visual acuity is normal [75]. Ocular symptoms are common in both primary and secondary headache disorders (e.g., idiopathic intracranial hypertension). Many patients with primary and secondary headache disorders present with photophobia, blurred vision, tearing, ptosis, or ocular pain. Eye strain due to uncorrected vision is extremely unlikely to cause severe headache in the ED setting [76].

## Glaucoma

Acute primary angle-closure glaucoma is caused by a sudden increase in intraocular pressure. It is an ophthalmic emergency that without treatment causes severe visual loss. Signs and symptoms usually include conjunctival injection, corneal edema, mid-dilated nonreactive or oval pupil, blurry vision with halos

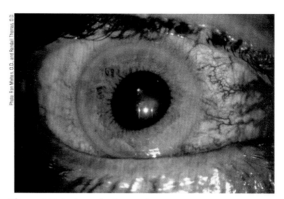

**Figure 6.7** Acute angle-closure glaucoma.

around lights, severe eye pain and headache, and nausea and vomiting (Figure 6.7). The globe feels firm and intraocular pressure is usually elevated (usually 40–80 mmHg). Cluster headache, unlike angle-closure glaucoma, has no effect on visual acuity, intraocular pressure, or pupil reactivity, but may be associated with miosis/Horner's syndrome. Other more common forms of glaucoma are less likely to cause headache, although subacute angle-closure glaucoma may be associated with migrainous (photophobia, nausea) symptoms [77].

## Cervicogenic Headache

Neck pain is a common symptom in patients with migraine, but occasionally headache may result from cervical spine disease. The upper cervical neurons provide sensory input to the trigeminal nucleus caudalis, the lower brainstem/upper cervical spine relay nucleus central to migraine nociception. Degenerative disease (arthritis) of the uncovertebral joints and facet joints, and other spinal pathology, can therefore cause pain that will be perceived as a headache or migraine. Cervicogenic headache tends to be unilateral, usually occipital, is associated with poor range of motion, and worsens with provocative maneuvers [23]. Occasionally patients may present to the ED with acute cervicogenic headache, with or without significant neck pain [78]. Diagnosis should be considered with reproduction of pain when the upper neck is palpated or the head is repositioned. Definitive diagnosis requires confirmation by relieving the pain with cervical nerve blockade. NSAIDs, muscle relaxants, and even opioids may be used to control pain in the ED [79].

## Autonomic Dysreflexia

In patients with acute or chronic spinal cord injuries, and in those who have recently undergone a carotid procedure (e.g., endarterectomy, angioplasty/stenting), a severe, sudden-onset (thunderclap) headache with a paroxysmal rise in blood pressure suggests autonomic dysreflexia [23] or baroreceptor dysfunction. Clinical signs may include diaphoresis, tachycardia as well as blood pressure well above baseline. The usual triggers include bladder distension or infection, bowel distension, or pressure ulcers [80]. Reversible cerebral vasoconstriction syndrome (RCVS) has been associated with autonomic dysreflexia (Figure 6.8) [81]. CT of the head to rule out subarachnoid hemorrhage, as in all thunderclap headaches, is indicated. Subarachnoid blood in the sulci of the brain may be seen, especially in the presence of RCVS. Non-invasive angiography (CT angiography, MR angiography) may be indicated to rule out RCVS since the risk of hemorrhagic and ischemic stroke from RCVS within the first two weeks mandates that it be diagnosed as early as possible.

## Headaches due to Substances or Withdrawal

Many substances can generate acute headache with routine use. In most of these cases, the relationship between exposure and headache is obvious if elicited. Atropine, digitalis, hydralazine, lithium, and cyclosporine are a few of the many medications that may produce headache [82]. Monosodium glutamate and alcohol can also trigger headache. Carbon monoxide exposure can initiate severe throbbing headache, and should be suspected in colder months once home heating has begun [83]. Headache can be a prominent symptom of substance withdrawal, such as with caffeine, opioids, antidepressants, or exogenous hormones such as estrogen.

Medication overuse headache (MOH) is a complication of chronic analgesic use which worsens headache severity and frequency over time [23]. Opioid or barbiturate-containing medications and migraine-specific drugs, such as triptans, are more likely than simple analgesics to cause MOH. The International Classification of Headache Disorders suggests that the use of opioids, barbiturate-containing and other combination analgesics, or triptans over ten days per month may lead to medication overuse or "rebound" headache [24]. Likewise, the use of simple analgesics, including non-steroidal anti-inflammatory medications, acetaminophen-containing

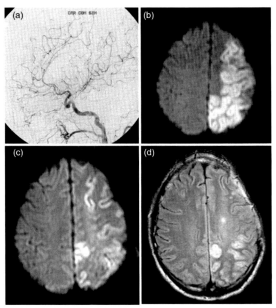

**Figure 6.8** Reversible cerebral vasoconstriction syndrome occurring in the context of autonomic dysreflexia following a spinal cord injury. (a) Multiple intracranial blood vessel caliber changes on a selective cerebral angiogram in a patient with spastic quadriparesis from a remote C5–C6 fracture, presenting with reversible cerebral vasoconstriction syndrome in the context of an episode of autonomic dysreflexia. (b) Diffusion-weighted MRI sequence performed two weeks after the patient's admission showing acute ischemia in the left hemisphere. (c) Repeat diffusion-weighted MRI sequence three weeks after admission. (d) T2-weighted MRI sequence three weeks after admission showing expected evolution of the prior ischemic changes. Source: reprinted from [81].

compounds and acetylsalicylic acid, over fifteen days per month may lead to medication overuse headache. Often acute migraine medications are initially helpful but lead to tolerance or tachyphylaxis. Seizures are a not-uncommon complication of barbiturate withdrawal [84]. It is essential to determine recent medication use among patients presenting to an ED with headache.

## Trigeminal Neuralgia

Trigeminal neuralgia (TN) is a painful disorder of the face characterized by short-lasting electric pain in one or more divisions of the trigeminal nerve. The prevalence of TN is approximately 0.2 per 1000 and generally increases with age, with a peak prevalence in the sixth decade of life [85]. About 150,000 new cases of TN are diagnosed each year in the United States. Pain is commonly evoked by trivial stimuli (e.g., washing, shaving, smoking, talking, or brushing teeth) but also may occur spontaneously. The attacks typically start in a small trigger zone, last less than two minutes, and occur in the V2 and/or V3 distribution. Patients may freeze and grimace with facial contortions during attacks [24]. Most patients experience a refractory period (i.e., further stimulation does not evoke an attack) after stimulation, especially after severe attacks [86].

Although some patients with TN will present to the ED for frequent attacks, the presentation of either short-lasting unilateral neuralgiform headache with conjunctival injection and tearing (SUNCT) or short-lasting unilateral neuralgiform headache with cranial autonomic features (SUNA) may mimic TN. In most cases SUNCT and SUNA cause ocular pain. SUNCT and SUNA can also be distinguished from TN by the following: (1) characteristic and robust parasympathetic (lacrimation, conjunctival injection, nasal congestion, rhinorrhea) features; (2) lack of refractory period; (3) spontaneous attacks without clear triggers; and (4) pain confined to first (V1) division of trigeminal nerve (occurs in less than 5 percent of TN sufferers).

A useful categorization divides TN into patients with symptomatic TN, which is caused by lesions including malignancy and white matter abnormalities, and classical TN, in which neuroimaging is unremarkable [87]. Neurovascular contact between the trigeminal nerve root and local vasculature (usually the superior cerebellar artery) is common among patients referred for MRI, often causing displacement or atrophy of the trigeminal root [88]. This neurovascular contact is now believed to cause many cases of TN. The microvascular compression of the trigeminal nerve by the vascular contact produces a chronic focal demyelination of the trigeminal nerve.

Progressive symptoms and facial numbness suggest a secondary cause, such as neoplasm, brainstem infarct, or infection such as herpes zoster. Demyelinating disease, such as multiple sclerosis, is of greatest concern in young patients or in those with bilateral disease. MRI is indicated in previously undiagnosed patients, particularly when sensory loss or motor dysfunction is present. Routine MRI has identified a non-vascular cause of pain in 15 percent of cases [87], but MRI with 3D volume acquisition is necessary to document the presence of a vascular loop or compression of the trigeminal nerve root. MRI verification of compression on the side of the pain may predict good surgical outcomes [89].

The treatment of TN includes medications such as carbamazepine, oxcarbazepine, baclofen, topiramate, and gabapentin. In the ED setting, intravenous phenytoin or phosphenytoin may be effective [90]. An initial dose of 15–20 mg/kg can be given with a plan to continue oral dosing after discharge. Facial nerve blocks with a long-acting local anesthetic such as bupivacaine can also provide patients with relief until oral medications begin to take effect. Medications for the treatment of TN may become less effective over time, and up to 50 percent of patients eventually require surgical treatment such as microvascular decompression. Constant pain between attacks predicts a worse prognosis [91].

## Primary (Idiopathic) Stabbing Headache

Primary stabbing headache often coexists with other primary headache disorders such as migraine. Most attacks are brief, unilateral, and last 1–10 seconds. Attacks commonly occur in the orbital, temporal, parietal, and occipital areas. Most patients do not experience clear triggers or autonomic features. Many patients respond to indomethacin 25–150 mg/day [92].

## Conclusion

We have discussed a number of secondary headaches that may present to an acute care setting. These various diagnoses should be on the differential diagnosis for patients who present to an emergency department with headache.

## References

1. Boiardi A, Salmaggi A, Eoli M, Lamperti E, Silvani A. Headache in brain tumours: a symptom to reappraise critically. *Neurol Sci.* 2004;25(Suppl. 3):S143–7.

2. Valentinis L, Tuniz F, Valent F, et al. Headache attributed to intracranial tumours: a prospective cohort study. *Cephalalgia.* 2010;30(4):389–98.

3. Pfund Z, Szapary L, Jaszberenyi O, Nagy F, Czopf J. Headache in intracranial tumors. *Cephalalgia.* 1999;19(9):787–90; discussion 765.

4. Schankin CJ, Ferrari U, Reinisch VM, et al. Characteristics of brain tumour-associated headache. *Cephalalgia.* 2007;27(8):904–11.

5. Lanphear J, Sarnaik S. Presenting symptoms of pediatric brain tumors diagnosed in the emergency department. *Pediatr Emerg Care.* 2014;30(2):77–80.

6. Forsyth PA, Posner JB. Headaches in patients with brain tumors: a study of 111 patients. *Neurology.* 1993;43(9):1678–83.

7.  Wilne SH, Ferris RC, Nathwani A, Kennedy CR. The presenting features of brain tumours: a review of 200 cases. *Arch Dis Child*. 2006;91(6):502–6.

8.  Kernick D, Stapley S, Goadsby PJ, Hamilton W. What happens to new-onset headache presented to primary care? A case-cohort study using electronic primary care records. *Cephalalgia*. 2008;28(11):1188–95.

9.  Yung WK, Albright RE, Olson J, et al. A phase II study of temozolomide vs. procarbazine in patients with glioblastoma multiforme at first relapse. *Br J Cancer*. 2000;83(5):588–93.

10. Rogers LR. Neurologic complications of radiation. *Continuum (Minneap Minn)*. 2012;18(2):343–54.

11. Ryzenman JM, Pensak ML, Tew JM, Jr. Headache: a quality of life analysis in a cohort of 1,657 patients undergoing acoustic neuroma surgery, results from the Acoustic Neuroma Association. *Laryngoscope*. 2005;115(4):703–11.

12. Navi BB, Reichman JS, Berlin D, et al. Intracerebral and subarachnoid hemorrhage in patients with cancer. *Neurology*. 2010;74(6):494–501.

13. Barnholtz-Sloan JS, Yu C, Sloan AE, et al. A nomogram for individualized estimation of survival among patients with brain metastasis. *Neuro Oncol*. 2012;14(7):910–18.

14. Nutt SH, Patchell RA. Intracranial hemorrhage associated with primary and secondary tumors. *Neurosurg Clin N Am*. 1992;3(3):591–9.

15. Jayson GC, Howell A. Carcinomatous meningitis in solid tumours. *Ann Oncol*. 1996;7(8):773–86.

16. Johnston JL. Parasellar syndromes. *Curr Neurol Neurosci Rep*. 2002;2(5):423–31.

17. Capobianco DJ, Brazis PW, Rubino FA, Dalton JN. Occipital condyle syndrome. *Headache*. 2002;42(2):142–6.

18. Levy MJ, Matharu MS, Meeran K, Powell M, Goadsby PJ. The clinical characteristics of headache in patients with pituitary tumours. *Brain*. 2005;128(Pt 8):1921–30.

19. Edvardsson B. Cluster headache associated with a clinically non-functioning pituitary adenoma: a case report. *J Med Case Rep*. 2014;8:451.

20. Levy A. Pituitary disease: presentation, diagnosis, and management. *J Neurol Neurosurg Psychiatry*. 2004;75(Suppl. 3):iii47–52.

21. Mohr G, Hardy J. Hemorrhage, necrosis, and apoplexy in pituitary adenomas. *Surg Neurol*. 1982;18(3):181–9.

22. Muthukumar N, Rossette D, Soundaram M, Senthilbabu S, Badrinarayanan T. Blindness following pituitary apoplexy: timing of surgery and neuro-ophthalmic outcome. *J Clin Neurosci*. 2008;15(8):873–9.

23. Oh K, Kim JH, Choi JW, Kang JK, Kim SH. Pituitary apoplexy mimicking meningitis. *Brain Tumor Res Treat*. 2013;1(2):111–15.

24. Headache Classification Committee of the International Headache Society (IHS). The International Classification of Headache Disorders, 3rd edition (beta version). *Cephalalgia*. 2013;33(9):629–808.

25. Centers for Disease Control and Prevention. Rates of TBI-related emergency department visits, hospitalizations, and deaths — United States, 2001–2010. Available at: www.cdc.gov/traumaticbraininjury/data/rates.html.

26. Nampiaparampil DE. Prevalence of chronic pain after traumatic brain injury: a systematic review. *JAMA*. 2008;300(6):711–19.

27. Sigurdardottir S, Andelic N, Roe C, Jerstad T, Schanke AK. Post-concussion symptoms after traumatic brain injury at 3 and 12 months post-injury: a prospective study. *Brain Inj*. 2009;23(6):489–97.

28. Lucas S, Hoffman JM, Bell KR, Dikmen S. A prospective study of prevalence and characterization of headache following mild traumatic brain injury. *Cephalalgia*. 2014;34:93–102.

29. Lucas S, Hoffman JM, Bell KR, Walker W, Dikmen S. Characterization of headache after traumatic brain injury. *Cephalalgia*. 2012;32(8):600–6.

30. De Benedittis G, De Santis A. Chronic post-traumatic headache: clinical, psychopathological features and outcome determinants. *J Neurosurg Sci*. 1983;27(3):177–86.

31. Lipton ML, Gulko E, Zimmerman ME, et al. Diffusion-tensor imaging implicates prefrontal axonal injury in executive function impairment following very mild traumatic brain injury. *Radiology*. 2009;252(3):816–24.

32. Yuh EL, Hawryluk GWJ, Manley G. Imaging concussion: a review. *Neurosurgery*. 2014;75:S50–63.

33. Aoki Y, Inokuchi R, Gunshin M, et al. Diffusion tensor imaging studies of mild traumatic brain injury: a meta-analysis. *J Neurol Neurosurg Psychiatry*. 2012;83:870–6.

34. Huang YL, Kuo YS, Tseng YC, et al. Susceptibility-weighted MRI in mild traumatic brain injury. *Neurology*. 2015;84:580–5.

35. Stiell IG, Clement CM, Rowe BH, et al. Comparison of the Canadian CT Head Rule and the New Orleans Criteria in patients with minor head injury. *JAMA*. 2005;294(12):1511–18.

36. Miller J, Lieberman L, Nahab B, et al. Delayed intracranial hemorrhage in the anticoagulated patient: a systematic review. *J Trauma Acute Care Surg*. 2015;79(2):310–13.

37. Haydel MJ, Preston CA, Mills TJ, et al. Indications for computed tomography in patients with minor head injury. *N Engl J Med.* 2000;343(2):100–5.

38. Stiell IG, Wells GA, Vandemheen K, et al. The Canadian CT Head Rule for patients with minor head injury. *Lancet.* 2001;357(9266):1391–6.

39. Smits M, Dippel DW, de Haan GG, et al. External validation of the Canadian CT Head Rule and the New Orleans Criteria for CT scanning in patients with minor head injury. *JAMA.* 2005;294(12):1519–25.

40. Bazarian JJ, Blyth B, Mookerjee S, He H, McDermott MP. Sex differences in outcome after mild traumatic brain injury. *J Neurotrauma.* 2010;27(3):527–39.

41. Nakao JH, Jafri FN, Shah K, Newman DH. Jolt accentuation of headache and other clinical signs: poor predictors of meningitis in adults. *Am J Emerg Med.* 2014;32(1):24–8.

42. Thigpen MC, Whitney CG, Messonnier NE, et al. Bacterial meningitis in the United States, 1998–2007. *N Engl J Med.* 2011;364(21):2016–25.

43. Attia J, Hatala R, Cook DJ, Wong JG. The rational clinical examination: does this adult patient have acute meningitis? *JAMA.* 1999;282(2):175–81.

44. Tamune H, Takeya H, Suzuki W, et al. Absence of jolt accentuation of headache cannot accurately rule out meningitis in adults. *Am J Emerg Med.* 2013;31(11):1601–4.

45. Pachner AR, Steiner I. Lyme neuroborreliosis: infection, immunity, and inflammation. *Lancet Neurol.* 2007;6(6):544–52.

46. Edlow JA, Panagos PD, Godwin SA, Thomas TL, Decker WW. Clinical policy: critical issues in the evaluation and management of adult patients presenting to the emergency department with acute headache. *Ann Emerg Med.* 2008;52(4):407–36.

47. Brouwer MC, McIntyre P, Prasad K, van de Beek D. Corticosteroids for acute bacterial meningitis. *Cochrane Database Syst Rev.* 2015;9:CD004405.

48. Durcan FJ, Corbett JJ, Wall M. The incidence of pseudotumor cerebri: population studies in Iowa and Louisiana. *Arch Neurol.* 1988;45(8):875–7.

49. Jones JS, Nevai J, Freeman MP, McNinch DE. Emergency department presentation of idiopathic intracranial hypertension. *Am J Emerg Med.* 1999;17(6):517–21.

50. Wall M, George D. Idiopathic intracranial hypertension: a prospective study of 50 patients. *Brain.* 1991;114(Pt 1A):155–80.

51. Wall M, Kupersmith MJ, Kieburtz KD, et al. The idiopathic intracranial hypertension treatment trial: clinical profile at baseline. *JAMA Neurol.* 2014;71(6):693–701.

52. Yri HM, Jensen RH. Idiopathic intracranial hypertension: Clinical nosography and field-testing of the ICHD diagnostic criteria. A case-control study. *Cephalalgia.* 2015;35(7):553–62.

53. Hingwala DR, Kesavadas C, Thomas B, Kapilamoorthy TR, Sarma S. Imaging signs in idiopathic intracranial hypertension: are these signs seen in secondary intracranial hypertension too? *Ann Indian Acad Neurol.* 2013;16(2):229–33.

54. Committee NIIHSGW, Wall M, McDermott MP, et al. Effect of acetazolamide on visual function in patients with idiopathic intracranial hypertension and mild visual loss: the idiopathic intracranial hypertension treatment trial. *JAMA.* 2014;311(16):1641–51.

55. Yri HM, Ronnback C, Wegener M, Hamann S, Jensen RH. The course of headache in idiopathic intracranial hypertension: a 12-month prospective follow-up study. *Eur J Neurol.* 2014;21(12):1458–64.

56. Bezov D, Lipton RB, Ashina S. Post-dural puncture headache: part I diagnosis, epidemiology, etiology, and pathophysiology. *Headache.* 2010;50(7):1144–52.

57. Schievink WI, Maya MM, Moser F, Tourje J, Torbati S. Frequency of spontaneous intracranial hypotension in the emergency department. *J Headache Pain.* 2007;8(6):325–8.

58. Schievink WI. Spontaneous spinal cerebrospinal fluid leaks and intracranial hypotension. *JAMA.* 2006;295(19):2286–96.

59. Chung SJ, Kim JS, Lee MC. Syndrome of cerebral spinal fluid hypovolemia: clinical and imaging features and outcome. *Neurology.* 2000;55(9):1321–7.

60. Russo A, Tessitore A, Cirillo M, et al. A transient third cranial nerve palsy as presenting sign of spontaneous intracranial hypotension. *J Headache Pain.* 2011;12(4):493–6.

61. Basurto Ona X, Osorio D, Bonfill Cosp X. Drug therapy for treating post-dural puncture headache. *Cochrane Database Syst Rev.* 2015;7:CD007887.

62. Mokri B. Spontaneous CSF leaks: low CSF volume syndromes. *Neurol Clin.* 2014;32(2):397–422.

63. Brill CB, Gutierrez J, Mishkin MM. Chiari I malformation: association with seizures and developmental disabilities. *J Child Neurol.* 1997;12(2):101–6.

64. Arnautovic A, Splavski B, Boop FA, Arnautovic KI. Pediatric and adult Chiari malformation Type I surgical series 1965–2013: a review of demographics, operative treatment, and outcomes. *J Neurosurg Pediatr.* 2015;15(2):161–77.

65. Loch-Wilkinson T, Tsimiklis C, Santoreneaos S. Trigeminal neuralgia associated with Chiari 1 malformation: symptom resolution following

craniocervical decompression and duroplasty: case report and review of the literature. *Surg Neurol Int.* 2015;6(Suppl. 11):S327–9.

66. Solomon GD, Kunkel RS, Jr, Frame J. Demographics of headache in elderly patients. *Headache.* 1990;30(5):273–6.

67. Kermani TA, Schmidt J, Crowson CS, et al. Utility of erythrocyte sedimentation rate and C-reactive protein for the diagnosis of giant cell arteritis. *Semin Arthritis Rheum.* 2012;41(6):866–71.

68. Parikh M, Miller NR, Lee AG, et al. Prevalence of a normal C-reactive protein with an elevated erythrocyte sedimentation rate in biopsy-proven giant cell arteritis. *Ophthalmology.* 2006;113(10):1842–5.

69. Nesher G, Rubınow A, Sonnenblick M. Efficacy and adverse effects of different corticosteroid dose regimens in temporal arteritis: a retrospective study. *Clin Exp Rheumatol.* 1997;15(3):303–6.

70. Moore PM, Calabrese LH. Neurologic manifestations of systemic vasculitides. *Semin Neurol.* 1994;14(4):300–6.

71. de Groot K, Schmidt DK, Arlt AC, Gross WL, Reinhold-Keller E. Standardized neurologic evaluations of 128 patients with Wegener granulomatosis. *Arch Neurol.* 2001;58(8):1215–21.

72. Baumann RJ, Robertson WC, Jr. Neurosarcoid presents differently in children than in adults. *Pediatrics.* 2003;112(6 Pt 1):e480–6.

73. Singhal AB. Diagnostic challenges in RCVS, PACNS, and other cerebral arteriopathies. *Cephalalgia.* 2011;31(10):1067–70.

74. Scolding NJ, Jayne DR, Zajicek JP, et al. Cerebral vasculitis: recognition, diagnosis and management. *QJM.* 1997;90(1):61–73.

75. Behrens MM. Headaches associated with disorders of the eye. *Med Clin North Am.* 1978;62(3):507–21.

76. Vincent AJ, Spierings EL, Messinger HB. A controlled study of visual symptoms and eye strain factors in chronic headache. *Headache.* 1989;29(8):523–7.

77. Nesher R, Epstein E, Stern Y, Assia E, Nesher G. Headaches as the main presenting symptom of subacute angle closure glaucoma. *Headache.* 2005;45(2):172–6.

78. Antonaci F, Fredriksen TA, Sjaastad O. Cervicogenic headache: clinical presentation, diagnostic criteria, and differential diagnosis. *Curr Pain Headache Rep.* 2001;5(4):387–92.

79. Edmeads J. The cervical spine and headache. *Neurology.* 1988;38(12):1874–8.

80. Furlan JC. Headache attributed to autonomic dysreflexia: an underrecognized clinical entity. *Neurology.* 2011;77(8):792–8.

81. Edvardsson B, Persson S. Reversible cerebral vasoconstriction syndrome associated with autonomic dysreflexia. *J Headache Pain.* 2010;11(3):277–80.

82. Toth C. Medications and substances as a cause of headache: a systematic review of the literature. *Clin Neuropharmacol.* 2003;26(3):122–36.

83. Sykes OT, Walker E. The neurotoxicology of carbon monoxide: Historical perspective and review. *Cortex.* 2015;74:440–8.

84. Katsarava Z, Fritsche G, Muessig M, Diener HC, Limmroth V. Clinical features of withdrawal headache following overuse of triptans and other headache drugs. *Neurology.* 2001;57(9):1694–8.

85. Zakrzewska JM, Linskey ME. Trigeminal neuralgia. *BMJ.* 2014;348:g474.

86. Lain AH, Caminero AB, Pareja JA. SUNCT syndrome: absence of refractory periods and modulation of attack duration by lengthening of the trigger stimuli. *Cephalalgia.* 2000;20(7):671–3.

87. Cruccu G, Gronseth G, Alksne J, et al. AAN-EFNS guidelines on trigeminal neuralgia management. *Eur J Neurol.* 2008;15(10):1013–28.

88. Antonini G, Di Pasquale A, Cruccu G, et al. Magnetic resonance imaging contribution for diagnosing symptomatic neurovascular contact in classical trigeminal neuralgia: a blinded case-control study and meta-analysis. *Pain.* 2014;155(8):1464–71.

89. Kress B, Schindler M, Rasche D, et al. MRI volumetry for the preoperative diagnosis of trigeminal neuralgia. *Eur Radiol.* 2005;15(7):1344–8.

90. Tate R, Rubin LM, Krajewski KC. Treatment of refractory trigeminal neuralgia with intravenous phenytoin. *Am J Health Syst Pharm.* 2011;68(21):2059–61.

91. Gronseth G, Cruccu G, Alksne J, et al. Practice parameter: the diagnostic evaluation and treatment of trigeminal neuralgia (an evidence-based review): report of the Quality Standards Subcommittee of the American Academy of Neurology and the European Federation of Neurological Societies. *Neurology.* 2008;71(15):1183–90.

92. Pareja JA, Ruiz J, de Isla C, al-Sabbah H, Espejo J. Idiopathic stabbing headache (jabs and jolts syndrome). *Cephalalgia.* 1996;16(2):93–6.

# The Migraine Patient in the Emergency Department

Serena L. Orr

Brian H. Rowe

## Abstract

Migraine is the most common primary headache disorder seen in the emergency department (ED). Patients with migraine present to the ED for a variety of reasons, including intolerable pain severity, failure of at-home treatment strategies, and debilitating associated symptoms. The diagnosis and management of migraine in the ED can be challenging. In this chapter, the epidemiology of migraine in the ED will be reviewed. A detailed and practical approach to the diagnosis and management of migraine in the ED will be outlined, followed by a discussion of discharge planning issues in this population.

## Epidemiology of Migraine

Migraine is a very common disorder. In the United States, the prevalence of migraine is estimated to be between 16.6 percent and 22.7 percent when considering the number of respondents reporting migraine in the past three months [1]. Comparable prevalence estimates have been calculated for Canada [2] and Europe [3]. A study commissioned by the World Health Organization found migraine to be the third most prevalent disorder worldwide, and the eighth most common cause of disability [4].

## Prevalence of Migraine Visits to the Emergency Department

Acute migraine attacks can often be aborted or successfully managed with early self-management; however, in some cases management fails, the headache pain is more severe, or debilitating associated symptoms occur, resulting in a presentation to the emergency department (ED). In the United States, head pain is estimated to be between the third and fifth most common reason for visiting the ED [1]. Annually, approximately five million of the ED visits in the United States

are related to headache, with approximately half of the visits having headache as the first-listed diagnosis and migraine accounting for over one-third of headache visits [5,6]. In one study, among all pain-related ED visits, headache and migraine were associated with the third highest pain scores [7].

Patients with migraine utilize the ED more frequently than controls [8]. The proportion of migraine patients who utilize ED services varies widely from country to country. In the first International Burden of Migraine (IBMS) study, rates of ED use in the past three months varied considerably across the five European countries assessed, with Spain having the highest rate at 16 percent, and France having the lowest rate at 2 percent [9]. In the second IBMS, which assessed migraine-related resource utilization in the United States, Canada, the United Kingdom, Germany, France, and Australia, anywhere from 8 percent to 35 percent of episodic migraine patients and 14 percent to 52 percent of chronic migraine patients reported ever having visited the ED for migraine. The highest rates of ED use were in Canada, the United States, and Australia and the lowest rates were in the UK [10]. Another multinational study estimated an average of 0.53 ED visits per migraine patient annually across the European, North American, and Latin American countries surveyed, with the highest rates being in Latin America (0.92 ED visits per patient annually) and the lowest being in Europe (0.35 ED visits per patient annually) [11]. Thus, migraine patients visit the ED frequently and rates vary considerably from country to country.

A large proportion of ED visits are due to a small subset of migraine patients. This issue was examined in the American Migraine Prevalence and Prevention Study (AMPP), which is a US-based study that identified a large cohort of severe headache sufferers, the majority of whom had migraine. In AMPP, 19 percent of the patients surveyed reported using the ED four or more times in the past year, and those patients accounted for 51 percent of the reported ED visits. Most of these frequent ED users had chronic migraine [12].

## Factors Influencing Prevalence of Migraine Visits to the Emergency Department

The frequency of ED use among migraine patients is dependent on a range of factors in addition to country of residence.

Patients visiting the ED for migraine seem to have a more severe headache disorder at baseline as compared to the general population of migraine patients. In the AMPP study, several markers of a severe headache disorder were predictive of ED use in multivariate models, including the migraine disability score, history of consultation with a headache specialist and prescription medication use [12].

As alluded to above, patients with chronic migraine have more frequent visits to the ED than patients with episodic migraine [10,12,13]. This is reflective of the general trend seen in patients with chronic migraine, whereby healthcare resource utilization tends to exceed that of patients with episodic migraine. In the AMPP study, patients with chronic migraine had total annual healthcare costs that were four times higher than those of patients with episodic migraine [13].

Outpatient medication usage patterns appear to be related to the frequency of ED use. Migraine patients with a history of opioid use are significantly more likely to visit the ED than migraine patients who are opioid-naïve, even when a series of important confounders such as socioeconomic status, migraine frequency, and psychiatric and medical comorbidities are accounted for in multivariate regression models [14]. In addition, patients prescribed opiates in the ED for acute migraine also return more frequently [15]. This patient population is particularly challenging to manage in the ED setting, especially given the overwhelming evidence that opioids should be avoided in the acute treatment of migraine. Conversely, patients using triptans for acute migraine relief, as well as those taking prophylactic migraine medications, appear to visit the ED less frequently as compared to the general migraine population [16].

General patterns of ED use appear to predict ED use for migraine. Several studies have found that the frequency of ED use for other health conditions is predictive of the frequency of ED use for migraine [12,17].

Socioeconomic status is inversely related to the frequency of ED use for migraine. This trend has been uncovered in studies based both in the United States [12] and Canada [18], whereby low socioeconomic status was found to be related to a higher frequency of ED visits for migraine. In the United States, insurance status appears to mediate the proportion of migraine care provided in the ED. In one study, uninsured patients received 34.1 percent of their migraine care in the ED, as compared to patients with private insurance who received only 13.2 percent of their migraine care in the ED [19]. Therefore, low socioeconomic status leads to more ED visits, and patients without healthcare insurance, who are of lower socioeconomic status than their insured counterparts, receive a greater proportion of their migraine care in the ED.

There is also evidence to suggest that among migraine patients, those with psychiatric comorbidities are more likely to visit the ED [20]. In addition, the subset of patients with migraine and psychiatric comorbidities appears to have more frequent ED visits as compared to patients with psychiatric diagnoses alone. Figure 7.1 lists the factors associated with frequent ED visits for migraine.

## Costs Associated With Emergency Department Visits for Migraine

Migraine is a very costly disorder, both in terms of direct costs accrued through health resource utilization, as well as through indirect costs, namely loss of productivity and work absenteeism. The majority of patients with migraine headache are discharged home after their ED care, and most often generic/low-cost medications are prescribed; however, other costs are incurred during the stay, including, but not limited to, laboratory testing, advanced imaging, and staff resources. A surprisingly high percentage of patients with migraine headache receive a computerized tomography (CT) of the brain, and in some severe cases patients receive a lumbar puncture to rule out malignant causes of headache (e.g., subarachnoid hemorrhage and meningitis).

Costs associated with ED visits among migraine patients vary greatly from country to country, primarily given differences in the structure of healthcare systems. In the first IBMS study, the mean cost of ED

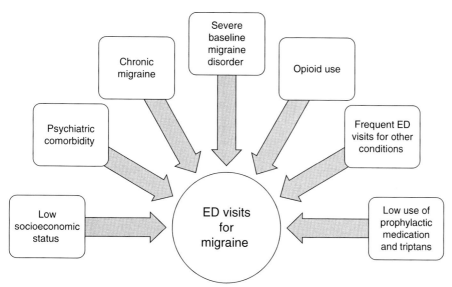

**Figure 7.1** Factors associated with frequent ED visits for migraine.

visits for the past three months, standardized to the 2010 euro (€2010), varied between €0.79 and €45.6 per patient for episodic migraine patients and between €0.43 and €93.6 per patient for chronic migraine patients, with the lowest costs in France and the highest costs in Spain [9]. In Spain, ED visits account for approximately 20.5 percent of the total direct costs associated with migraine, for an annual cost of €40.98 per patient, totaling over €70 million annually [21].

In the United States, costs associated with ED use for migraine are also impressive. One study found that migraine patients had higher ED visit costs in the past six months as compared to matched non-migraine patients, with an average of $33 spent on ED visits for each migraine patient vs. $18 for the matched non-migraine patients ($p < 0.001$) over the six-month period [22]. The cost of each ED visit in the United States is very high. In one study, ED visits for migraine totaled an average of $1799 per patient per visit, with 53 percent of the cost attributed to the ED charge and neuroimaging representing over one-third of the remaining costs associated with the visit [23]. The total annual cost of ED visits for migraine in the United States is estimated at $700 million [24].

Healthcare costs associated with ED visits for migraine are also high in Canada. Data from the IBMS found the costs associated with visiting the ED in the past three months to be $12 per episodic migraine patient vs. $78 per chronic migraine patient

in Canada, and $29 per episodic migraine patient vs. $22 per chronic migraine patient in the United States [25].

## Characteristics of Patients Visiting the ED with Migraine

There is a lack of information in the literature on the particular profile of patients who visit the ED for migraine, and about what motivates ED use in this population. What is known from the literature is that more women present than men, the median visual analogue score (VAS, ranging 0–10) is high, and that most patients have failed abortive medications and self-management strategies prior to their ED visit.

A cross-sectional study based in a US ED revealed several interesting facts about patients using ED services for migraine [26]. Over half of the patients had previously been diagnosed with migraines and had previously seen a physician for headaches. Just over one-fifth had already sought medical care for this particular migraine prior to visiting the ED. The majority of patients were not on migraine prophylaxis: only 27 percent reported daily use of a preventive medication. Fifty-five percent of the patients had taken medication to acutely relieve the migraine prior to presenting to the ED, though only 6 percent had used a triptan that day. Patients tended to have a protracted migraine: less than 10 percent had a migraine lasting five hours or less at presentation, and the median duration was 24 hours. Half of the patients screened positive for depression. This finding is congruent with previous studies that revealed higher rates of ED use among migraine patients with psychiatric comorbidities [12,20].

When questioned about their reason for visiting the ED, one-third of the patients in this US study reported that they were concerned about a life-threatening condition or that a physician referred them to the ED. Just under one-third attributed the visit to lack of access to their usual physician because of office closure or inability to book an expedient appointment. Several other reasons were given among the remaining patients, including financial concerns and personal preference for care in the ED [26].

## Diagnosing Migraine in the ED

### The Importance of Excluding Secondary Headache

Patients presenting to the ED with acute headache may have one of many possible diagnoses, some of which are benign and self-limiting, while others are more serious. The priority in the ED is to identify malignant causes and initiate treatment for migraine once these secondary causes of headache are excluded. For example, clinicians must consider infectious causes (e.g., viral and bacterial meningitis, encephalitis) when fever, chills, and/or myalgias are associated with the headache. Sudden-onset severe headaches suggest a vascular cause and may be associated with serious and life-threatening diseases such as subarachnoid or intracerebral hemorrhage, reversible cerebral vasoconstriction syndrome, cerebral venous sinus thrombosis, and arterial dissection. Finally, acute angle-closure glaucoma (unilateral severe ocular pain), temporal arteritis (older patients with headache, temporal artery tenderness, and elevated inflammatory biomarkers), and neoplasms are rare causes of headache in the ED, which must be excluded.

### How to Diagnose Migraine in the ED

Once the malignant causes of headache are excluded, migraine can be classified using criteria established by the International Headache Society (ICHD) [27]. Migraines come in several types; some are more common than others. A migraine headache preceded by an aura (e.g., a set of self-limited sensory [visual, tactile, and/or olfactory] symptoms) is referred to as a migraine with aura (previously known as classic migraine). Headaches not preceded by an aura are referred to as migraine without aura (previously known as common migraine). A diagnosis of migraine headache can be made when the patient meets the following criteria for migraine [27]:

- recurrent (>5 attacks in lifetime)
- prolonged (lasting 4–72 hours)
- associated with more than two of the following:
  ◦ unilateral location
  ◦ pulsating quality
  ◦ moderate or severe pain intensity
  ◦ aggravated by or causing avoidance of routine physical activity
- associated with one or more of the following:
  ◦ nausea and/or vomiting
  ◦ photophobia and phonophobia/sonophonia

Migraines that occur more than 15 days per month for at least three months are referred to as chronic migraines [27].

The ICHD criteria are considered the gold standard for the diagnosis of migraine, but they are not without issues when applied in the ED setting. Perhaps the most significant limitation on the sensitivity of the ICHD in the ED is Criterion A, that is, the criterion that requires that the patient report at least five similar headache episodes. This criterion is challenging in the ED setting as many patients will present with migraine prior to having experienced five episodes. In the pediatric population, it has been shown that removal of Criterion A significantly improves the sensitivity of the ICHD criteria for the diagnosis of migraine in the ED, as compared to diagnosis by a neurologist [28]. However, because of the overlap of the clinical features (severe throbbing headache, which is worse with movement and associated with photophobia, phonophobia, and nausea) of migraine with many serious secondary causes, taking Criterion A into account becomes crucial in an effort to avoid missing a sinister secondary cause of headache in a patient presenting for the first time with what looks phenotypically like migraine. In other words, patients presenting for the first time with headache that meets the pain and associated symptom criteria for migraine should be carefully and thoroughly evaluated for red flags and appropriate investigations should be pursued.

In addition, the ID-Migraine™ instrument may prove useful for the diagnosis of migraine in the ED once secondary headaches have been excluded. This instrument was developed to facilitate the diagnosis of migraine in the primary care setting and comprises three questions: the first pertains to nausea and vomiting, the second pertains to photosensitivity, and the third pertains to disability related to the headaches [29]. Although only one study has assessed its validity in the ED, results were promising: as compared to the gold standard of ICHD criteria, the ID-Migraine™ had a sensitivity of 94 percent and a specificity of 83 percent [30]. These findings have not yet been replicated, but future studies should address the use of ID-Migraine™ in the ED, given that it could theoretically reduce the proportion of patients diagnosed with headache not otherwise specified, a phenomenon that occurs very frequently in the ED. A simple mnemonic based on ID-Migraine™, *PIN* (*p*hotophobia, *i*mpaired function, *n*ausea), has been used to assist in the diagnosis of migraine.

## Recognizing Secondary Headaches in Patients with Migraine

Although a patient may have a history of migraines, it is important to recognize when they may be presenting with a secondary headache, rather than a migraine. The clinician must always take a detailed headache history and carry out a physical examination. If the characteristics of the headache differ significantly from the patient's usual migraines, other possibilities must be considered. In addition, if the neurologic exam is abnormal, further investigations are warranted even if the headache corresponds to the patient's typical migraine.

## Differentiating Tension-Type Headache from Migraine in the ED

### Epidemiology of Tension-Type Headache in the ED

Tension-type headache is very common, with a lifetime prevalence estimated at 78 percent [31]. Although it is more prevalent than migraine in the general population, tension-type headache is less common than migraine in the ED setting.

Whereas migraine underlies over one-third of ED visits for headache and 60 percent of ED visits for primary headache, tension-type headache accounts for approximately 7 percent of all ED visits for headache, and 11 percent of ED visits for primary headache, based on data from a US center [6]. This is true despite the fact that tension-type headache is more prevalent than migraine in the general population. This discrepancy occurs because patients with tension-type headaches are less likely to visit the ED for acute headache than are migraine patients. Data from the AMPP study highlight this trend: whereas 7.3 percent of patients with episodic migraine had visited the ED in the past year, only 3 percent of patients with episodic tension-type headache had done so (OR 0.4, 95 percent CI 0.3–0.6) [12].

Therefore, patients presenting to the ED with a primary headache are much more likely to have migraine than tension-type headache.

## Diagnosing Tension-Type Headache in the ED

Since the headache associated with brain tumors and other space-occupying lesions most often resembles tension-type headache [32], and because tension-type headache as a primary headache disorder rarely brings patients to the ED, the *diagnosis of tension-type headache in the emergency department should be a diagnosis of exclusion*. Tension-type headache, like migraine, is subdivided into episodic and chronic forms. The International Classification of Headache Disorders (ICHD-3, beta version) outlines diagnostic criteria for three core types of tension-type headache [27]: infrequent episodic, frequent episodic, and chronic tension-type headache. The ICHD-3 also recognizes that tension-type headache may or may not be associated with pericranial muscle tenderness, and also accounts for cases in which one diagnostic criterion is lacking, under the umbrella of the probable tension-type headaches.

The ICHD defines five diagnostic criteria that need to be met to make the diagnosis of tension-type headache. Criterion A describes the frequency of the headaches and thereby defines whether the disorder is classified as infrequent episodic, frequent episodic, or chronic. Criterion B outlines the usual duration of tension-type headaches. Criterion C is invariable between the three types of tension-type headache and outlines the pain characteristics associated with this type of headache. Criterion D refers to associated symptoms, with more lenience in chronic tension-type

**Table 7.1** ICHD-3 (beta version) Diagnostic Criteria for Tension-Type Headache [27]

| Criterion | Infrequent episodic TTH | Frequent episodic TTH | Chronic TTH |
|---|---|---|---|
| A | At least ten headaches, occurring less than once per month (less than 12 days per year), that meet criteria B–D | At least ten headaches, occurring on average between 1 and 14 days per month for at least three months (between 12 and 180 days per year), that meet criteria B–D | Headaches occurring on at least 15 days per month for at least three months (more than 180 days per year), that meet criteria B–D |
| B | Headaches last between 30 minutes and 7 days | Headaches last between 30 minutes and 7 days | Lasting hours to days or constant |
| C | At least two of the following four characteristics are present:<br>• bilateral<br>• non-pulsating (pressing or tightening quality)<br>• mild or moderate pain intensity<br>• not aggravated by routine physical activity such as walking or climbing stairs | At least two of the following four characteristics are present:<br>• bilateral<br>• non-pulsating (pressing or tightening quality)<br>• mild or moderate pain intensity<br>• not aggravated by routine physical activity such as walking or climbing stairs | At least two of the following four characteristics are present:<br>• bilateral location<br>• pressing or tightening (non-pulsating) quality<br>• mild or moderate pain intensity<br>• not aggravated by routine physical activity such as walking or climbing stairs |
| D | Both of the following are present:<br>1. No nausea nor vomiting<br>2. No more than one of either photophobia or phonophobia | Both of the following are present:<br>1. No nausea nor vomiting<br>2. No more than one of either photophobia or phonophobia | Both of the following are present:<br>1. No more than one of mild nausea, photophobia, or phonophobia<br>2. Neither moderate or severe nausea or vomiting |
| E | Not better accounted for by another ICHD-3 diagnosis | Not better accounted for by another ICHD-3 diagnosis | Not better accounted for by another ICHD-3 diagnosis |

headache than in the episodic forms. Finally, Criterion E reminds clinicians that tension-type headache is a diagnosis of exclusion. The criteria for tension-type headache are described in detail in Table 7.1.

The vast majority of patients presenting to the ED with tension-type headache will have frequent episodic or chronic tension-type headache, seeing as most patients with infrequent episodic tension-type headache do not present to medical attention [27].

## Differentiation of Migraine and Tension-Type Headache in the ED

While there is some degree of overlap between migraine and tension-type headache, with some in the past even arguing that the two conditions are in fact variations of the same underlying disorder [33], they are considered to be separate disorders and should be diagnosed as such [27]. Often, patients with frequent headaches have both migraine and tension-type headache. For example, the diagnosis of chronic migraine only requires that eight of the headache days per month be phenotypically consistent with migraine [27], and many of these patients will have some headache days where the diagnostic criteria for tension-type headache are fulfilled. However, the headaches that meet criteria for tension-type headache in those with migraine often respond to triptans and are considered by many experts to be mild migraine from an underlying biological perspective [34].

The key to differentiating tension-type headache from migraine rests in identifying headache features that are specific to migraine, notably: unilateral pain, throbbing or pulsating pain quality, high pain intensity, worsening of the pain with routine activities, the presence of nausea or vomiting, and the presence of both photophobia and phonophobia. Many experts consider tension-type headache to be a *featureless* headache; pain is not throbbing and there are no associated symptoms of photophobia, phonophobia, nausea, or emesis. In addition, when either the pain or associated symptom criteria for migraine are missing, most experts would render a diagnosis of probable migraine rather than probable tension-type headache. Some headache triggers appear to occur more commonly with migraine than with tension-type headache. Whereas stress, fatigue, sleep deprivation, and an irregular eating schedule can trigger both migraine and tension-type headache, one study found that weather, light, smoke, and certain smells are more likely to trigger migraine than tension-type headache [35].

Although one should always refer to diagnostic criteria to distinguish between migraine and tension-type headache, pain intensity is a strong differentiating factor. In the ED, most cases of severe primary headache will be due to migraine given that tension-type headache is typically less severe and given that the other primary headache disorders are rare. One study found that migraine accounted for 95.1 percent of all severe primary headaches diagnosed in the ED [12]. Therefore, high pain intensity in a patient with a suspected primary headache should prompt the clinician to ask about migrainous features. Figure 7.2 summarizes the features of migraine and tension-type headache.

## Approach to the Treatment of Tension-Type Headache in the ED

The acute treatment of tension-type headache in the ED is an area that has been neglected in the literature. Although the typical approach to treating acute tension-type headache involves administration of oral nonsteroidal anti-inflammatory agents, this approach may be insufficient for patients presenting to the ED. Patients who present with an episode of severe tension-type headache often require parenteral therapy, and commonly respond to some of the same interventions that are used for acute migraine in this setting.

The European Federation of Neurological Societies has addressed the treatment of tension-type headache with guidelines that were released in 2010 [36]. Level A evidence (ascribed to interventions with at least one class I study or two class II studies supporting their efficacy) was given to the following interventions for the acute treatment of tension-type

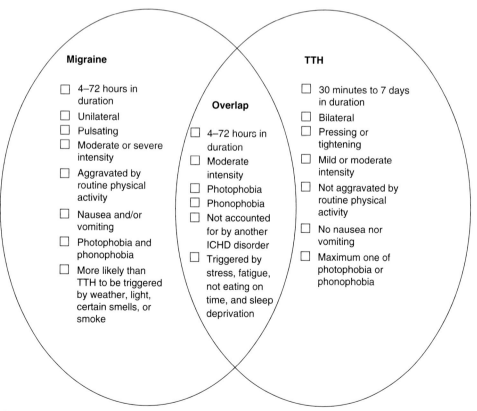

Migraine

☐ 4–72 hours in duration
☐ Unilateral
☐ Pulsating
☐ Moderate or severe intensity
☐ Aggravated by routine physical activity
☐ Nausea and/or vomiting
☐ Photophobia and phonophobia
☐ More likely than TTH to be triggered by weather, light, certain smells, or smoke

Overlap

☐ 4–72 hours in duration
☐ Moderate intensity
☐ Photophobia
☐ Phonophobia
☐ Not accounted for by another ICHD disorder
☐ Triggered by stress, fatigue, not eating on time, and sleep deprivation

TTH

☐ 30 minutes to 7 days in duration
☐ Bilateral
☐ Pressing or tightening
☐ Mild or moderate intensity
☐ Not aggravated by routine physical activity
☐ No nausea nor vomiting
☐ Maximum one of photophobia or phonophobia

**Figure 7.2** Features of migraine and tension-type headache (TTH).

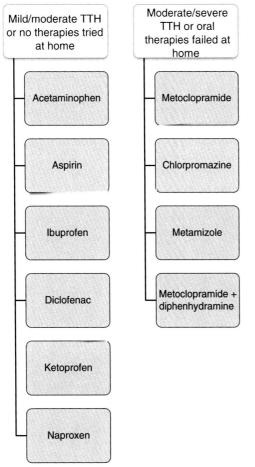

**Figure 7.3** Treatment options for acute tension-type headache in the ED.

ketorolac, intravenous chlorpromazine, and intravenous metamizole. A systematic review published in 2014 searched all major databases and identified only eight eligible studies that included a total of 486 patients, which assessed parenteral therapies for acute tension-type headache. The review concluded that the following medications have demonstrated efficacy based on the limited eligible studies: metoclopramide, chlorpromazine, metamizole, and the combination of metoclopramide and diphenhydramine [37].

Clinicians treating patients with tension-type headache in the ED have limited evidence to guide their decisions. A reasonable approach would involve stratifying the patients by headache severity, and determining which therapies have been ineffective at home for the headache. Patients with mild or moderate headache intensity who have not already failed oral therapies at home can be treated with oral or suppository nonsteroidal anti-inflammatory medications first-line. Those with moderate or severe headaches or those who have failed oral therapies at home may require parenteral therapy (see Figure 7.3).

## Approach to the Treatment of Migraine in the ED

### General Considerations When Choosing Acute Migraine Treatment in the ED

Because of the significant number and diversity of interventions at the clinician's disposal, it is important to take a number of patient factors into consideration when selecting an intervention. First and foremost, severity of the migraine is important. Patients with mild headache pain may simply require hydration and oral analgesics and antinauseants. Mild to moderate pain with the ability to tolerate oral agents may be treated with oral or intramuscular agents and hydration. Patients with more severe pain, in association with nausea/vomiting, usually require the establishment of an intravenous route for medication delivery. These patients represent the majority of patient presentations in EDs in most developed countries.

The timing of presentation to the ED is important when consideration is being given to treating the migraine with a triptan. Because triptans are more

headache: acetaminophen, aspirin, diclofenac, ibuprofen, ketoprofen, and naproxen. Level B evidence (ascribed to interventions with at least one "convincing" class II study or class III evidence that is "overwhelming") was given to combination medications containing caffeine. Although very useful in approaching the acute treatment of tension-type headaches, these guidelines did not outline parenteral treatment options, which are sometimes necessary for the patient presenting to the ED.

Several parenteral therapies for acute tension-type headache have been studied, albeit to a limited extent, and have been shown to have some efficacy for acute tension-type headache: intravenous metoclopramide, intramuscular pethidine, intravenous prochlorperazine, intramuscular/intravenous likely to be effective early in the course of an attack while pain intensity is mild [38], subcutaneous sumatriptan, the main triptan that has been studied in the ED setting, is most appropriate for the patient presenting to the ED early in their migraine attack. It is possible that other treatments also have differential efficacy based on the timing of their administration, though the evidence is less clear. For example, one of the trials assessing the efficacy of dexamethasone for persistent pain freedom at 24 hours found that the subgroup of patients presenting to the ED with prolonged migraine, defined as migraine lasting 72 hours or greater, were more likely to achieve this outcome than those with shorter durations of migraine at presentation [39].

Taking into account therapies that the patient has already tried at home for the present migraine is a rational approach to treatment. Triptans are to be limited to a maximum of two doses in a 24-hour period. Thus, if a patient has already reached the maximum number of triptan doses, subcutaneous sumatriptan would not be an appropriate treatment option. Triptans and ergot alkaloids (i.e., dihydroergotamine and ergotamine) should not be used within 24 hours of each other because of their vasoconstrictive properties.

Patients may have previous experience with ED migraine treatments. The clinician should inquire about previous successful migraine-specific parenteral interventions, their efficacy, and side-effects. It is important to understand what experience the patient has had with particular interventions, as they may influence patient preferences. The clinician may also choose to avoid interventions that have previously been ineffective or intolerable to the patient.

Because some of the ED migraine interventions have rare but serious potential adverse events, the clinician must consider the patient's risk of particular adverse events when selecting a medication. For example, dopamine receptor antagonists are best avoided in patients who have a higher baseline risk of extrapyramidal side-effects, such as individuals taking other anti-dopaminergic agents. In addition, because of their vasoconstrictive properties and association with chest symptoms, triptans and ergot alkaloids are contraindicated in patients with a history of ischemic heart disease, stroke, transient ischemic attack, basilar migraine, hemiplegic migraine, or peripheral vascular disease. Therefore, as with any treatment decision, the patient's baseline risk of adverse events should

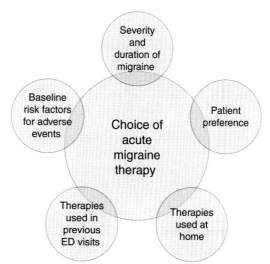

**Figure 7.4** Factors to consider when selecting a migraine intervention in the ED setting.

guide the clinician in selecting appropriate treatment options (Figure 7.4).

## Specific Interventions for Acute Migraine in the ED

There are multiple interventions that can be used for acutely treating migraines in the ED setting. Unfortunately, the evidence base for acute migraine interventions in this setting is relatively weak. Although the International Headache Society has released guidelines on controlled trials of drugs in migraine, many of the published randomized controlled trials that have been carried out in the ED setting have not followed these guidelines [40]. This compromises the quality of the evidence and the feasibility of pooling the evidence to generate more accurate estimates of effect that in turn can guide the formation of guidelines. Individual interventions will be reviewed here, and a proposed list of first-, second-, and third-line monotherapy interventions are displayed later in Figure 7.5, though in practice, clinicians often choose to administer combination agents (see section 'Combination Agents in Acute Migraine' on p. 75).

### Intravenous Crystalloid Solutions

Intravenous crystalloids (e.g., saline and Ringer's solutions) are often administered in the ED to manage migraine headaches. While many patients with migraine experience nausea and vomiting, decreased oral intake, and increased insensible losses through hyperventilation, the role of intravenous rehydration has been infrequently studied in the acute setting. Currently, there are no randomized controlled trials addressing this issue in adults. One post-hoc analysis of data from four clinical trials on migraine treatment in the ED compared treatment outcomes in patients who received IV fluids at the discretion of the treating physician and those who did not receive IV fluids [41]. Those who received IV fluids actually had less improvement on their pain scales as compared to those who did not receive IV fluids [41]. Clinicians are advised to treat based on the clinical assessment of hydration status (consensus recommendation).

## Metoclopramide in Acute Migraine

Intravenous metoclopramide (10 mg) is a common medication used in the ED for acute migraine, especially in Canada [42]. Metoclopramide is more effective than placebo in reducing migraine headache scores (measured on visual analog scales [VAS]) or in relieving pain [43]. In addition, metoclopramide has been compared to other agents for migraine headaches and has been found to be less effective than neuroleptics, and has a variable response compared to other agents as monotherapy. The agent is an excellent antinauseant; however, side-effects, including akathisia, are common [43]. In the Canadian Headache Society recommendations on the treatment of migraine pain in emergency settings, metoclopramide was given a strong recommendation to use based on moderate-quality evidence [44].

## Neuroleptics in Acute Migraine

Intravenous neuroleptics have been used for decades as specific anti-migraine medications in the ED for acute migraine. Although the first neuroleptic effectively employed in migraine was chlorpromazine, side-effects (i.e., hypotension and extrapyramidal symptoms) were concerning to both clinicians and patients. Since that time, prochlorperazine (10 mg) has been more commonly used. It is more effective than placebo in reducing migraine headache or relieving pain [43]. In addition, neuroleptics have been compared to other agents for migraine headaches and found to be more effective than metoclopramide, and most other agents as monotherapy [43]. While prochlorperazine is an excellent antinauseant, side-effects such as akathisia and sedation are common.

Diphenhydramine is often given simultaneously with the neuroleptics to prevent extrapyramidal side-effects; however, the evidence for this is weak [45]. Of note, diphenhydramine does not appear to be effective for the outcome of acute migraine pain relief, based on one high-quality trial [46]. The Canadian Headache Society recommendations provided a strong recommendation to use prochlorperazine for acute migraine based on high-quality evidence [44].

## Nonsteroidal Anti-Inflammatory Drugs (NSAIDs) in Acute Migraine

Intravenous NSAIDs have been widely studied in patients suffering from migraine headache. The most common agent is ketorolac, and it may be delivered via the intramuscular or oral route. It is superior to placebo, is as effective as meperidine, and more effective than sumatriptan [43]. In the Canadian Headache Society recommendations on the treatment of migraine pain in emergency settings, ketorolac was strongly recommended based on low-quality evidence [44].

## Triptans in Acute Migraine

Subcutaneous sumatriptan has been the best-studied triptan for the treatment of acute migraine in the ED setting. A large number of clinical trials have shown that subcutaneous sumatriptan is superior to placebo for acute migraine, but the majority of these trials were based in outpatient clinics, with a relatively small proportion having been carried out in ED settings [43,44]. Trials comparing subcutaneous sumatriptan to other active agents for migraine in the ED have yielded mixed results, and apart from metoclopramide, which has been compared to sumatriptan in two trials with one trial finding no difference [47] and the other suggesting superiority of metoclopramide [48], only single studies have compared sumatriptan to the other active comparators studied, making it difficult to draw conclusions about its efficacy in relation to other agents. Subcutaneous sumatriptan has more associated adverse events than placebo, with injection site reactions, paresthesias, and drowsiness being the most common, and chest symptoms being more rare but concerning adverse events. Because of the consistency of the evidence showing superiority of subcutaneous sumatriptan over placebo for acute migraine, the Canadian Headache Society has strongly recommended its use in the ED setting based on moderate-quality evidence [44].

## Dihydroergotamine in Acute Migraine

Dihydroergotamine (DHE) is an effective agent in patients in whom the agent is not contraindicated (e.g., those with coronary artery disease, previous stroke, etc.). Dihydroergotamine reduces VAS pain scores more effectively than placebo and has variable effectiveness compared to migraine-specific agents [49]. When parenteral (subcutaneous) DHE 1.0 mg was compared in a double-blind comparator trial to subcutaneous sumatriptan 6 mg in 295 evaluable patients, 73.1 percent of the patients treated with dihydroergotamine and 85.3 percent of those treated with sumatriptan had relief of headache at two hours ($p = 0.002$) [50]. Both were equally effective at four hours with 85.5 percent of those treated with dihydroergotamine and 83.3 percent of those treated with sumatriptan experiencing headache relief. While sumatriptan was more effective at the earliest time point, DHE was most effective at 24 hours, with 89.7 percent of dihydroergotamine-treated patients and 76.7 percent of sumatriptan-treated patients achieving headache relief ($p = 0.004$). Headache recurred within 24 hours after treatment in 45 percent of the sumatriptan-treated patients and in 17.7 percent of the dihydroergotamine-treated patients ($p \leq 0.001$). Dihydroergotamine may therefore be a more effective agent in the ED compared to subcutaneous sumatriptan in achieving and sustaining headache relief and reducing the potential for a return ED visit for a single attack. Dihydroergotamine is also an effective agent when used in combination with other migraine-specific agents (especially metoclopramide) [43]. In the Canadian Headache Society recommendations on the treatment of migraine pain in emergency settings, DHE was assigned a weak recommendation in favor of its use based on low-quality evidence [44].

## Opioids in Acute Migraine

A variety of opioid agents have been employed to treat migraine headache, and several studies have indicated an over-reliance on this medication class as first-line agents in acute migraine treatment in both Canadian [15] and US [51] EDs. Meperidine is the most commonly studied opioid in this setting; however, because of its addictive potential, safety concerns in the elderly, and the availability of alternative narcotic agents, many EDs have removed it as a therapeutic agent for pain relief. Notwithstanding these issues, evidence suggests that meperidine is an effective agent when compared to placebo and as effective as ketorolac [52]. Given the overall objective of complete pain relief in the ED setting, use of narcotics as third- or fourth-line agents may be an effective option for some patients. In the Canadian Headache Society recommendations on the treatment of migraine pain in emergency settings, a weak recommendation to use meperidine for this indication was made based on low-quality evidence [44].

## Other Agents in Acute Migraine

A number of other interventions have been studied for the management of migraine in the ED. Most of these interventions have only been studied in single, small, or poor-quality trials, and will not be discussed here.

Intravenous acetylsalicylic acid appears to be more effective than placebo and ergotamine for relief of acute migraine in the ED [43,44]. Based on single studies, intravenous acetaminophen was no different than placebo [53] or dexketoprofen [54], and showed some superiority over oral rizatriptan for one-hour pain outcomes, but this was not sustained at two hours [55]. Data on valproic acid thus far has suggested a lack of efficacy as compared to other active agents [43,56–58]. Propofol has emerged as an intervention of research interest in recent years, and small studies have hinted at its superiority over subcutaneous sumatriptan [59] and dexamethasone [60] for acute migraine relief. The evidence is sparse and weak, so the use of this agent is currently limited to specialists. Moreover, its side-effect profile, namely its sedating properties, and short half-life are concerning in the setting of migraine. Intravenous magnesium sulfate has been studied in several ED trials, with mixed results; however, it is an inexpensive alternative that can be tried in select patients. Based on the current evidence, the Canadian Headache Society has provided a weak recommendation against its use in this setting, based on moderate-quality evidence [44].

## Combination Agents in Acute Migraine [43]

Emergency physicians faced with patients in extreme pain from migraine headache and experiencing associated symptoms are reluctant to limit management to a single therapeutic agent. Combination agents have been investigated and appear to provide excellent relief compared to most agents used in monotherapy.

In Canada, the combination of metoclopramide and ketorolac appears popular [61]. Since the relative effectiveness of each combination remains unclear, it is premature to provide evidence-based recommendations on specific combination therapies.

### Comparative Effectiveness in Acute Migraine

A comprehensive and large network meta-analysis explored the comparative effectiveness of migraine agents [43]. This review ranked agents as first-line (e.g., prochlorperazine and combination agents), second-line (e.g., NSAIDs, opioids, and metoclopramide), and third-line (e.g., DHE, triptans, and other agents) agents on the basis of effectiveness with respect to reducing pain scores. Using similar methods, the same review ranked agents with respect to side-effects and identified metoclopramide and prochlorperazine as the most likely agents to cause akathisia. These methods provide insight for clinicians and reinforce the need to balance the treatment efficacy against the side-effects. Combining the evidence and conclusions from this meta-analysis with the recommendations made in the Canadian Headache Society systematic review [44], a proposed

approach to monotherapy for acute migraine in the ED is summarized in Figure 7.5.

## Recurrence of Migraine After Treatment in the ED

Despite efforts to resolve a migraine attack in the ED, repeat ED visits may occur due to return of headache or exacerbation of an existing headache. A variety of factors may be involved in relapses. First, despite few studies, some treatments (e.g., NSAIDs, metoclopramide, and neuroleptics) are associated with lower relapses after ED discharge as compared to others [43]. Second, while age and sex do not appear to influence migraine recurrence, certain factors have been associated with relapse. First, headache pain relief or near-relief (VAS < 2) is associated with fewer relapses. Second, a longer duration of symptoms (> 24 hours) prior to the ED visit has also been associated with relapse [61]. Third, use of narcotics has been associated with increased relapse, and whether this observation is due to failure of the treatment to address the pathophysiology of migraine or due to associated addictive behaviors has not yet been

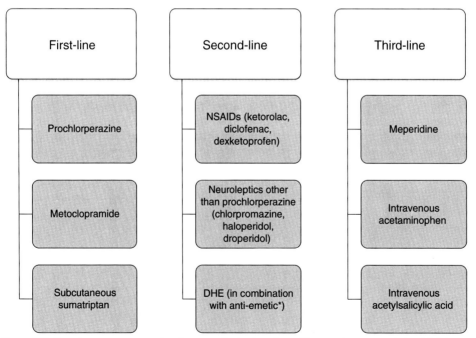

**Figure 7.5** Monotherapy treatment options for acute migraine based on evidence and recommendations [43,44].
* Given that DHE is frequently associated with precipitation or exacerbation of nausea, it should almost always be used in combination with an anti-emetic medication.

resolved [15]. Finally, non-pharmacological treatments to reduce the frequency of relapse (e.g., rest, hydration, etc.) may help resolve symptoms; however, few have been explored in sufficient detail to justify recommendations.

## Prevention of Recurrence After the ED Visit

There are a number of agents that have the potential to mitigate recurrence and relapse in the period immediately following an acute attack. For example, there are seven trials examining the role of dexamethasone on relapse following ED discharge. All studies reported on recurrence of pain or headache between 24 and 72 hours after discharge from the ED. The pooled results significantly favored the dexamethasone agents (RR = 0.68; 95 percent CI: 0.49, 0.96; $I^2$ = 63 percent). Overall, while not an effective acute headache treatment, patients receiving dexamethasone plus standard abortive therapy were less likely to report recurrence of pain or headache up to 72 hours after discharge compared with placebo plus standard abortive therapy (moderate strength of evidence) [43,62].

Different doses of dexamethasone have been employed. Studies that used less than 15 mg of dexamethasone reported a similar treatment effect (RR = 0.69; 95 percent CI: 0.40, 1.18) to those using 15 mg or more (RR = 0.65; 95 percent CI: 0.43 to 0.99) [43]. The difference between these two subgroups was not significant ($p$ = 0.16). Consequently, 10 mg seems an appropriate intravenous dose for most adults.

While acute side-effects are uncommon with systemic corticosteroids, chronic side-effects can be cumulative and clinicians should be discouraged from using the agent in all patients. One strategy espoused by trialists is to use dexamethasone for migraine attacks of prolonged duration (e.g., >24 hours), and in those who have contraindications to or have not achieved complete headache relief in the ED with other more commonly used acute medications [61].

## Follow-up

It is important for patients with frequent ED presentations for tension and/or migraine headache to be assessed by their primary care physicians. While a discussion of prophylaxis is beyond the scope of this chapter, considerations should be made regarding pharmacological and non-pharmacological efforts

to prevent or mitigate future headaches. Moreover, migraine action plans to abort acute headaches should be reviewed. Finally, failure of primary care management and recurrent ED visits present an opportunity to consider referral to a migraine specialist.

## References

1. Smitherman TA, Burch R, Sheikh H, Loder E. The prevalence, impact, and treatment of migraine and severe headaches in the United States: a review of statistics from national surveillance studies. *Headache.* 2013;53(3):427–36.

2. Cooke LJ, Becker WJ. Migraine prevalence, treatment and impact: the Canadian women and migraine study. *Can J Neurol Sci.* 2010;37(5):580–7.

3. Stovner LJ, Andree C. Prevalence of headache in Europe: a review for the Eurolight project. *J Headache Pain.* 2010;11(4):289–99.

4. Vos T, Flaxman AD, Naghavi M, et al. Years lived with disability (YLDs) for 1160 sequelae of 289 diseases and injuries 1990–2010: a systematic analysis for the Global Burden of Disease Study 2010. *Lancet.* 2012;380(9859):2163–96.

5. Lucado J, Paez K, Elixhauser A. Headaches in US Hospitals and Emergency Departments, 2008: Statistical Brief #111. *Healthcare Cost and Utilization Project (HCUP) Statistical Briefs.* 2011;24:1–12.

6. Friedman BW, Hochberg ML, Esses D, et al. Applying the International Classification of Headache Disorders to the emergency department: an assessment of reproducibility and the frequency with which a unique diagnosis can be assigned to every acute headache presentation. *Ann Emerg Med.* 2007;49(4):409–19.

7. Marco CA, Kanitz W, Jolly M. Pain scores among emergency department (ED) patients: comparison by ED diagnosis. *J Emerg Med.* 2013;44(1):46–52.

8. Lafata JE, Moon C, Leotta C, et al. The medical care utilization and costs associated with migraine headache. *J Gen Intern Med.* 2004;19(10):1005–12.

9. Bloudek LM, Stokes M, Buse DC, et al. Cost of healthcare for patients with migraine in five European countries: results from the International Burden of Migraine Study (IBMS). *J Headache Pain.* 2012;13(5):361–78.

10. Sanderson JC, Devine EB, Lipton RB, et al. Headache-related health resource utilisation in chronic and episodic migraine across six countries. *J Neurol Neurosurg Psychiatry.* 2013;84(12):1309–17.

11. Gerth WC, Carides GW, Dasbach EJ, Visser WH, Santanello NC. The multinational impact of migraine

symptoms on healthcare utilisation and work loss. *Pharmacoeconomics*. 2001;19(2):197–206.

12. Friedman BW, Serrano D, Reed M, Diamond M, Lipton RB. Use of the emergency department for severe headache: a population-based study. *Headache*. 2009;49(1):21–30.

13. Munakata J, Hazard E, Serrano D, et al. Economic burden of transformed migraine: results from the American Migraine Prevalence and Prevention (AMPP) Study. *Headache*. 2009;49(4):498–508.

14. Buse DC, Pearlman SH, Reed ML, et al. Opioid use and dependence among persons with migraine: results of the AMPP study. *Headache*. 2012;52(1):18–36.

15. Colman I, Rothney A, Wright S, Zilkalns B, Rowe BH. Use of narcotic analgesics in the emergency department treatment of migraine headache. *Neurology*. 2004;62(10):1695–700.

16. Lainez MJA. The effect of migraine prophylaxis on migraine-related resource use and productivity. *CNS Drugs*. 2009;23(9):727–38.

17. Lane P, Nituica C, Sorondo B. Headache patients: who does not come to the emergency department? *Acad Emerg Med*. 2003;10:528.

18. Chan BT, Ovens HJ. Chronic migraineurs: an important subgroup of patients who visit emergency departments frequently. *Ann Emerg Med*. 2004;43(2):238–42.

19. Wilper A, Woolhandler S, Himmelstein D, Nardin R. Impact of insurance status on migraine care in the United States: a population-based study. *Neurology*. 2010;74(15):1178–83.

20. Minen MT, Tanev K. Influence of psychiatric comorbidities in migraineurs in the emergency department. *Gen Hosp Psychiatry*. 2014;36(5):533–8.

21. Badia X, Magaz S, Gutierrez L, Galvan J. The burden of migraine in Spain: beyond direct costs. *Pharmacoeconomics*. 2004;22(9):591–603.

22. Edmeads J, Mackell JA. The economic impact of migraine: an analysis of direct and indirect costs. *Headache*. 2002;42(6):501–9.

23. Friedman D, Feldon S, Holloway R, Fisher S. Utilization, diagnosis, treatment and cost of migraine treatment in the emergency department. *Headache*. 2009;49(8):1163–73.

24. Insinga RP, Ng-Mak DS, Hanson ME. Costs associated with outpatient, emergency room and inpatient care for migraine in the USA. *Cephalalgia*. 2011;31(15):1570–5.

25. Stokes M, Becker WJ, Lipton RB, et al. Cost of health care among patients with chronic and episodic migraine in Canada and the USA: results from the International Burden of Migraine Study (IBMS). *Headache*. 2011;51(7):1058–77.

26. Minen MT, Loder E, Friedman B. Factors associated with emergency department visits for migraine: an observational study. *Headache*. 2014;54(10):1611–18.

27. Headache Classification Committee of the International Headache Society (IHS). The International Classification of Headache Disorders, 3rd edition (beta version). *Cephalalgia*. 2013;33(9):629–808.

28. Trottier ED, Bailey B, Lucas N, Lortie A. Diagnosis of migraine in the pediatric emergency department. *Pediatr Neurol*. 2013;49(1):40–5.

29. Lipton RB, Dodick D, Sadovsky R, et al. A self-administered screener for migraine in primary care: the ID Migraine validation study. *Neurology*. 2003;61(3):375–82.

30. Mostardini C, d'Agostino VC, Dugoni DE, Cerbo R. A possible role of ID-Migraine in the emergency department: study of an emergency department out-patient population. *Cephalalgia*. 2009;29(12):1326–30.

31. Rasmussen B, Jensen R, Schroll M, Olesen J. Epidemiology of headache in a general population: a prevalence study. *J Clin Epidemiol*. 1991;44(11):1147–57.

32. Forsyth PA, Posner JB. Headaches in patients with brain tumors: a study of 111 patients. *Neurology*. 1993;43(9):1678–83.

33. Marcus D. Migraine and tension-type headaches: the questionable validity of current classification systems. *Clin J Pain*. 1992;8:28–36.

34. Lipton RB, Cady RK, Stewart WF, Wilks K, Hall C. Diagnostic lessons from the spectrum study. *Neurology*. 2002;58(9 Suppl. 6):S27–31.

35. Spierings ELH, Ranke AH, Honkoop PC. Precipitating and aggravating factors of migraine versus tension-type headache. *Headache*. 2001;41(6):554–8.

36. Bendtsen L, Evers S, Linde M, et al. EFNS guideline on the treatment of tension-type headache: report of an EFNS task force. *Eur J Neurol*. 2010;17(11):1318–25.

37. Weinman D, Nicastro O, Akala O, Friedman BW. Parenteral treatment of episodic tension-type headache: a systematic review. *Headache*. 2014;54(2):260–8.

38. D'Amico D, Moschiano F, Bussone G. Early treatment of migraine attacks with triptans: a strategy to enhance outcomes and patient satisfaction? *Expert Rev Neurother*. 2006;6(7):1087–97.

39. Friedman BW, Greenwald P, Bania TC, et al. Randomized trial of IV dexamethasone for acute migraine in the emergency department. *Neurology*. 2007;69(22):2038–44.

40. Tfelt-Hansen P, Pascual J, Ramadan N, et al. Guidelines for controlled trials of drugs in migraine: third edition. A guide for investigators. *Cephalalgia*. 2012;32(1):6–38.

41. Friedman B. Intravenous fluids for migraine: a post-hoc analysis of clinical trial data [abstract]. *Headache*. 2015;55(Suppl. 3):127–87.

42. Colman I, Brown MD, Innes GD, et al. Parenteral metoclopramide for acute migraine: meta-analysis of randomised controlled trials. *BMJ*. 2004;329(7479):1369–72.

43. Sumamo Schellenberg E, Dryden DM, Pasichnyk D, et al. *Acute Migraine Treatment in Emergency Settings. Comparative Effectiveness Review No. 84*. Rockville, MD: Agency for Healthcare Research and Quality; 2012.

44. Orr SL, Aubé M, Becker WJ, et al. Canadian Headache Society systematic review and recommendations on the treatment of migraine pain in emergency settings. *Cephalalgia*. 2015;35(3):271–84.

45. Taggart E, Doran S, Kokotillo A, et al. Ketorolac in the treatment of acute migraine: a systematic review. *Headache*. 2013;53(2):277–87.

46. Friedman BW, Cabral L, Adewunmi V, et al. Diphenhydramine as adjuvant therapy for acute migraine: an emergency department-based randomized clinical trial. *Ann Emerg Med*. 2016;67(1):32–9.

47. Friedman BW, Corbo J, Lipton RB, et al. A trial of metoclopramide vs sumatriptan for the emergency department treatment of migraines. *Neurology*. 2005;64(3):463–8.

48. Talabi S, Masoumi B, Azizkhani R, Esmailian M. Metoclopramide versus sumatriptan for treatment of migraine headache: a randomized clinical trial. *J Res Med Sci*. 2013;18(8):695–8.

49. Colman I, Brown MD, Innes GD, et al. Parenteral dihydroergotamine for acute migraine headache: a systematic review of the literature. *Ann Emerg Med*. 2005;45(4):393–401.

50. Winner P, Ricalde O, Le Force B, Saper J, Margul B. A double-blind study of subcutaneous dihydroergotamine vs subcutaneous sumatriptan in the treatment of acute migraine. *Arch Neurol*. 1996;53:180–4.

51. Vinson DR. Treatment patterns of isolated benign headache in US emergency departments. *Ann Emerg Med*. 2002;39(3):215–22.

52. Friedman BW, Kapoor A, Friedman MS, Hochberg ML, Rowe BH. The relative efficacy of meperidine for the treatment of acute migraine: a meta-analysis of randomized controlled trials. *Ann Emerg Med*. 2008;52(6):705–13.

53. Leinisch E, Evers S, Kaempfe N, et al. Evaluation of the efficacy of intravenous acetaminophen in the treatment of acute migraine attacks: a double-blind, placebo-controlled parallel group multicenter study. *Pain*. 2005;117(3):396–400.

54. Turkcuer I, Serinken M, Eken C, et al. Intravenous paracetamol versus dexketoprofen versus morphine in acute mechanical low back pain in the emergency department: a randomised double-blind controlled trial. *EMJ*. 2014;31(3):177–81.

55. Zhang A, Jiang T, Luo Y, et al. Efficacy of intravenous propacetamol hydrochloride in the treatment of an acute attack of migraine. *Eur J Intern Med*. 2014;25(7):629–32.

56. Leniger T, Pageler L, Stude P, Diener HC, Limmroth V. Comparison of intravenous valproate with intravenous lysine-acetylsalicylic acid in acute migraine attacks. *Headache*. 2005;45(1):42–6.

57. Foroughipour M, Ghandehari K, Khazaei M, et al. Randomized clinical trial of intravenous valproate (Orifil) and dexamethasone in patients with migraine disorder. *Iran J Med Sci*. 2013;38(Suppl. 2):150–5.

58. Friedman BW, Garber L, Yoon A, et al. Randomized trial of IV valproate vs metoclopramide vs ketorolac for acute migraine. *Neurology*. 2014;82(11):976–83.

59. Moshtaghion H, Heiranizadeh N, Rahimdel A, et al. The efficacy of propofol vs. subcutaneous sumatriptan for treatment of acute migraine headaches in the emergency department: a double-blinded clinical trial. *Pain Pract*. 2014;15(8)701–5.

60. Soleimanpour H, Ghafouri RR, Taheraghdam A, et al. Effectiveness of intravenous dexamethasone versus propofol for pain relief in the migraine headache: a prospective double blind randomized clinical trial. *BMC Neurol*. 2012;12:114.

61. Rowe BH, Colman I, Edmonds ML, et al. Randomized controlled trial of intravenous dexamethasone to prevent relapse in acute migraine headache. *Headache*. 2008;48(3):333–40.

62. Colman I, Friedman BW, Brown MD, et al. Parenteral dexamethasone for acute severe migraine headache: meta-analysis of randomised controlled trials for preventing recurrence. *BMJ*. 2008;336(7657):1359–61.

**Chapter**

**8**

# The Patient with a Trigeminal Autonomic Cephalalgia in the Emergency Department

Anne Ducros

## Abstract

Trigeminal autonomic cephalalgias (TACs) are primary headaches responsible for unilateral facial and/or cranial pain with ipsilateral autonomic signs. In the absence of any radiological or biological marker, diagnosis relies upon clinical history. Patients are often misdiagnosed as having secondary headaches due to sinus, dental, or eye disorders or as having migraine, leading to inadequate management. Efficient treatments do exist, and differ among the various TACs. Patients with TACs often present to the emergency department (ED) with excruciating headache. These are pain urgencies that require quick diagnosis and tailored treatment. Therefore, management of TACs, and especially of cluster headache (CH), the most common TAC, should be well known by ED physicians.

## Introduction

Headache affects about 90 percent of the general population. The most common causes are migraine and episodic tension-type headache. TACs are less common primary headaches. Patients with TACs may present acutely to the ED for many reasons [1]. The correct headache diagnosis may not have been made previously. In CH – the most common TAC – the delay between the first attack and the diagnosis is often several years. Patients without a previous correct diagnosis may present to the ED because they have very severe pain and no efficient treatment. Patients with a known TAC may also visit the ED given the urgent need for a prescription because they have used their last specific treatment, had a recent increase in the number of daily attacks, or due to a fear of adverse reactions because they have escalated the doses of their treatments above recommended limits. Finally, a patient with a TAC may be affected by another disorder causing secondary headaches. Such cases will present to the ED for a recent new-onset headache, different from the usual TAC attacks, requiring investigations to search for the underlying cause.

The main objectives of this chapter are to describe the diagnosis and management of patients with TACs in the ED.

## What are TACs?

These forms of primary headaches are defined by severe and debilitating unilateral facial or cranial pain with ipsilateral autonomic signs. Trigeminal autonomic cephalalgias constitute Chapter 3 of the International Classification of Headache Disorders (ICHD-3) and include CH, paroxysmal hemicrania, SUNCT (short unilateral neuralgiform headache with conjunctival injection and tearing), and hemicrania continua [2]. Most TACs – namely CH, paroxysmal hemicrania, and SUNCT – manifest as daily short-lived recurrent attacks, and can be distinguished from each other by the duration of each attack (Table 8.1). Only hemicrania continua manifests as a continuous daily unilateral pain without attacks. Diagnosis of TACs is purely clinical, based on the diagnostic criteria from the International Classification of Headache Disorders-3 Beta (ICHD-3β). Precise diagnosis is necessary to initiate appropriate treatment, since TACs are not responsive to analgesics and the different subforms of TACs respond to different specific acute and preventive treatments.

## How to Recognize a Primary Headache in the ED

Primary headaches account for the vast majority of ED visits for headache. After excluding a secondary cause of the headache with which the patient presents, the most important part of the interview is thus to diagnose the specific primary headache disorder – the

**Table 8.1** Trigeminal autonomic cephalalgias (TACs) responsible for attacks

|  | Cluster headache | Paroxysmal hemicrania | SUNCT |
|---|---|---|---|
| Sex ratio M:F | 3:1 | 1:2 | 2:1 |
| **Duration of attacks** | 15–180 min | 2–30 min | 5–240 sec |
| Frequency of attacks | 1 every 2 days to 8 per day | 5–40/day | 3–200/day |
| Periodicity | Episodic form may be seasonal | Episodic or chronic | Episodic or chronic |
| Prophylactic treatment | Verapamil Lithium Steroids | Indomethacin | Anticonvulsants |

most frequent being migraine, episodic, or chronic tension-type headache and CH [1]. The first two questions to ask the patient are the following:

1. How quickly did this headache peak in intensity? (Thunderclap – maximal intensity within 60 seconds.)
2. Have you ever had this same type of headache before, and if so, when did they begin to occur? (An unusual headache or an attack different from their known headache pattern.)

According to the responses to these two questions, there are three different situations. First, the patient is able to say that he/she has already suffered from several similar headaches for months or years. In such cases, a primary headache disorder is the most likely cause and the description of headache characteristics – age of onset, duration of headache attacks, pain location, associated signs and symptoms, trigger factors – will help in making a precise diagnosis. Second, the patient may deny a previous headache history and report having headaches for the first time in his/her life for some hours, days, weeks, or months. In such cases, a secondary headache has to be excluded and investigations have to be performed. Finally, the patient reports a history of definite primary headaches but states that his/her acute headache is different from his/her usual headaches attacks. In such cases, a secondary headache has to be suspected and investigations are noteworthy. This is especially true if the headache began and peaked suddenly (less than 60 seconds – i.e., thunderclap headache).

## How to Recognize a TAC in the ED

Once determined that the patient already had several similar headaches in the past, and is thus most likely having a primary headache, the next step is to make a precise diagnosis: Is it a migraine attack? Is it an exacerbation of tension-type headaches? Or is it a CH or another TAC? Patients have to be carefully interviewed because the diagnosis is based on the description of the characteristics of headache attacks and on a normal physical and neurological examination. Consequently, emergency physicians have to be familiar with the diagnostic criteria of these primary headache disorders [3].

First, ask the patient precisely how long the pain is lasting during each attack and how frequently the attacks occur (one or more per day, per week, or per month).

Second, ask the patient about the location of the pain. Trigeminal autonomic cephalalgias are responsible for strictly unilateral facial or cranial pain in the distribution of the first division of the trigeminal nerve, affecting the orbital, frontal, and temporal regions.

Third, ask the patient for the presence of ipsilateral autonomic signs during the pain attacks [2]. Parasympathetic hyperactivity signs include ipsilateral lacrimation, redness of the eye, and nasal congestion. The affected side of the face may be red and sweaty. Sympathetic hypoactivity is responsible for an ipsilateral Horner syndrome with miosis and/or ptosis.

Fourth, ask the patient how she/he behaves during the pain attack. Patients with CH, the most frequent TAC, are typically restless. They are alert, but may be irritable and aggressive, especially if they have to wait in the ED with an ongoing attack.

Finally, examine the patient. Clinical examination is normal in patients with TACs except during an ongoing attack or just after the end of an attack, where autonomic signs may be observed. A Horner sign (droopy eye and smaller pupil) can be present during an attack or just after.

Finally, ask the patient which acute and preventive treatments she/he has already tried, and what the effects were.

**Box 8.1 Diagnostic Criteria for Cluster Headache According to the ICHD-3β**

Cluster Headache

A. At least five attacks fulfilling criteria B–D

B. Severe or very severe unilateral orbital, supraorbital, and/or temporal pain lasting 15–180 minutes (when untreated)

C. Either or both of the following:

  1. at least one of the following symptoms or signs, ipsilateral to the headache:

    a. conjunctival injection and/or lacrimation

    b. nasal congestion and/or rhinorrhea

    c. eyelid edema

    d. forehead and facial sweating

    e. forehead and facial flushing

    f. sensation of fullness in the ear

    g. miosis and/or ptosis

  2. a sense of restlessness or agitation

D. Attacks have a frequency between one every other day and eight per day for more than half of the time when the disorder is active

E. Not better accounted for by another ICHD-3 diagnosis

After this clinical assessment, the precise diagnosis of the type of TAC can be made according to the ICHD-3β criteria (Table 8.1 and Box 8.1) [2].

# When is Imaging Necessary in a Patient with a Suspected TAC?

Diagnosis of TACs is based on clinical criteria and exclusion of a secondary cause. Features suggesting a secondary TAC are: a new-onset TAC-like pain; a persistent or worsening pain; abnormal signs on neurological examination; persistence of Horner syndrome after the end of the attack; and a first attack after 50 years old.

When features suggesting a secondary TAC are present, the rule is to consider the headache as being potentially secondary to a serious secondary cause and to perform investigations. Disorders to consider first-line include internal carotid artery dissection and acute bacterial sinusitis. Other causes include benign or malignant intracranial tumors, especially pituitary tumors [4–7], orbital tumors or infections, cervical

tumors [8], and rarely strategically located aneurysms or arteriovenous malformations. Therefore, any new-onset case of CH deserves imaging.

*Internal carotid artery dissection* is the main differential diagnosis to rule out. An isolated head or neck pain can be the sole clinical manifestation of an internal carotid artery dissection [9]. Headache caused by carotid dissection is mostly unilateral, ipsilateral to the dissected artery, severe, and persistent (a mean of four days). The headache can be accompanied by ipsilateral unilateral cervical and facial pain, has no specific features, and can mimic CH attacks, except that cluster attacks last between 15 minutes and three hours, whereas the pain related to a carotid artery dissection can persist well beyond three hours. Distinguishing a painful carotid artery dissection from a first episode of CH may be challenging, because the pain characteristics may be similar, a Horner syndrome may be present in both disorders, and both headaches may respond to triptans [10]. Any patient with a painful Horner syndrome has to be screened for an ipsilateral internal carotid artery dissection. Since local signs precede ischemic complications, urgent investigations are required, based on CT or MR angiography of the cervical vessels, and cervical MRI with T1 fat-saturated (FAT SAT) sequences. Treatment requires antithrombotics, either heparin or aspirin [11], together with symptomatic pain treatment.

*Acute sinusitis* is another differential diagnosis to consider. Acute frontal, maxillary, and sphenoid sinusitis can manifest as severe ipsilateral facial pain, sometimes following a pseudo-attack rhythm. Typically, acute sinusitis is responsible for pain over the cheek and radiating to the frontal region or teeth, increasing with straining or bending, and nasal symptoms including postnasal discharge, blocked nose, persistent coughing, or pharyngeal irritation and hyposmia. Fever is rare (<5 percent of cases). However, nasal signs may be absent in some cases. An acute sphenoid sinusitis may be responsible for a severe unilateral headache with periorbital edema and eye redness, mimicking a TAC. Diagnosis relies on sinus and head CT. Treatment relies on amoxicillin with or without clavulanate as first-line therapy for 5–10 days in most adults if acute bacterial rhinosinusitis has to be treated with an antibiotic [12]. Some cases require local drainage.

*Other causes of secondary TACs* can be found in patients with atypical clinical features, or sometimes in patients with typical features of a primary TAC, fulfilling all ICHD-3β diagnosis criteria [8,13,14]. Therefore, any refractory case of TAC should be imaged with an MRI to exclude a treatable cause. The pituitary, orbit, and trigeminal pathway have to be specifically examined on MRI studies. An association between CH and pituitary tumors has been suspected [4]. Therefore, some guidelines have suggested that any patient with CH or another TAC should have a brain MRI with and without gadolinium and MR angiography [15]. When the history is typical with numerous cluster periods, periods over years, and no interictal abnormalities on neurological examination, emergency MRI is not mandatory in cases of TACs in the ED. In these cases, the imaging studies can be done on an outpatient basis.

## How to Differentiate a TAC from Other Primary Headaches in the ED?

### Migraine

The only way to differentiate CH from migraine is with a thorough headache history. Table 8.2 presents a clinical comparison of CH and migraine [2]. Migraine attacks start more progressively, and are longer than CH attacks. In the ED, patients with a severe migraine attack tend to stay quiet and avoid any movement, preferring to lie down in the dark. Pain is moderate to severe, but is usually not described as intolerable or excruciating. The presence of nausea and/or photophobia and phonophobia is a main clinical criterion but is not specific for migraine, as such "migraine" signs are found in up to 50 percent of CH patients [16].

**Table 8.2** Comparison of migraine and cluster headache

| Migraine | Cluster headache | Common characteristics |
|---|---|---|
| **No periodicity** (except menses) | **Periodicity** (annual and daily) | Incapacitating |
| **Attacks >4 h** | **Attacks <3 h** | Alcohol is a trigger |
| Female > Male | Male > Female | Triptan effect (spray and subcutaneous) |
| **Prostration, quietness** | **Restlessness, agitation** | Dysautonomic symptoms typical in CH, but may occur in migraine |
| Pain moderate to severe | Pain is severe | |
| Pain can be bilateral | Unilateral | NB. Migraine and CH may coexist |
| Nausea and photophobia typical | Nausea and photophobia in 50% | |
| Dietary and hormonal triggers | No dietary trigger except alcohol | |

However, photophobia and phonophobia are often ipsilateral to the side of the pain in patients with CH and other TACs. Conversely, autonomic/parasympathetic signs are not exclusive or unique to cluster and other TACs, since up to 30 percent of migraine patients have cranial parasympathetic signs. Moreover, both CH and migraine may awaken patients from sleep, though CH usually does so with more consistency and generally at the same time each night – usually 90 minutes after falling asleep.

In case of doubt when trying to differentiate migraine and CH, further observation of attacks by the patient is warranted. The clinician in the ED may ask the patient to complete a diary of the next attacks, to further qualify their duration, autonomic symptoms, triggers, response to treatment, and daily rhythmicity. These cases should be referred to a headache specialist.

### Trigeminal Neuralgia

Table 8.3 describes the clinical features helpful to distinguish trigeminal neuralgia (TN) from CH [16]. Trigeminal neuralgia is more frequent in women in their fifties or older. Attacks are centered on the maxillary and/or mandibular area, are more frequent, much briefer, electric-like, and are triggered by touching specific zones of the face or buccal cavity (trigger

**Table 8.3** Comparison of cluster headache and trigeminal neuralgia

| | Cluster headache | Trigeminal neuralgia |
|---|---|---|
| Age | Starts around 20–30 | 60 |
| Sex | Male | Female |
| Pain localization | Orbital, temporal | Nasal, maxillary, dental |
| Attack duration | 15–180 minutes | Seconds, but repeated shocks |
| Pain character | Knife-like, stabbing, lancinating | Electric shocks, burning, stinging |
| Trigger zone | No | Yes |
| Neurovegetative signs | Yes | No |
| Refractory period after attack | Not typical | Yes |
| Frequency per day | 1–8 | Highly variable but may be dozens or more |

zones). Eating, laughing, talking, shaving, and brushing the teeth may all trigger the shocks. Patients may lose weight because they avoid eating. There is no clustering in periods, and mostly it is persistent and chronic until a treatment is started. Trigeminal neuralgia responds very well to carbamazepine.

## Hypnic Headache

In an elderly patient with exclusively nocturnal attacks, hypnic headache may be diagnosed, but it is very rare and the pain is usually bilateral, diffuse, mild or moderate, and without cranial autonomic signs. Attacks occur exclusively during sleep [17] and usually at the same time during a 24-hour period.

# How to Diagnose and Manage Cluster Headache in the ED

## Detailed Description of Cluster Headache

Cluster headache has a prevalence of 0.5–1/1000 and predominantly affects males and young adults [18,19]. It can start at any age, but the first attacks usually begin in the third decade. Tobacco smoking is frequent among CH patients. The mechanisms of CH are still poorly understood.

CH attacks are so typical that one can make the diagnosis in less than five minutes by asking a few questions, and some patients make their own diagnosis by entering the key clinical features (headache, severe, unilateral) on a web search engine, and present saying "I have cluster headache" [3,18].

Attacks are characterized by excruciating unilateral facial, orbital, or temporal pain lasting 15 minutes to three hours, accompanied by signs of autonomic dysfunction (Box 8.1). The fact that attacks end after one or two hours must not be attributed to the success of analgesics, which are ineffective in CH. The unilateral pain is mostly located in the territory of the first trigeminal branch, centered on the eye itself. It can involve the maxillary, ear, teeth, and occipital-cervical regions. Patients may express suicidal ideations because of the intensity of the pain.

The typical autonomic signs (Box 8.1) are subtle or even absent in 3 percent of CH patients. In their absence, CH can be diagnosed if the patient describes a sense of restlessness or is agitated during attacks.

They may pace back and forth in the room, rock to and fro, hit their heads, hit objects with their fist, or even hit their head against the wall. Cluster headache patients are alert, but may be irritable, aggressive, and agitated.

Symptoms such as nausea, vomiting, photophobia, and phonophobia are reported by 50 percent of CH patients and must not detract from the diagnosis of CH if other criteria are fulfilled [20].

CH attacks can be triggered by alcohol, nitrates, odors (solvents), cigarette smoke, napping, exertion, and heat.

One of the main characteristics of CH is its circannual and circadian cyclicity. Peaks of CH bouts and attacks have been described around solstices. During bouts, CH attacks occur every day, and can happen at a precise time during the sleep-cycle, with dramatic regularity reported by patients. This rhythmicity is not observed in all CH patients.

CH has two clinical forms. Most patients (80 percent) have episodic CH (ICHD-3 code 3.1.1) and may have one or two periods with recurrent attacks every year, or even go into remission for many years. About 20 percent of patients have chronic CH (ICHD-3 code 3.1.2), and have ongoing attacks for one year or more without more than one month of remission. Patients with CH need to be referred to a headache specialist after a visit to the ED.

## Treatment of Cluster Headache

Acute treatments are used to alleviate pain during attacks and preventive treatments are used with the aim of reducing the daily number of attacks [21]. No curative treatment exists. Several American and European guidelines exist to guide the management of CH [15,22–24].

### Acute Management of Attacks

In the ED, patients with an ongoing CH attack should be treated as soon as possible with one of the two most effective acute treatments, namely with subcutaneous sumatriptan or with high-flow inhaled oxygen, because of the excruciating character of the pain [22,24].

Subcutaneous sumatriptan 6 mg is effective in relieving CH pain [25]. After the injection, the patient may feel a rush of heat and chest tightness, lasting a few minutes, followed by rapid relief of the pain. Intranasal sumatriptan 20 mg [26] and zolmitriptan 5 mg [27] may be tried if the patient refuses to use injections. Scientific contraindications to subcutaneous sumatriptan include ischemic heart disease, vasospastic angina, peripheral arterial disease, stroke, severe hepatic failure, moderate or severe arterial hypertension, use of ergots within the previous 24 hours, or use of monoamine oxidase inhibitors (MAO inhibitors). Marketing contraindications are age under 18 or over 65. Close monitoring is necessary when prescribing subcutaneous sumatriptan to patients with Raynaud's phenomenon, allergy to sulfa medications, and treatment with drugs that increase the release or block the reuptake of serotonin (e.g., tramadol). Maximal doses per 24-hour period (sumatriptan 12 mg subcutaneous or 40 mg intranasal, zolmitriptan 10 mg intranasal) have to be explained to the patient to avoid dangerous side-effects like coronary or peripheral artery spasm.

Inhaled oxygen with high-flow (10–15 liters per minute) delivered as 100 percent normobaric oxygen and breathed in through a non-rebreathing face mask is effective, and useful especially when contraindications to triptans exist [28]. There are very few contraindications to the use of oxygen and it is widely available in all EDs.

### Preventive Treatment

The aim of preventive treatment is to reduce the frequency of attacks during the bout in the case of episodic CH. In chronic CH, treatments are used long term, and the goal is to achieve a low attack rate, while always considering potentially serious and incapacitating side-effects.

The calcium-channel blocker verapamil remains the main treatment of CH [15,22–24]. Doses range from 360 mg to 960 mg per day, and the maximal tolerated dose should be reached before making conclusions about efficacy. Side-effects include weakness, fatigue, lower extremity edema, and conduction block in the heart. An electrocardiogram should be performed at baseline and for every dose increase when the dose exceeds 480 mg per day, because of the risk of heart block. Treatment can be initiated in the ED, with 120 mg twice per day, to be increased up to 120 mg three times per day after 2–7 days. Higher doses can be prescribed when attacks continue to occur at 480 mg per day.

A short course of tapering-dose oral prednisone (starting at 1 mg/kg) may be used to end a bout refractory to verapamil, but recurrence is frequent as the dose is decreased. Long-term side-effects of corticosteroid therapy restrict the use of steroids for the long-term treatment of chronic CH.

Greater occipital nerve blocks can be used to end a bout, or at least diminish the number of attacks per day [29,30]. The block is performed with a long-acting injectable steroid, sometimes combined with a local anesthetic.

Lithium is used in selected cases with chronic CH [15,22–24]. Because of its side-effects, it should not be initiated in the ED.

Other CH treatments include topiramate, for which usual dosing for this indication is 100 mg per day (range 25–200 mg). Escalation has to be slow (25 mg every 10–15 days).

Refractory chronic cases should be sent to a headache specialist after ED presentation in order to refine the medical treatment, consider surgical treatments, and provide long-term care.

## How to Recognize and Manage Paroxysmal Hemicrania in the ED

Paroxysmal hemicrania (PH) is a rare TAC, predominantly affecting adult women, which differs from CH by the shorter length (2–30 minutes) of attacks, the higher frequency of daily attacks (usually 10–20), the quiet attitude of patients during the pain, and the absolute response to an adequate dose of indomethacin (150 mg or more per day) [2,31].

The dose of indomethacin should be increased to at least 200 mg/day for 3–4 days. A beneficial effect is usually seen within 48 hours, but may take as long as 14 days.

Maintenance dosage is usually 25–100 mg/day but may range from 12.5 mg/day to 300 mg/day. After discontinuation of the medication, symptoms usually reappear within 12 hours to a few days. However, remission periods lasting years have been described.

About 10 percent of patients may experience adverse effects of indomethacin, including dyspepsia, nausea, vomiting, vertigo, gastric bleeding, purpura, and other conditions.

It is necessary to take precautions to prevent serious gastrointestinal and renal complications secondary to the long-term use of indomethacin. Adverse gastric effects may be prevented by the co-administration of antacids, misoprostol, or an H2 antagonist or proton pump inhibitor when indomethacin is being used for longer periods. In older patients, renal function and blood pressure should be monitored.

## How to Recognize and Manage Paroxysmal SUNCT in the ED

SUNCT is a very rare TAC characterized by short-lived (5–240 seconds), orbital/periorbital, painful attacks accompanied by autonomic symptoms, generally conjunctival injection and lacrimation. SUNCT shares many similarities with trigeminal neuralgia, namely unilaterality, sting-like character, abrupt short paroxysms, and precipitation of attacks by mechanical stimuli acting on trigeminal and extratrigeminal areas [2,31].

None of the current available therapies is consistently effective for SUNCT, and treatment is often disappointing. There is no available abortive treatment for the individual SUNCT attacks. Intravenous infusion of lidocaine (1–4 mg kg$^{-1}$ hr$^{-1}$) may be indicated in periods of significant exacerbation of SUNCT attacks to attenuate the flow of attacks [31]. Greater occipital nerve (GON) blockade with a combination of lidocaine and a steroid was beneficial in some cases. Long-term preventive treatment is based on the use of antiepileptics, with lamotrigine being the drug of first choice, followed by others such as carbamazepine, gabapentin, and topiramate. Patients with SUNCT should be referred to a headache specialist.

## How to Recognize and Manage Hemicrania Continua in the ED

Hemicrania continua (HC) is a rare condition that predominantly affects adult women [31]. It is a primary headache disorder, characterized by a continuous, fluctuating, strictly unilateral pain which is mild to moderate in intensity, with episodes of severe exacerbations [2]. During these exacerbations, patients may experience a variable combination of ipsilateral autonomic features. Migraine symptoms such as photophobia and phonophobia are often seen.

The hallmark of this syndrome is the absolute positive response to indomethacin. The positive response to this drug is an essential criterion for the diagnosis. The dose and strategy for use of indomethacin for HC is similar to PHs.

## Conclusion

TACs are extremely disabling primary headaches. Patients with TACs might present to the ED with excruciating headache, requiring prompt management. Diagnosis of TACs is purely clinical, based on the diagnostic criteria from the ICHD-3β. Effective treatments are different according to the specific type of TAC, and comprise acute treatments to alleviate an ongoing attack, and preventive treatment to prevent further attacks. These treatments can respectively be delivered and initiated in the ED, in order to relieve headache, and also reduce risk of readmission to the ED because of recurrent attacks.

## References

1. Valade D, Ducros A. Acute headache in the emergency department. *Handb Clin Neurol.* 2010;97:173–81.

2. Headache Classification Committee of the International Headache Society (IHS). The International Classification of Headache Disorders, 3rd edition (beta version). *Cephalalgia.* 2013;33(9):629–808.

3. Kernick D, Matharu MS, Goadsby PJ. Cluster headache in primary care: unmissable, underdiagnosed and undertreated. *Br J Gen Pract.* 2006;56(528):486–7.

4. Levy MJ, Matharu MS, Meeran K, Powell M, Goadsby PJ. The clinical characteristics of headache in patients with pituitary tumours. *Brain.* 2005;128(8):1921–30.

5. Porta Etessam J, Ramos-Carrasco A, Berbel-Garcia A, Martinez-Salio A, Benito-Leon J. Clusterlike headache as first manifestation of a prolactinoma. *Headache.* 2001;41(7):723–5.

6. Milos P, Havelius U, Hindfelt B. Clusterlike headache in a patient with a pituitary adenoma: with a review of the literature. *Headache.* 1996;36(3):184–8.

7. Sarov M, Valade D, Jublanc C, Ducros A. Chronic paroxysmal hemicrania in a patient with a macroprolactinoma. *Cephalalgia.* 2006;26(6):738–41.

8. Malissart P, Ducros A, Labauge P, De Champfleur NM, Carra-Dalliere C. Carotid paraganglioma mimicking a cluster headache. *Cephalalgia.* 2014;34(13):1111.

9. Arnold M, Cumurciuc R, Stapf C, et al. Pain as the only symptom of cervical artery dissection. *J Neurol Neurosurg Psychiatry.* 2006;77(9):1021–4.

10. Leira EC, Cruz-Flores S, Leacock RO, Abdulrauf SI. Sumatriptan can alleviate headaches due to carotid artery dissection. *Headache.* 2001;41(6):590–1.

11. Georgiadis D, Arnold M, von Buedingen HC, et al. Aspirin vs anticoagulation in carotid artery dissection: a study of 298 patients. *Neurology.* 2009;72(21):1810–15.

12. Brook I. Acute and chronic bacterial sinusitis. *Infect Dis Clin North Am.* 2007;21(2):427–48.

13. Carter DM. Cluster headache mimics. *Curr Pain Headache Rep.* 2004;8(2):133–9.

14. Favier I, van Vliet JA, Roon KI, et al. Trigeminal autonomic cephalgias due to structural lesions: a review of 31 cases. *Arch Neurol.* 2007;64(1):25–31.

15. Donnet A, Demarquay G, Ducros A, et al. [French guidelines for diagnosis and treatment of cluster headache (French Headache Society).]. *Rev Neurol (Paris)*. 2014;170(11):653–70.

16. Bahra A, May A, Goadsby PJ. Cluster headache: a prospective clinical study with diagnostic implications. *Neurology*. 2002;58(3):354–61.

17. Lanteri-Minet M. Hypnic headache. *Headache*. 2014;54(9):1556–9.

18. Leroux E, Ducros A. Cluster headache. *Orphanet J Rare Dis*. 2008;3:20.

19. Nesbitt AD, Goadsby PJ. Cluster headache. *BMJ*. 2012;344:e2407.

20. Goadsby PJ. Lacrimation, conjunctival injection, nasal symptoms... cluster headache, migraine and cranial autonomic symptoms in primary headache disorders: what's new? *J Neurol Neurosurg Psychiatry*. 2009;80(10):1057–8.

21. Halker R, Vargas B, Dodick DW. Cluster headache: diagnosis and treatment. *Semin Neurol*. 2010;30(2):175–85.

22. May A, Leone M, Afra J, et al. EFNS guidelines on the treatment of cluster headache and other trigeminal-autonomic cephalalgias. *Eur J Neurol*. 2006;13(10):1066–77.

23. Sarchielli P, Granella F, Prudenzano MP, et al. Italian guidelines for primary headaches: 2012 revised version. *J Headache Pain*. 2012;13(Suppl. 2):S31–70.

24. Becker WJ, Findlay T, Moga C, et al. Guideline for primary care management of headache in adults. *Can Fam Physician*. 2015;61(8):670–9.

25. The Sumatriptan Cluster Headache Study Group. Treatment of acute cluster headache with sumatriptan. *N Engl J Med*. 1991;325(5):322–6.

26. Schuh-Hofer S, Reuter U, Kinze S, Einhaupl KM, Arnold G. Treatment of acute cluster headache with 20 mg sumatriptan nasal spray: an open pilot study. *J Neurol*. 2002;249(1):94–9.

27. Cittadini E, May A, Straube A, et al. Effectiveness of intranasal zolmitriptan in acute cluster headache: a randomized, placebo-controlled, double-blind crossover study. *Arch Neurol*. 2006;63(11):1537–42.

28. Cohen AS, Burns B, Goadsby PJ. High-flow oxygen for treatment of cluster headache: a randomized trial. *JAMA*. 2009;302(22):2451–7.

29. Ambrosini A, Vandenheede M, Rossi P, et al. Suboccipital injection with a mixture of rapid- and long-acting steroids in cluster headache: a double-blind placebo-controlled study. *Pain*. 2005;118(1–2):92–6.

30. Leroux E, Ducros A. Occipital injections for trigemino-autonomic cephalalgias: evidence and uncertainties. *Curr Pain Headache Rep*. 2013;17(4):325.

31. Goadsby PJ, Cittadini E, Cohen AS. Trigeminal autonomic cephalalgias: paroxysmal hemicrania, SUNCT/SUNA, and hemicrania continua. *Semin Neurol*. 2010;30(2):186–91.

# Other Primary Headache Disorders That Can Present to the Emergency Department

Yasmin Idu Jion

Brian M. Grosberg

## Abstract

Although other primary headache disorders such as cough headache, exercise headache, headache associated with sexual activity, thunderclap headache, hypnic headache, and new daily persistent headache are less common than migraine and tension-type headache, these disorders can be severe, disabling, and misdiagnosed. A good proportion of them coexist with other primary headache disorders. In addition, they may be associated with underlying structural pathology, and it is paramount that they are investigated for secondary causes. Diagnosis of the other primary headache disorders requires exclusion of secondary mimics, as stipulated in the International Classification of Headache Disorders, third edition beta version [1]. Treatment and prognosis are dependent on the diagnosis, and the majority are indomethacin responsive.

This chapter reviews the epidemiology, clinical features, pathophysiology, and management of these less common headache disorders that may present to the emergency department (ED).

## Primary Cough Headache

Primary headaches occurring during cough, exertion, and sexual activity have clear provoking factors, respond to indomethacin, and can be idiopathic or symptomatic (Box 9.1).

Previously thought to be an ominous symptom, primary cough headache was first described by Symonds in 1956 as benign cough headache [2]. It can be triggered by other Valsalva maneuvers including sneezing, straining during stool, vigorous weightlifting, and laughing. Primary cough headache is not typically triggered by sustained physical exercise [3]. The lifetime prevalence is estimated to be 1 percent [4].

Cough headache typically occurs in the older adult, with a mean age of onset of 67 years. The headache is usually of sudden onset, occurring within seconds of coughing or other Valsalva maneuvers. The pain is usually described as sharp and stabbing, peaking almost immediately with rapid improvement usually over several seconds to minutes. The pain may be transient for a few minutes or up to 120 minutes, and may occur one to multiple times in a day [3,5,6]. There is typically no associated nausea, vomiting, or autonomic features. There is a correlation between the frequency of the cough and the severity of the headache [7]. There have also been reports of Valsalva-induced cluster headaches and cough headache coexisting with chronic paroxysmal hemicrania, and both headaches respond to indomethacin [8,9].

Although the precise etiology of cough headache is unknown, it has been postulated that these headaches may be the result of a sudden transient increase in intracranial pressure (ICP) with resulting traction upon pain-sensitive vascular and dural structures from downward displacement of the cerebellar tonsils [10]. Other hypotheses include pain resulting from stretching of the walls of the dural venous sinuses and their tributaries, heightened sensitivity of unidentified receptors, a crowded posterior cranial fossa space, cerebrospinal fluid (CSF) hypervolemia, associations with internal jugular or transverse vein stenosis, and a form of adhesive arachnoiditis [2,11,12].

Differentiating primary from secondary cough headache can be difficult. In Pascual et al.'s review of 72 cases, 57 percent of cough headaches were symptomatic [5]. Symptomatic cases tend to begin earlier in life (mean age 39), last longer (up to days), lack indomethacin response, and have posterior fossa manifestations. Imaging is especially paramount in those with the following red flags: onset less than 50 years old, headaches lasting more than a minute, occipital headaches, headache duration of more than a year, presence of posterior fossa signs and symptoms (i.e., dizziness, unsteadiness, numbness, vertigo,

**Table 9.1** Summary of epidemiology and headache features in other primary headache disorders

| | Primary cough headache | Primary exercise headache | Primary headache associated with sexual activity | Primary thunderclap headache | Hypnic headache | New daily persistent headache |
|---|---|---|---|---|---|---|
| Prevalence | 1% | 12% | 1% | 43/100,000 per year | 0.07–0.3% | 0.1% |
| Age of onset | 60s | 20s | 20s–40s | Not available | 60s | 20s–30s |
| Gender | M > F | M > F | M > F | Not available | F > M | F > M |
| **Headache features** | | | | | | |
| Onset | Sudden | Sudden | Gradual or explosive | Explosive | Abrupt, wakes patient from sleep | Starts within 24 hours |
| Character | Sharp, stabbing | Dull, diffuse, pulsatile | Dull and with increasing intensity with sexual activity or Severe in intensity, throbbing | Severe intensity | Dull, throbbing | Tension or migraine phenotype |
| Typical location | Vertex Frontal Occipital Temporal | Bilateral | Frontal Occipital Diffuse | Diffuse Occipital | Diffuse, bilateral Frontotemporal | Unilateral or generalized |
| Duration | Seconds to minutes | Hours | Minutes to hours | Hours to few days | Minutes to few hours | Daily and continuous for ≥3 months |
| Triggers | Coughing Sneezing Straining Laughing | Sustained physical exertion Short burst of physical exertion | Sexual activity Masturbation | Spontaneous Valsalva maneuvers Sex Exertion Stress | Sleep (120–480 min into sleep) | Antecedent viral illness Cranial surgery Menarche Stressful life events |

**Box 9.1 ICHD-3 Beta Diagnostic Criteria for Primary Cough Headache**

**Description**

Headache precipitated by coughing or other Valsalva (straining) maneuver, but not by prolonged physical exercise, in the absence of any intracranial disorder.

**Diagnostic Criteria**

A. At least two headache episodes fulfilling criteria B–D

B. Brought on by and occurring only in association with coughing, straining, and/or other Valsalva maneuver

C. Sudden onset

D. Lasting between one second and two hours

E. Not better accounted for by another ICHD-3 diagnosis

syncope), precipitants other than cough, and lack of response to indomethacin [12,13]. Unfortunately, headache location and characteristics did not reliably distinguish between primary and symptomatic forms [6,14]. A modified Valsalva test involving exhalation into the connecting tube of a sphygmomanometer to 60 mmHg for 10 s positively identified secondary causes in a small series if the maneuver provoked headache [14]. Common secondary causes for cough-induced headache include Chiari malformation, posterior fossa tumors, posterior fossa crowding, subarachnoid hemorrhage (SAH), midbrain cyst, pinealoma, basilar impression, obstructive hydrocephalus, low CSF pressure, reversible cerebral vasoconstriction syndrome (RCVS), cerebral aneurysm, meningitis, and sphenoid sinusitis. Confusion may arise with other headache disorders that can potentially be aggravated but not consistently and specifically precipitated by cough; this is why it is important for the clinician to clearly differentiate between headache worsened by cough and headache that is consistently triggered by cough. Headaches worsened by cough include headache attributed to intracranial hypertension, postictal headache, high-altitude headache, migraine, tension-type headache, and cluster headache. Diagnostic testing should include magnetic resonance imaging (MRI) of the brain with gadolinium (including visualization of the craniocervical junction) and magnetic resonance angiography (MRA) of the head [3,7,12].

Treatment of primary cough headache is mainly prophylactic. Indomethacin is the treatment of choice in those patients who frequently experience cough headache. The usual effective dose ranges from 50 mg to 200 mg per day [6,15]. Indomethacin has both an analgesic effect and also reduces intracranial pressure. Other therapies with reported efficacy include acetazolamide 1–2 g/day, methysergide 2 mg/day, topiramate, propranolol, naproxen, intravenous dihydroergotamine (DHE) and metoclopramide, and lumbar puncture [3,6,7,12]. It is important to note that a positive response to therapy does not distinguish between benign and secondary forms, as secondary forms may also respond to medications [16]. In earlier descriptions, 80–90 percent had improvement or eventual recovery when followed up to 12 years. Improvement was either spontaneous, or occurred after lumbar puncture or air encephalography [2,17]. Most remit in four years, though cases lasting longer than 12 years have also been described [12].

## Primary Exercise Headache

Primary exercise headache, formerly known as exertional headache, shares similar characteristics as headache associated with sexual activity. There are two types of exertional headache: Type 1 occurs with sustained physical exertion in weightlifters,

> **Box 9.2 ICHD-3 Beta Diagnostic Criteria for Primary Exercise Headache**
>
> **Description**
>
> Headache precipitated by any form of exercise in the absence of any intracranial disorder.
>
> **Diagnostic Criteria**
>
> A. At least two headache episodes fulfilling criteria B and C
>
> B. Brought on by and occurring only during or after strenuous physical exercise
>
> C. Lasting <48 hours
>
> D. Not better accounted for by another ICHD-3 diagnosis

swimmers, and runners; Type 2 occurs with brief physical exertion such as bending, straining, laughing, singing, and coughing [18]. The prevalence is estimated to be 12.3 percent [19], though a higher prevalence can be found in adolescents (30 percent) and athletes (up to 45 percent) [20,21]. Prevalence decreases with age, with a mean age of onset at 24 years old [5]. Approximately 40 percent of patients have other primary headache syndromes, especially migraine. Benign exertional headache was first recognized by the International Headache Society (IHS) classification in 1988, and was later renamed primary exercise headache in the International Classification of Headache Disorders second edition (ICHD-2) in 2004 (see Box 9.2).

The pain of primary exercise headache is typically bilateral or diffuse, throbbing or pulsating, and can be associated with nausea, photophobia, phonophobia, and neck soreness. The vast majority (80 percent) last less than one hour, although they may be prolonged for up to two days [5,20]. They may occur daily or as infrequently as once every two months [5]. Risk factors include extreme or sustained physical exertion, low fluid intake, high altitude, and warm weather [7].

Primary exercise headache has a female predominance [22]. These headaches are associated with headache related to sexual activity in 40 percent of cases. Exercise can also be a trigger for migraine in about 40 percent of migraineurs. These exercise-triggered migraines can be similar to a patient's usual migraine attacks or can be more severe in intensity [20,23].

The underlying mechanism behind primary exertional headache is poorly understood, and mirrors that of primary cough headache. It has been postulated that these headaches may be the result of transmission of intra-abdominal and intra-thoracic pressure up to the cranium via the venous system, with subsequent traction on pain-sensitive vascular and meningeal structures. In the presence of structural disease, the raised ICP may cause cerebral herniation into the foramen magnum. Other postulated mechanisms include transient venous congestion, internal jugular valve incompetence, lowered pain threshold in primary and secondary nociceptive trigeminocervical neurons, alterations in central pain processing, and impaired autoregulation of cerebrovascular smooth muscles resulting in an inability to respond to increased blood pressure during exercise [7]. In primary exercise headache, internal jugular vein valve incompetence and a valveless internal jugular vein have been put forward as potential causes, but this etiological hypothesis remains unproven [18].

Exertional headaches are benign in 80 percent of cases, though the study by Pascual et al. found that 43 percent of patients with exertional headache had an intracranial abnormality, the majority of which were SAH [5]. Other structural abnormalities that have been found to cause exertional headaches include Chiari malformation, posterior fossa lesions, craniovertebral junction abnormalities, post-traumatic sequelae, sinus disease, cerebral aneurysm, craniocervical artery dissection, arterial venous malformation (AVM), RCVS, pheochromocytoma, intermittent CSF obstruction, and cardiac cephalalgia. The suggested work-up for exertional headache includes imaging of the brain (with visualization of the craniocervical junction) and intracranial vessels by MRI and MRA of the brain [7,18]. Symptomatic exertional headache tends to occur later in life, with a mean age of 42, and lasts longer (weeks to months) than the primary form. In addition, secondary exertional headaches may be associated with meningismus or symptoms indicative of raised ICP [5].

Management is usually prophylactic due to its brief duration, and includes treatment with indomethacin. The vast majority (80 percent) respond to this pharmacological therapy administered at doses of 25–150 mg per day prior to starting exercise, though a maximum dose of 250 mg per day is infrequently required for benefit. There are also reports of beta-blockers (i.e., nadolol, propranolol), naproxen, phenelzine, and

ergonovine being effective [7]. Triptans may be effective if the primary exercise headache has migrainous features [22]. Other possible treatments include proper warm-up prior to exercise, sports training, and maintaining adequate hydration [18]. In children, head cooling was found to be effective [24]. The prognosis is generally good as 73 percent achieve headache freedom in ten years [18]. Unfortunately, 2 percent of patients with primary exercise headache give up sports due to their headaches [19].

# Headache Associated with Sexual Activity

**Box 9.3 ICHD-3 Beta Diagnostic Criteria for Primary Headache Associated with Sexual Activity**

**Description**
Headache precipitated by sexual activity, usually starting as a dull bilateral ache as sexual excitement increases and suddenly becoming intense at orgasm, in the absence of any intracranial disorder.

**Diagnostic Criteria**
A. At least two episodes of pain in the head and/or neck fulfilling criteria B–D
B. Brought on by and occurring only during sexual activity
C. Either or both of the following:
   1. Increasing in intensity with increasing sexual excitement
   2. Abrupt explosive intensity just before or with orgasm
D. Lasting from 1 minute to 24 hours with severe intensity, and/or up to 72 hours with mild intensity
E. Not better accounted for by another ICHD-3 diagnosis

Headache associated with sexual activity, as its name suggests, is headache brought on by sexual exertion (see Box 9.3). The lifetime prevalence is estimated to be 1 percent [4]. Traditionally it was classified into three types: Type 1 (24 percent) is the dull pre-orgasmic type which increases with increasing sexual excitement from excessive muscular contraction of the neck and jaw muscles; Type 2 (69 percent) is the explosive orgasmic type which occurs just before or at the moment of orgasm; Type 3 (7 percent) is a generalized postural headache which is a form of low CSF pressure headache after sexual activity, presumably from a CSF leak. The IHS subsequently reclassified Type 3 as a low-pressure headache in ICHD-2. In the latest ICHD-3 beta version, Types 1 and 2 are not differentiated as there are no significant differences in patient characteristics and prognosis between the two types of headache. The explosive orgasmic headache is the more common presentation, occurring in 70 percent of cases. Thirty percent of patients have coexisting migraine and 40 percent also fulfill criteria for primary exercise headache [7,25].

Headache associated with exertion and headache associated with sexual activity have fairly similar patient characteristics. Both disorders have a male preponderance, share similar headache characteristics (duration, frequency, persistence, and quality) and treatment response. Patients with sexual activity-associated headaches tend to be older [5]. Some associated risk factors include hypertension, obesity, psychosocial stress, migraine, exertional headache, family history of headache, kneeling position during sexual activity, occlusive arterial disease, and poor physical health [18].

There is a bimodal distribution for age of onset, with headaches occurring between ages 20 and 24 years and between ages 35 and 44 years [26]. The mean age of onset is 36.7 years old. There are two temporal courses, an episodic form with remitting bouts of headaches and a chronic form. The bouts last a mean of three months, but may last more than a year [27]. The pain is typically bilateral, diffuse, or occipital, and can be dull, throbbing, or stabbing. Pain can be severe for a median of four hours, and can be followed by milder pain for up to 72 hours. The headache may not necessarily be precipitated by every sexual encounter, though masturbation and nocturnal penile tumescence may precipitate it.

Preorgasmic headache is regarded as a variant of tension-type headache. The pathophysiology of orgasmic headache is presumed to be of vascular origin with impaired cerebrovascular autoregulation and an abnormal increase of systemic blood pressure during exertion [22,25]. Some postulate that a transient increase in ICP due to a Valsalva maneuver during coitus might play a role in the pathophysiology of orgasmic headache [26].

Headache associated with sexual activity must be investigated, as SAH occurs in 4–11 percent of all cases [26]. Sexual activity has been reported to be a precipitating cause of bleeding from cerebral aneurysmal rupture in 3.8–12 percent of cases [18]. Red flags that warrant investigations include onset greater than 40 years old, presentation in women, duration lasting more than 24 hours, loss of consciousness, raised ICP, and nuchal rigidity. Diagnostic testing should include neuroimaging and sometimes lumbar puncture and cerebral angiography [13]. Testing for pheochromocytoma should be considered in patients with prominent flushing or tachycardia [7]. Differential diagnoses include RCVS, cervicocranial artery dissection, stroke, encephalitis, meningitis, hemorrhage into a tumor, myocardial ischemia, hydrocephalus, drugs (amiodarone, cannabis, pseudoephedrine, oral contraceptive pills), and other non-neurological conditions (glaucoma, sinusitis, abdominal aorta occlusion, chronic obstructive pulmonary disease, anemia, myxedema, Cushing's disease). Reversible cerebral vasoconstriction syndrome has been found to be a common finding in patients thought to have primary sexual headache. In a study of 30 patients (16 men, 14 women, mean age at onset 40.2 ± 10.0 years) 20 patients (67 percent) had secondary causes, including one subarachnoid hemorrhage, one basilar artery dissection, and 18 cases of RCVS. Only ten patients (33 percent) had primary headache associated with sexual activity. This study underscored the need for thorough neurovascular imaging for all patients with presumed primary headache associated with sexual activity [28].

Management of headache associated with sexual activity involves avoidance of sexual activity until secondary causes have been excluded [18]. Primary preorgasmic headaches can be eased by stopping sexual activity, muscle relaxation, or assuming a more passive role (e.g., kneeling, supine, fellatio) [18,26]. Triptans might be a treatment option to shorten primary orgasmic headache attacks after SAH and RCVS have been excluded [29]. Pharmacological prophylactic treatment of headache associated with sexual activity includes preemptive treatment with indomethacin 30–60 minutes prior to sexual activity. Prophylaxis with oral triptans 30–60 minutes before sexual activity might be a therapeutic option in those not responsive to or not tolerating indomethacin. Beta-blockers such as propranolol at a dose of 60–240 mg/day can be helpful but may potentially interfere with sexual function. Other therapeutic agents with anecdotal benefit include diltiazem, methysergide, and ergotamine. The prognosis is generally good, with most patients having only single episodes or bouts. About 80 percent are headache-free after a mean follow-up of three years [27].

# Primary Thunderclap Headache

> **Box 9.4  ICHD-3 Beta Diagnostic Criteria for Primary Thunderclap Headache**
>
> **Description**
>
> High-intensity headache of abrupt onset, mimicking that of ruptured cerebral aneurysm, in the absence of any intracranial pathology.
>
> **Diagnostic Criteria**
>
> A.  Severe head pain fulfilling criteria B and C
> B.  Abrupt onset, reaching maximum intensity in <1 minute
> C.  Lasting for ≥5 minutes
> D.  Not better accounted for by another ICHD-3 diagnosis

Primary thunderclap headache is a controversial diagnosis of exclusion. Though in the ICHD classification since 2004 (see Box 9.4), most headache specialists question its existence and believe that secondary causes were missed due to insensitive, incomplete, or poor timing of investigations [30]. A better terminology suggested would be "thunderclap headache of undefined origin." Nonetheless, a thunderclap headache presentation is a neurologic emergency and should be evaluated and treated urgently. As with the rest of the other primary headache disorders, up to 40 percent have coexistent migraine or tension-type headache.

As its name suggests, thunderclap headache has an abrupt explosive onset, with intense pain (>7/10) reaching its peak intensity within one minute. Patients often describe it as the worst headache of their life. Pain lasts from minutes to hours, and can linger for days to weeks [31]. They can recur over the next two weeks, and less commonly over months to years. Thunderclap headache can occur spontaneously or be provoked by Valsalva maneuvers, sex, exertion, or stress. The incidence of thunderclap headache is estimated to be 43 per 100,000 adults per year, with recurrence of thunderclap headache occurring in up to one-quarter of patients with non-SAH thunderclap headache [30].

The pathophysiologic mechanism of primary thunderclap headache is believed to be sympathetic nervous system dysfunction or autonomic dysreflexia with a heightened response to endogenous catecholamines and resultant vasospasm [32].

Thunderclap headache is a neurological emergency, as up to 11 percent of cases can be found to have SAH. Mortality may be as high as 50 percent from SAH [33]. The vast majority of SAH (85 percent) arise from aneurysmal bleeds. Risk factors for aneurysmal SAH include hypertension, smoking, alcohol use, family history of aneurysm, genetic predisposition for connective tissue disorders, and autosomal dominant polycystic kidney disease. Aneurysmal SAH may present with a sentinel headache in 10 percent to 43 percent of patients days to weeks before the ictus, presumptively from stretching of the aneurysm wall or from an earlier bleed [32]. In the general population, the rate of unruptured aneurysm is 3.6–6 percent. Other causes of SAH include perimesencephalic SAH, AVM, tumors, cervicocranial artery dissection, primary angiitis of the central nervous system (PACNS), RCVS, cerebral venous thrombosis (CVT), and dural-arterial venous fistula (dAVF).

Diagnostic testing is mandatory to exclude SAH and other secondary disorders. Computed tomography (CT) of the brain is 98 percent sensitive in detecting intracranial blood if performed within 12 hours of ictal onset. Subsequently, diagnostic sensitivity of a CT brain performed one week after ictal onset decreases to 50 percent and almost 0 percent at three weeks out [34]. An MRI of the brain is equally sensitive in the acute phase and more sensitive in the subacute phase [35]. Lumbar puncture may have to be performed if the suspicion of SAH is high despite negative neuroimaging studies, and may remain positive for xanthochromia for up to three weeks. Cerebral angiography performed by either CT, MR, or conventional angiogram may be required to look for aneurysms.

The differential diagnosis for thunderclap headache is vast. Unfortunately, clinical features do not reliably distinguish between primary and secondary forms. Other neurovascular disorders that may present in a similar manner include arterial dissection, CVT, and RCVS. Reversible cerebral vasoconstriction syndrome, previously known as Call Fleming syndrome or benign angiopathy of the CNS, may present with thunderclap headache, with angiography demonstrating beading of cerebral arteries from vasoconstriction and normalization of the affected vessels within three months. They typically present with recurrent thunderclap headache over a mean of one week. Reversible cerebral vasoconstriction syndrome has a female predominance, affecting those usually between the ages of 20 and 50 years old. Up to 37 percent have no precipitating cause. Reversible cerebral vasoconstriction syndrome needs to be differentiated from PACNS, which presents insidiously with progressive signs and other abnormal imaging and laboratory abnormalities. It is important to note that imaging may be normal early in RCVS, and that repeat imaging may be required three weeks after onset [32]. Other causes of thunderclap headache include intracranial infection, intracranial hyper- and hypotension, pituitary apoplexy, hemorrhage of intracranial tumors, colloid cyst of the third ventricle, posterior reversible leukoencephalopathy syndrome (PRES), cardiac cephalalgia, retroclival hematoma, temporal arteritis, pheochromocytoma, and complicated sinusitis.

Management of thunderclap headache is directed to its underlying cause. In cases where no cause can be found despite extensive investigations, treatment is mainly symptomatic. There are reports of good symptomatic relief with oral nimodipine 30–60 mg every four hours or IV nimodipine 0.5–2 mg per hour when vasoconstriction is demonstrated [36].

# Hypnic Headache

> **Box 9.5 ICHD-3 Beta Diagnostic Criteria for Hypnic Headache**
>
> **Description**
>
> Frequently recurring headache attacks developing only during sleep, causing awakening and lasting for up to four hours, without characteristic associated symptoms and not attributed to other pathology.
>
> **Diagnostic Criteria**
>
> A. Recurrent headache attacks fulfilling criteria B–E
>
> B. Developing only during sleep, and causes wakening
>
> C. Occurring on ≥10 days per month for >3 months
>
> D. Lasting ≥15 minutes and for up to 4 hours after waking
>
> E. No cranial autonomic symptoms or restlessness
>
> F. Not better accounted for by another ICHD-3 diagnosis

Hypnic headache is a rare primary headache disorder that was first described by Raskin in 1988 [37]. It has an estimated prevalence of 0.07–0.3 percent at tertiary headache centers [38]. It was included in the ICHD-2 criteria in 2004 (see Box 9.5). Hypnic headaches are strictly sleep-dependent attacks and share similar features of periodicity with cluster headaches, often occurring at the same time every night and awakening the patient. Referred to as alarm clock headaches, they occur typically within 120–480 minutes after falling asleep, mostly between 1 a.m. and 3 a.m. [39]. Rarely, they may occur during daytime naps. About 40 percent have comorbid migraine and 30 percent have comorbid tension-type headache. Hypnic headache primarily affects the elderly, with a mean age of onset of 63 years. There is a female predominance, with women affected in 63 percent of cases.

The pain is typically moderate in intensity, dull in character, and bilateral or diffuse in location, though it can be unilateral in 39 percent of patients. The pain can also be sharp, stabbing, or pulsating in character. The average duration of headache is 67 minutes, with a range of 15–180 minutes. The frequency ranges from once per week to six times per night. Raskin's original description did not describe autonomic features, but subsequent descriptions demonstrated that 10 percent of cases have autonomic symptoms and up to 20 percent have migrainous features of nausea, photophobia, or phonophobia [39]. Almost all patients have some motor activity when awoken, though not the restlessness noted in patients with cluster headache [40].

The etiology of hypnic headache remains an enigma [41]. It was initially thought to be associated with the rapid eye movement (REM) stage of sleep, which is associated with dorsal raphe, locus ceruleus, and periaqueductal gray matter antinociceptive dysfunction. However, hypnic headaches can occur in other sleep stages as well. Considered a chronobiological disorder, the circadian periodicity suggests the involvement of the hypothalamus and the suprachiasmatic nucleus, the pacemaker of circadian rhythm. The function of the suprachiasmatic nucleus and the hypothalamic-pineal axis are also impaired with age, resulting in reduction of melatonin secretion. This explains the higher prevalence in older adults. Lithium, which is used to treat hypnic headache, indirectly raises the melatonin level and increases serotonin release, supporting the role of melatonin and serotonin in this disorder.

The differential diagnosis of nocturnal headache includes cluster headache, paroxysmal hemicrania, nocturnal occurrence of migraine, obstructive sleep apnea, restless legs syndrome, periodic limb movement disorder, nocturnal arterial hypertension, psychiatric comorbidity with sleep disturbances, chronic pain states, exploding head syndrome, and turtle headache. In contrast to hypnic headache, cluster headache has prominent autonomic signs and is side locked. Migraine tends to occur at other times of the day as well, and may be provoked by specific triggers other than sleep. Nocturnal hypertension may be associated with the occurrence of headache during sleep at night and is treated with antihypertensives. Turtle headache, a condition of hypoxia inducing headache when lying retracted beneath a blanket, is transient and resolves after emergence from the blanket. There are reports of pituitary tumors, posterior fossa space-occupying pathology, intracranial hypotension, and pontine infarction presenting with hypnic headache symptoms. A thorough diagnostic work-up is mandatory to exclude secondary causes of hypnic headache, such as structural intracranial pathology, nocturnal hypertension, and obstructive sleep apnea.

Treatment of hypnic headache is derived from single treatment reports or case series. Only three drugs have shown efficacy in preventing hypnic headache. They are lithium carbonate, caffeine, and indomethacin [40]. The therapeutic serum concentration of lithium in hypnic headache is 0.5–1 mmol per liter, which is usually attained with doses ranging from 150 mg to 600 mg daily. Lithium is efficacious in 64 percent of patients as a prophylactic medication. Lithium levels must be monitored regularly, especially in the elderly, as lithium has an extremely narrow therapeutic window and the potential for many side-effects. Baseline kidney and thyroid function tests should be obtained before initiating treatment and should be periodically monitored along with a serum lithium level. Lithium works by increasing melatonin and serotonin levels. Caffeine and caffeine-containing analgesics are effective in about 70 percent of patients, both as an acute and prophylactic treatment [42]. Drinking a cup of coffee when awoken by a headache or prophylactically drinking a cup of coffee before bedtime may treat and prevent the occurrence of hypnic headache, respectively. The mechanism behind the efficacy of caffeine lies in it being a competitive antagonist at the adenosine receptor. Adenosine is a potent cerebral vasodilator and reduces cortical hyperexcitability. Therefore,

caffeine alters cerebral excitability and causes cerebral vasoconstriction. Indomethacin at a dose of 25–150 mg/day successfully treats hypnic headache in up to 70 percent of patients [39]. Indomethacin is believed to work for hypnic headache by lowering CSF pressure. Indomethacin is preferentially helpful in patients with unilateral hypnic headache [43]. Other treatments with anecdotal benefit in hypnic headache include topiramate, verapamil, flunarizine, antidepressants, benzodiazepines, gabapentin, prednisone, clonidine, melatonin, and botulinum neurotoxin type A.

# New Daily Persistent Headache

**Box 9.6 ICHD-3 Beta Diagnostic Criteria for New Daily Persistent Headache**

**Description**

Persistent headache, daily from its onset, which is clearly remembered. The pain lacks characteristic features, and may be migraine-like or tension-type-like, or have elements of both.

**Diagnostic Criteria**

A.  Persistent headache fulfilling criteria B and C
B.  Distinct and clearly remembered onset, with pain becoming continuous and unremitting within 24 hours
C.  Present for >3 months
D.  Not better accounted for by another ICHD-3 diagnosis

New daily persistent headache (NDPH) is a type of chronic daily headache of long duration [44]. It is characterized by its continuous or near-continuous pain from onset. Patients can recall the date and circumstances of pain onset. Though it can only be diagnosed after excluding secondary causes and after a duration of three months, it usually presents first to the emergency room with new-onset headache. It was first described by Vanast in 1986 and was initially included in the ICHD-2 criteria in 2004 as a feature-less headache with no migrainous characteristics, although his original description included patients with migrainous features [45]. In the ICHD-3 classification, the criteria were refined to not include pain characteristics and associated features (see Box 9.6). The one-year population prevalence is reported to be

0.1 percent, though prevalence in a tertiary headache center can be as high as 20 percent [46]. A quarter of patients with NDPH have other preexisting primary headache disorders, including migraine and tension-type headache [47].

NDPH typically affects people in their twenties and thirties [48]. The pain is bilateral and moderate in intensity at baseline, though it can be unilateral in about 10 percent of patients. The median age of onset is 28 years old, affecting women more than men. Roughly half of all patients can recall a specific trigger prior to the onset of pain, commonly an antecedent viral or systemic illness, menarche, thunderclap headache, intracranial surgery, or a stressful life event. More than half of patients have migrainous features such as nausea, vomiting, photophobia, phonophobia, throbbing quality of pain, or aggravation by physical activity. Those with migrainous features were more likely to be women, have a greater association with depression, and have headaches that were more responsive to triptans. Concomitant auras were rare [47]. Cranial autonomic symptoms occurred with exacerbations in 20 percent of patients. Cutaneous allodynia was present in another quarter of these patients [48].

The etiology of NDPH is poorly understood. A post-infectious phenomenon due to Epstein–Barr virus, cytomegalovirus, adenovirus, herpes simplex, salmonella, toxoplasmosis, or E. coli has been suspected as a causative factor. Studies also found raised inflammatory cytokines and tumor necrosis factor alpha in the CSF but not in the serum, suggesting a central inflammatory process. Other hypothesized clues to the etiology of NDPH include a remote CSF leak secondary to cervical joint hypermobility and defective internal jugular venous drainage [48,49].

Investigations need to be performed in all acute cases of new-onset continuous headache. When the headache has been present for more than three months with a normal neurological examination, the yield of testing is low [50].

The differential diagnosis of NDPH includes meningitis, post-meningitis headache, brain tumors, leptomeningeal metastasis, intracranial hypo- and hypertension, temporal arteritis, chronic subdural hematomas, post-traumatic headache, medication overuse headache, cervicocranial artery dissection, CVT, dAVF, RCVS, sphenoid sinusitis, and hypertension. Secondary pathology should especially be considered when NDPH occurs over the age of 50. Other primary headache syndromes such as chronic migraine, tension-type headache, hemicrania continua, and bifocal nummular headache are also considerations [51]. Chronic migraine may occur abruptly and appear continuous or near-continuous in children with a history of episodic migraine [52].

Blood tests including a complete blood count, thyroid function tests, renal function, and electrolytes are usually required. Collagen vascular and infectious screen (such as erythrocyte sedimentation rate, antinuclear antibody, Lyme antibody, and HIV testing) may be carried out if a systemic cause is suspected. Lumbar puncture may also be indicated in selected cases in those immunocompromised patients with suspected chronic meningitis, or in those with symptoms suggestive of low or high CSF pressures [50]. MRI of the brain with gadolinium should be performed to exclude structural pathology, infections, and low CSF pressure headaches.

There is insufficient evidence to make specific treatment recommendations for NDPH. Treatment is often based on the phenotype of the headache [49]. Suggested treatments for suspected post-infectious causes of NDPH include intravenous methylprednisolone up to 1 g/day for 2–3 days and intravenous acyclovir for 3–5 days with or without corticosteroids [53]. Alternatively, doxycycline has been tried based on its inhibition of tumor necrosis factor alpha. For patients with suspected cervical joint hypermobility, nerve blocks and physical therapy have been suggested. Suggested treatments for a postsurgical cause include nerve blocks and a combination of muscle relaxants and nonsteroidal anti-inflammatory drugs (NSAIDs), tetracycline derivatives, or anticonvulsants. For those with no clear cause found, pharmacological therapies that can be considered include muscle relaxants (baclofen or tizanidine), tricyclic antidepressants (amitriptyline, nortriptyline), anticonvulsants (topiramate, valproic acid, gabapentin), beta-blockers (propranolol), selective serotonin reuptake inhibitors (SSRIs), mexiletine, onabotulinum toxin type A, and clonazepam [48,53]. Triptans and nerve blocks may provide relief in some patients [47]. If outpatient therapy fails, inpatient treatment with intravenous dihydroergotamine, which has been used in those with migrainous features, can be considered [54]. Other intravenous agents used include intravenous haloperidol and intravenous magnesium [48].

The prognosis in Vanast's initial series was good, with the majority of patients having a remission within two years [45]. Unfortunately, subsequent studies note that NDPH can have a chronic and persisting form with continuous headache from onset in about 75 percent of patients, the majority of which will have headaches that persist for at least two years. Less commonly, they may have complete remission or a relapsing remitting form of variable duration [47].

## Conclusion

Other primary headache disorders are generally uncommon. However, they may present initially to the ED. As a significant proportion of them have underlying secondary causes, it is imperative that due diligence is taken to exclude secondary causes.

## References

1. Headache Classification Committee of the International Headache Society (IHS). The International Classification of Headache Disorders, 3rd edition (beta version). *Cephalalgia.* 2013;33(9):629–808.

2. Symonds C. Cough headache. *Brain.* 1956;79(4):557–68.

3. Boes CJ, Matharu MS, Goadsby PJ. Benign cough headache. *Cephalalgia.* 2002;22(10):772–9.

4. Rasmussen BK, Olesen J. Symptomatic and nonsymptomatic headaches in a general population. *Neurology.* 1992;42(6):1225–31.

5. Pascual J, Iglesias F, Oterino A, Vazquez-Barquero A, Berciano J. Cough, exertional, and sexual headaches: an analysis of 72 benign and symptomatic cases. *Neurology.* 1996;46(6):1520–4.

6. Chen PK, Fuh JL, Wang SJ. Cough headache: a study of 83 consecutive patients. *Cephalalgia.* 2009;29(10):1079–85.

7. Cutrer FM, DeLange J. Cough, exercise, and sex headaches. *Neurol Clin.* 2014;32(2):433–50.

8. Ko J, Rozen TD. Valsalva-induced cluster: a new subtype of cluster headache. *Headache.* 2002;42(4):301–2.

9. Mateo I, Pascual J. Coexistence of chronic paroxysmal hemicrania and benign cough headache. *Headache.* 1999;39(6):437–8.

10. Williams B. Cerebrospinal fluid pressure changes in response to coughing. *Brain.* 1976;99(2):331–46.

11. Chen YY, Lirng JF, Fuh JL, et al. Primary cough headache is associated with posterior fossa crowdedness: a morphometric MRI study. *Cephalalgia.* 2004;24(9):694–9.

12. Cordenier A, De Hertogh W, De Keyser J, Versijpt J. Headache associated with cough: a review. *J Headache Pain.* 2013;14:42.

13. Alvarez R, Ramón C, Pascual J. Clues in the differential diagnosis of primary vs secondary cough, exercise, and sexual headaches. *Headache.* 2014;54(9):1560–2.

14. Lane RJ, Davies PT. Modified Valsalva test differentiates primary from secondary cough headache. *J Headache Pain.* 2013;14(1):31.

15. Raskin NH. The cough headache syndrome: treatment. *Neurology.* 1995;45(9):1784.

16. Buzzi MG, Formisano R, Colonnese C, Pierelli F. Chiari-associated exertional, cough, and sneeze headache responsive to medical therapy. *Headache.* 2003;43(4):404–6.

17. Rooke ED. Benign exertional headache. *Med Clin North Am.* 1968;52(4):801–8.

18. Queiroz LP. Symptoms and therapies: exertional and sexual headaches. *Curr Pain Headache Rep.* 2001;5(3):275–8.

19. Sjaastad O, Bakketeig LS. Exertional headache: I. Vaga study of headache epidemiology. *Cephalalgia.* 2002;22(10):784–90.

20. Chen SP, Fuh JL, Lu SR, Wang SJ. Exertional headache: a survey of 1963 adolescents. *Cephalalgia.* 2009;29(4):401–7.

21. van der Ende-Kastelijn K, Oerlemans W, Goedegebuure S. An online survey of exercise-related headaches among cyclists. *Headache.* 2012;52(10):1566–73.

22. Wang SJ, Fuh JL. The "other" headaches: primary cough, exertion, sex, and primary stabbing headaches. *Curr Pain Headache Rep.* 2010;14(1):41–6.

23. Koppen H, van Veldhoven PL. Migraineurs with exercise-triggered attacks have a distinct migraine. *J Headache Pain.* 2013;14:99.

24. Singh RK, Martinez A, Baxter P. Head cooling for exercise-induced headache. *J Child Neurol.* 2006;21(12):1067–8.

25. Evers S, Schmidt O, Frese A, Husstedt I-W, Ringelstein EB. The cerebral hemodynamics of headache associated with sexual activity. *Pain.* 2003;102(1):73–8.

26. Frese A, Eikermann A, Frese K, et al. Headache associated with sexual activity: demography, clinical features, and comorbidity. *Neurology.* 2003;61(6):796–800.

27. Frese A, Rahmann A, Gregor N, et al. Headache associated with sexual activity: prognosis and treatment options. *Cephalalgia.* 2007;27(11):1265–70.

28. Yeh Y-C, Fuh J-L, Chen S-P, Wang, S-J. Clinical features, imaging findings and outcomes of headache associated with sexual activity. *Cephalalgia.* 2010;30:1329–35.

29. Frese A, Gantenbein A, Marziniak M, et al. Triptans in orgasmic headache. *Cephalalgia*. 2006;26(12):1458–61.

30. Dilli E. Thunderclap headache. *Curr Neurol Neurosci Rep*. 2014;14(4):437.

31. Dodick DW. Thunderclap headache. *Curr Pain Headache Rep*. 2002;6(3):226–32.

32. Ducros A, Bousser MG. Thunderclap headache. *BMJ*. 2013;346:e8557.

33. Linn FHH. Primary thunderclap headache. *Handb Clin Neurol*. 2010;97:473–81.

34. van Gijn J, van Dongen KJ. The time course of aneurysmal haemorrhage on computed tomograms. *Neuroradiology*. 1982;23(3):153–6.

35. Mitchell P, Wilkinson ID, Hoggard N, et al. Detection of subarachnoid haemorrhage with magnetic resonance imaging. *J Neurol Neurosurg Psychiatry*. 2001;70(2):205–11.

36. Lu SR, Liao YC, Fuh JL, Lirng JF, Wang SJ. Nimodipine for treatment of primary thunderclap headache. *Neurology*. 2004;62(8):1414–16.

37. Raskin NH. The hypnic headache syndrome. *Headache*. 1988;28(8):534–6.

38. Obermann M, Holle D. Hypnic headache. *Expert Rev Neurother*. 2010;10(9):1391–7.

39. Evers S, Goadsby PJ. Hypnic headache: clinical features, pathophysiology, and treatment. *Neurology*. 2003;60(6):905–9.

40. Holle D, Naegel S, Obermann M. Hypnic headache. *Cephalalgia*. 2013;33(16):1349–57.

41. Holle D, Naegel S, Obermann M. Pathophysiology of hypnic headache. *Cephalalgia*. 2014;34(10):806–12.

42. Holle D, Naegel S, Krebs S, et al. Clinical characteristics and therapeutic options in hypnic headache. *Cephalalgia*. 2010;30(12):1435–42.

43. Dodick DW, Jones JM, Capobianco DJ. Hypnic headache: another indomethacin-responsive headache syndrome? *Headache*. 2000;40(10):830–5.

44. Bigal ME, Lipton RB. The differential diagnosis of chronic daily headaches: an algorithm-based approach. *J Headache Pain*. 2007;8(5):263–72.

45. Vanast WJ. New daily persistent headaches: definition of a benign syndrome. *Headache*. 1986;26(6):318.

46. Pascual J, Colás R, Castillo J. Epidemiology of chronic daily headache. *Curr Pain Headache Rep*. 2001;5(6):529–36.

47. Robbins MS, Grosberg BM, Napchan U, Crystal SC, Lipton RB. Clinical and prognostic subforms of new daily-persistent headache. *Neurology*. 2010;74(17):1358–64.

48. Evans RW. New daily persistent headache. *Headache*. 2012;52(Suppl. 1):40–4.

49. Goadsby PJ. New daily persistent headache: a syndrome, not a discrete disorder. *Headache*. 2011;51(4):650–3.

50. Evans RW, Seifert TD. The challenge of new daily persistent headache. *Headache*. 2011;51(1):145–54.

51. Robbins MS, Evans RW. The heterogeneity of new daily persistent headache. *Headache*. 2012;52(10):1579–89.

52. Mack KJ. What incites new daily persistent headache in children? *Pediatr Neurol*. 2004;31(2):122–5.

53. Rozen TD. New daily persistent headache: clinical perspective. *Headache*. 2011;51(4):641–9.

54. Nagy AJ, Gandhi S, Bhola R, Goadsby PJ. Intravenous dihydroergotamine for inpatient management of refractory primary headaches. *Neurology*. 2011;77(20):1827–32.

# Chapter 10

# Medication Overuse Headache in the Emergency Department

Chia-Chun Chiang
Todd J. Schwedt
Shuu-Jiun Wang
David W. Dodick

## Abstract

Medication overuse headache (MOH) is defined as headache occurring on 15 or more days per month developing as a consequence of regular overuse of acute or symptomatic headache medication (on 10 or more, or 15 or more days per month, depending on the medication) for more than three months. Triptans, NSAIDs, acetaminophen, ergotamine, barbiturates, and opioids can all cause MOH. Although the optimal treatment strategy for MOH is debated, treatments include discontinuing the overused medications and treating with preventive migraine medications. In the ED, it is important to recognize patients who have MOH to provide appropriate treatment recommendations for MOH and to avoid perpetuating the patient's medication overuse. In general, ED treatment of the patient with frequent headaches should not include narcotics or butalbital-containing medications as they are associated with the highest risk of developing MOH as well as the potential to create drug-seeking behavior. Proper follow-up should be arranged prior to discharge from the ED.

## The Concept of Medication Overuse Headache

Medication overuse headache, previously known as rebound headache, drug-induced headache, or medication-misuse headache, is a common and disabling neurological disorder that has an enormous impact on patients, families, and society.

## Diagnostic Criteria for Medication Overuse Headache

In 2004, operational diagnostic criteria for MOH were formally introduced in the International Classification of Headache Disorders (second edition) (ICHD-2). Criteria were revised in 2006 [1–3], and again in 2013 (ICHD-3 beta version) (ICHD-3 beta) [4]. Currently, MOH is defined as headache occurring on 15 or more days per month developing as a consequence of regular overuse of acute or symptomatic headache medication (on 10 or more, or 15 or more days per month, depending on the medication) for more than three months (see Box 10.1). It usually, but not invariably, resolves after the overuse is stopped [4].

In the ICHD-2, MOH excluded a concomitant diagnosis of a primary headache such as chronic migraine (CM). However, according to the ICHD-3β, patients meeting criteria for both a primary headache (e.g., CM) and for MOH can be given both diagnoses [4,5] (see Table 1 in Current Diagnostic Criteria from 2013 ICHD-3 Beta).

## Epidemiology of Medication Overuse Headache

The true prevalence of MOH is unknown as in some cases the drug is involved in generating frequent headache, whereas in others the frequent use of medication is a reflection of frequent headache [5]. In 2008, a series of articles was published to characterize MOH in different countries, including Canada, Germany, India, Japan, Moldova, Spain, Scandinavia, and Taiwan [6–12]. Population-based studies for chronic daily headache were also done in the United States [13,14]. In general, the prevalence of MOH ranges from 1 to 2 percent worldwide. There is a female predominance; migraine is the most common underlying primary headache type; and patients with MOH have a mean age around 40–50 years. Longer duration of chronic daily headache, higher psychological distress, and

**Box 10.1 Current Diagnostic Criteria for MOH from 2013 ICHD-3 Beta**

**Medication Overuse Headache**

A. Headache occurring on ≥15 days per month in a patient with a preexisting headache disorder

B. Regular overuse for >3 months of one or more drugs that can be taken for acute and/or symptomatic treatment of headache[1]

C. Not better accounted for by another ICHD-3 diagnosis

MOH subtypes

Ergotamine overuse headache

Regular intake of ergotamine on ≥10 days per month for >3 months.

Triptan overuse headache

Regular intake of one or more triptans in any formulation, on ≥10 days per month for >3 months

Simple analgesic overuse headache

Paracetamol (acetaminophen) overuse headache

Regular intake of paracetamol on ≥15 days per month for >3 months.

Acetylsalicylic acid overuse headache

Regular intake of acetylsalicylic acid on ≥15 days per month for >3 months.

Other nonsteroidal anti-inflammatory drug (NSAID) overuse headache

Regular intake of one or more NSAIDs other than acetylsalicylic acid on ≥15 days per month for >3 months

Opioid overuse headache

Regular intake of one or more opioids on ≥10 days per month for >3 months

Combination-analgesic overuse[2] headache

Regular intake of one or more combination-analgesic medications[2] on ≥10 days/month for 3 months

Medication overuse headache attributed to multiple drug classes not individually overused

Regular intake of any combination of ergotamine, triptans, simple analgesics, NSAIDs, and/or opioids on a total of ≥10 days per month for >3 months without overuse of any single drug or drug class alone

Medication overuse headache attributed to unverified overuse of multiple drug classes

Both of the following:

1. Regular intake of any combination of ergotamine, triptans, simple analgesics, NSAIDs, and/or opioids on ≥10 days per month for >3 months

2. The identity, quantity, and/or pattern of use or overuse of these classes of drug cannot be reliably established

Medication overuse headache attributed to other medication

Regular overuse, on ≥10 days per month for >3 months, of one or more medications other than those described above, taken for acute or symptomatic treatment of headache.

---

[1] Patients should be coded for one or more subtype of 8.2 MOH according to the specific medication(s) overused and the criteria for each above.

[2] The term combination-analgesic is used specifically for formulations combining drugs of two or more classes, each with analgesic effect or acting as adjuvants.

other pain comorbidities are associated with MOH. Due to geographical differences in the types of medications available and restrictions on medications such as opioid analgesics, the types of medication overused and treatments are slightly different among different countries.

# Pathophysiology of Medication Overuse Headache

The true pathophysiology of MOH is still unclear; however, both human and animal research indicates that central sensitization plays a key role.

Green et al. used a rat model of MOH and compared the cortical spreading depression (CSD) threshold of rats following treatment with sumatriptan or saline continuous subcutaneous pump infusion for six days. Cortical spreading depression is believed to be the bioelectrical homologue of migraine aura. Two weeks after pump removal, the sumatriptan-treated group had a significantly lower threshold of electrical stimulation for CSD generation compared with the saline-treated control group. Treating rats with topiramate prior to recording normalized the CSD threshold in the sumatriptan group. In addition, immunohistochemistry studies showed that Fos expression in the trigeminal nucleus caudalis (TNC) was increased in the sumatriptan group, suggesting amplification mechanisms to promote central sensitization of the trigeminal nociceptive pathway. The trigeminal nociceptive pathway, including the TNC, is believed to be involved in the pathophysiology of migraine through its role in nociception, sensitization, and releasing vasoactive neuropeptides such as substance P and calcitonin gene-related peptide (CGRP). This study concluded that lower CSD threshold and amplification of the effects of CSD (Fos expression) may represent the mechanism of triptan-related MOH [15].

Meng et al. reviewed the pathophysiology of MOH from preclinical studies and indicated that exposure to triptans in rats resulted in: (1) behavioral responses indicating increased sensitivity to environmental stress and tactile stimulation; (2) elevated expression of CGRP and of neuronal nitric oxide synthase (nNOS) in dural afferents of the trigeminal ganglion; and (3) significant increase in plasma CGRP levels [16]. CGRP is a potent vasodilator of cerebral and dural vessels that is expressed in the trigeminal ganglia nerves. Neuronal nitric oxide synthase (nNOS) is an enzyme that produces nitric oxide (NO) that controls vascular tone and neurotransmission. There has been ample evidence supporting CGRP and NO playing key roles in migraine pathogenesis.

Okada-Ogawa et al. reported a possible mechanism of opioid-induced chronic pain, which may be an explanation for opioid overuse headache. In this study, rats were given sustained subcutaneous administration of morphine or control vehicle for 6–7 days. Electrodes placed at the dorsal brainstem recorded the activation of medullary dorsal horn neurons, where nociceptive input from orofacial regions and the intracranial blood vessels are received. When compared to vehicle controls, the electrical and mechanical activation thresholds were significantly lower in chronic morphine-treated animals. Furthermore, diffuse noxious inhibitory controls (DNIC), an inhibitory pain modulation pathway that is activated when another noxious stimulus is present, were also impaired [17,18].

Research demonstrates clinical and fMRI evidence of alterations in pain processing and pain perception in MOH patients. Munksgaard et al. examined pain perception in MOH patients before and 12 months after discontinuation of the overused medication. The changes in cephalic pressure-pain thresholds, cephalic supra-threshold pain scores, and temporal summation demonstrated that patients with MOH had altered pain perception. In addition, the alterations in pain perception were reversible and could improve substantially after discontinuation of the overused medication [19]. Grazzi et al. collected fMRI data from a group of patients suffering from CM with medication overuse and evaluated those patients prior to, and six months following, discontinuation of the overused medication. The results also indicated that there exists a modification of the pain network in CM with medication overuse patients which is reversible with discontinuation [20].

## Medications That Commonly Cause MOH

It is possible that all classes of acute headache medications have the potential to cause MOH. According to the ICHD-3 beta, MOH has the following subtypes: ergotamine overuse headache (regular intake of ergotamine on more than ten days per month for more than three months); triptan overuse headache (regular intake of one or more triptans, in any formulation, on more than ten days per month for more than three months); simple analgesic overuse headache (regular intake of paracetamol/acetaminophen, acetylsalicylic acid, or other NSAIDs on more than 15 days per month for more than three months); opioid overuse headache (regular intake of one or more opioids on more than ten days per month for more than three months); combination-analgesic overuse headache (regular intake of one or more combination-analgesic medications on more than ten days per month for more than three months); MOH attributed to multiple drug classes not individually overused (regular intake of any combination of ergotamine, triptans, simple analgesics, NSAIDs, and/or opioids on more than ten days per month for more than three months); MOH attributed to unverified overuse of multiple drug classes; MOH attributed to other medication (regular overuse, on more than ten days per month for more than three months, of one or more medications other than those described above, taken for acute or symptomatic treatment of headache).

The specific acute headache medication overused is also reported to associate with migraine progression from episodic migraine to chronic migraine. Specific classes of medications and the critical frequency of exposure associated with migraine progression have been estimated in a population-based study. Bigal et al. reported that: (1) Opiates are associated with migraine progression; critical dose of exposure is around eight days per month, and the effect is more pronounced in men. (2) Barbiturates are also associated with migraine progression; critical dose of exposure is around five days per month, and the effect is more pronounced in women. (3) Triptans induced migraine progression in those with high frequency of migraine at baseline (10–14 days per month), but not overall. (4) Nonsteroidal anti-inflammatory medications were protective in those with <10 days of headache at baseline, and, as triptans, induced migraine progression in those with high frequency of headaches [21].

In addition to migraine progression, other longitudinal studies have suggested that medications containing opioids and barbiturates are associated with the highest risk of developing MOH, while NSAIDs and triptans are associated with lower risk [22–24].

The medications that are overused have changed significantly in the past 20 years. The relative proportion of patients overusing ergotamine and combination analgesics has decreased, and the use of triptans and simple analgesics has increased, and continues to do so [22,23]. Of note, the most commonly overused medications vary among different countries.

In our systematic review of the literature [5] we concluded that patients overusing different medications may have variable prognoses. Triptan overusers account for 10–40 percent of the MOH population, and the frequency of triptan overuse has been increasing over the past 20 years [22]. Some studies showed that triptan overusers, after discontinuing their triptan with or without adding a preventive medication, have a greater reduction in headache frequency, shorter headache resolution time, and lower relapse rate compared to patients overusing other types of acute headache medications [25–29]. In the studies reviewed, approximately 3–13 percent of MOH patients were overusing ergotamine [22], and conflicting prognostic outcomes were reported from different studies after discontinuing ergotamine with or without adding preventive medication [30,31]. Simple and combined analgesic overusers account for more than 50 percent of the medication overuse population [22]. Some studies indicate that patients overusing simple and combined analgesics might have higher relapse rates compared to patients overusing different types of acute headache medication after discontinuation, especially when combination analgesics are being overused [32]. Although less than 10 percent of MOH patients overused opioids in the studies reviewed, the true prevalence is likely much higher since most MOH studies intentionally excluded opioid overusers. Patients with opioid overuse tend to have a less favorable outcome with regards to headache frequency, relapse rate, and pain improvement compared to patients overusing other kinds of medications [32–34].

## How to Recognize Medication Overuse Headache in the ED

To recognize MOH in the ED, obtaining a precise history is crucial. All patients presenting to the ED with headache should be screened for MOH: determine how many days per month they have headache of any severity and the number of days per month they take acute headache medication. For patients who have at least 15 headache days per month and meet criteria for medication overuse, determine the duration of this headache and the medication use pattern. Knowing the type(s) of medication they are overusing is helpful when formulating treatment plans and prognosticating patient outcomes. For patients overusing opioids, government-sponsored prescription monitoring programs, such as the Controlled Substances Prescription Monitoring Program that list all previous pharmacy-filled prescriptions, should be checked. Understanding whether the patient has been given opioid prescriptions from different providers and the frequency of those prescriptions provides important information to evaluate whether drug-seeking behavior may be present.

For patients with MOH, it is important to identify "red flags" for headache and, when present, to arrange for appropriate lab and imaging tests, as delineated in previous chapters. Depending upon the medication that is being overused, blood tests might be indicated to check for renal or hepatic dysfunction that could develop secondary to medication overuse. In Figure 10.1 we summarize an algorithm for recognizing and treating MOH patients in the ED.

## Approach to Treating Medication Overuse Headache

Once MOH is identified in the ED, treatment should focus on alleviating the patient's headache pain and associated symptoms while not exacerbating the MOH. Prior to discharge, one should ensure follow-up with a specialist for further evaluation and treatment, commonly including the initiation of preventive migraine medication and the discontinuation of overused medication. Patients should be educated

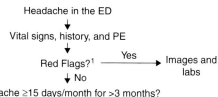

Headache in the ED

↓

Vital signs, history, and PE

↓

Red Flags?[1] ———Yes——→ Images and labs

↓ No

Headache ≥15 days/month for >3 months?
Overuse of acute headache medication on
≥10 (or 15)[2] days/month?

↓

MOH diagnosed

↓

Treat current headache according to the underlying headache phenotype
Avoid using the same class of drug as the overused medication
Check labs or signs of side-effects of the overused medication

↓

If opioid addiction is present,
referral to detoxification program may also be necessary

↓

Arrange OPD Neurology/Headache Clinic follow-
up prior to discharge from the ED

↓

Patient education, discontinuation of the overused medication, and
addition of preventive medication

**Figure 10.1** Algorithm for the recognition and management of MOH in the ED.
[1] Red flags as outlined in Chapter 3.
[2] Depending on the types of medications overused.

that appropriate outpatient evaluation and treatment is the key to avoid worsening of medication overuse headache and frequent ED visits.

The major reasons for ED visits by MOH patients include acute exacerbation of headache or suffering from withdrawal headache. Currently, there are no data from controlled clinical trials to determine which treatments are most effective for treating breakthrough headaches among patients with MOH. We recommend treating acute headache exacerbations according to the underlying headache phenotype, with the treatment options discussed in previous chapters. It is important to avoid treating a patient who has MOH with a medication that is in the same drug class as the overused medication. Use of opioid analgesics and butalbital should generally be avoided when treating patients who have frequent headaches.

When the overused medications are discontinued, MOH patients might experience worsening of their headache before having improvement. Headache might be accompanied by nausea, vomiting, restlessness, and sleep disturbance – symptoms that might account for some ED visits.

Several studies investigated the efficacy of steroids for treating worsening headaches after discontinuing the overused medication in MOH patients. Bøe et al.

compared the effect of oral prednisolone for six days (60 mg on days 1 and 2, 40 mg on days 3 and 4, and 20 mg on days 5 and 6) vs. placebo for six days, in a double-blind, placebo-controlled study in hospitalized patients with MOH. The results showed that the headache intensity and the number of headache days were similar in both groups [35]. In contrast, there was a double-blind, placebo-controlled, randomized, single-center pilot study conducted by Pageler et al. reporting the effect of prednisone 100 mg once daily for the first five days of inpatient discontinuation. The results showed that the total number of hours with severe or moderate headache within the first 72 (primary endpoint) and 120 hours was significantly lower in the prednisone group than in the placebo group (18.1 vs. 36.7 h, $p = 0.031$, and 27.22 vs. 42.67 h, $p = 0.05$) [36]. There are other studies with similar results, suggesting that prednisone helps to decrease the frequency and intensity of withdrawal headaches and associated symptoms [37]. As already suggested in the European Federation of Neurological Sciences guideline, treatment with a corticosteroid (at least 60 mg of prednisone) is possibly effective in treating worsening headaches after discontinuation of the overused medication, but large randomized controlled trials are needed [38].

Other studies have reported possible beneficial effects from the short-term use of oral naproxen, or tizanidine plus a long-acting NSAID, in treating the worsening headaches after discontinuing the overused medication on MOH patients. However, the studies were limited due to small patient groups or retrospective study designs [39]. In addition, intravenous dihydroergotamine, valproic acid, and prochlorperazine might be effective for treating withdrawal headaches – however, the evidence for these interventions is derived from studies done on patients with CM or chronic daily headache with or without medication overuse [39]. More randomized treatment studies are needed for MOH patients with acute headache.

For MOH patients that might have opioid dependence or opioid withdrawal symptoms, it may be helpful to treat patients with a once-weekly clonidine patch (0.1–0.2 mg/24 hours) for one to two weeks [39]. For patients that are overusing butalbital, a phenobarbital taper can be used to help with withdrawal symptoms [39].

Appropriate follow-up should be arranged prior to discharge from the ED to address discontinuation of the overused medication and the decision of giving headache preventive medication.

The treatment of medication overuse headache primarily involves discontinuation of the overused medication and adding preventive medication. It was previously believed that early discontinuation of the overused medication is mandatory because it may increase the responsiveness to preventive medication [33,38,40,41]. However, discontinuation alone is often complicated by high rates of relapse [25,26]. Recent well-designed randomized controlled clinical trials have shown that migraine-preventive medication, especially onabotulinumtoxinA and topiramate, may be effective in patients with CM with medication overuse even when acute medications are not discontinued [42,43]. There are ongoing debates as to whether patients should be initially managed with early discontinuation of the overused medication alone, early discontinuation of the overused medication plus preventive therapy, or preventive therapy without early discontinuation of the overused medication [5].

In 2011, the European Federation of Neurological Sciences published a guideline on medication overuse headache. The recommendations are listed in Box 10.2. In this guideline, abrupt discontinuation or tapering down of overused medication is recommended. Whether medication discontinuation is performed in the inpatient or outpatient setting does not influence

---

**Box 10.2 Recommendations for the Treatment of MOH from the EFNS Guideline [38]**

The level of recommendation is classified as follows

Level A: established as effective, ineffective, or harmful by at least one convincing class I study or at least two consistent, convincing class II studies

Level B: probably effective, ineffective, or harmful by at least one convincing class II study or overwhelming class III evidence

Level C: possibly effective, ineffective, or harmful by at least two convincing class III studies

Good practice point: lack of evidence but consensus within the taskforce

1. Patients with MOH should be offered advice and teaching to encourage withdrawal treatment. (B)

2. There is no general evidence whether abrupt or tapering withdrawal treatment should be preferred. For the overuse of analgesics, ergotamine derivatives, or triptans, abrupt withdrawal is recommended. For the overuse of opioids, benzodiazepines, or barbiturates, tapering down of the medication should be offered. (Good practice point)

3. The type of withdrawal treatment (inpatient, outpatient, advice alone) does not influence the success of the treatment and the relapse rate in general. (A)

4. In patients with opioid, benzodiazepine, or barbiturate overuse, with severe psychiatric or medical comorbidity or with failure of a previous outpatient withdrawal treatment, inpatient withdrawal treatment should be offered. (Good practice point)

5. Individualized preventive medication should be started at the first day of withdrawal treatment or even before if applicable. (C)

6. Topiramate 100 mg (up to 200 mg maximum) per day is probably effective in the treatment of MOH. (B)

7. Corticosteroids (at least 60 mg prednisone or prednisolone) and amitriptyline (up to 50 mg) are possibly effective in the treatment of withdrawal symptoms. (Good practice point)

8. After withdrawal therapy, patients should be followed up regularly to prevent relapse of medication overuse. (Good practice point)

---

the success of treatment. Nonetheless, inpatient discontinuation may be necessary in some patients overusing opioids, benzodiazepines, or barbiturates. It is further recommended to start individualized prophylactic drug treatment at the first day of withdrawal therapy or even beforehand. In addition, following discontinuation of the overused medication, patients should be seen regularly to prevent relapse of medication overuse [38].

Our recent systematic review on treatment of MOH analyzed and discussed literature published from 2004, when the diagnostic criteria were introduced, to August 2014 [5]. The level of evidence to support each study was framed using the American Academy of Neurology Clinical Practice Guideline Manual [44]. Important studies are summarized below.

Zeeberg et al. assessed the effect of discontinuing the overused medication and adhering to a two-month medication-free period for 337 patients with probable MOH. Only 64 percent of the patients completed the two-month study. Among the completers, 45 percent improved, 48 percent had no changes, and 7 percent experienced an increase in headache frequency [26]. Although nearly half of the patients improved, this study did not include a control group and therefore can only be graded as class III evidence.

A recent multinational study involving centers from Europe and Latin America enrolled 376 MOH subjects and reported a consensus protocol for the management of MOH [45]. Patients were included for either inpatient or outpatient early discontinuation, with anti-emetics (metoclopramide, chlorpromazine, prochlorperazine, or domperidone) and analgesics (acetaminophen or naproxen) cautiously given for rescue medication. Preventive treatment (beta-blockers, valproic acid, topiramate, flunarizine, amitriptyline, and candesartan) was started during day 1 to day 7 of early discontinuation, and was chosen based on the patients' underlying primary headache, comorbid disorders, and the side-effect profiles. Patients were not allowed to use the same drug that he/she previously overused as their symptomatic medication. At the end of the study protocol, nearly two-thirds of the patients were no longer overusing medications, and nearly half had reverted to an episodic headache pattern [45]. Although the results are encouraging, the limitation of this study is that no control groups were included, and therefore this study is also graded as class III evidence [5].

The results from recent randomized controlled trials showed that patients with CM with medication overuse may have pain relief and decreased headache burden from preventive therapy, specifically onabotulinumtoxinA or topiramate, without discontinuing the overused medication. Merged data from two placebo-controlled RCTs of onabotulinumtoxinA revealed that in the CM with medication overuse subgroup, after 24 weeks of treatment, mean changes from baseline favored onabotulinumtoxinA vs. placebo for headache days and other secondary outcomes [46–49]. Studies for topiramate also reported similar results. Two randomized, multicenter trials established the efficacy of topiramate in patients who have CM with or without medication overuse [50]. The post-hoc analysis on patients with medication overuse showed that without early discontinuation, topiramate significantly reduced the mean number of monthly migraine days compared to placebo. Limitations for the onabotulinumtoxinA and topiramate studies include that the outcomes for medication overuse patients were analyzed as post-hoc analyses, as the studies were initially designed for patients with CM instead of specifically for MOH.

Recommendations for treatment of MOH with early discontinuation of the overused medication and initiation of preventive medication are summarized in Box 10.3. Considering current available evidence, the recommendations from established guidelines, and the toxicity of acute headache medications, we suggest discontinuation of the overused medication with the addition of preventive medication. Further studies on preventive medications plus early discontinuation vs. preventive treatment alone vs. early discontinuation alone for the treatment of MOH are needed.

---

**Box 10.3 Conclusions and Recommendations for Early Discontinuation and for Preventive Medication When Treating MOH [5]**

The evidence class (I, II, III, IV) was based on the "Classification of Evidence Matrix for Therapeutic Questions" AAN guideline, Appendix 3.

The Conclusions and Recommendations were based on p.13 and Appendix 6 of the same manual, "Synthesizing Evidence: Formulating Evidence-based Conclusions." The suggested verbiages are:

Multiple Class I studies: Are highly likely to be effective…

Multiple Class II studies or a single Class I study: Are likely effective…

Multiple Class III studies or a single Class II study: Are possibly effective…

Multiple Class IV studies or a single Class III study: There is insufficient evidence to support or refute the effectiveness…

## Conclusion and Recommendation for Early Discontinuation

1.  For patients with MOH, it is possible that early discontinuation of acute medications without giving preventive medication is effective in reducing headache frequency and acute medication consumption (three class III studies).

2.  For patients with MOH, it is possible that early discontinuation treatment with prophylactic medication is effective in reducing headache frequency and acute medication consumption, improving MIDAS score, quality of life, anxiety, and depression up to at least one year after discontinuation (19 class III studies).

3.  For patients with MOH, it is possible that preventive treatment alone is more effective than early discontinuation treatment alone in reducing total headache index (single class II).

## Conclusion and Recommendation for Preventive Medication

1.  For patients with CM plus medication overuse:
    a.  It is likely that onabotulinumtoxinA is effective in reducing headache days, migraine days, moderate/severe headache days, cumulative headache hours on headache days, headache episodes, migraine episodes, migraine-related disability (HIT-6), and triptan intake (two class II studies).
    b.  It is likely that onabotulinumtoxinA following discontinuation therapy is effective in reducing acute medication consumption (single class I).

2.  For patients with CM plus medication overuse:
    a.  It is likely that topiramate is effective in reducing mean number of monthly migraine days (three class II studies).
    b.  It is possible that topiramate is effective in reducing acute medication consumption (single class II).

3.  For patients with MOH, it is likely that nabilone is effective in reducing acute medication consumption, headache intensity, and quality of life (single class II); however, larger clinical trials are needed to support its efficacy.

4.  For patients with MOH, it is possible that acupuncture is effective in reducing headache frequency, acute medication consumption, and headache-related disability (single class II).

5.  For patients with MOH, there is insufficient evidence to support or refute the effectiveness of valproic acid in reducing headache days or improving VAS score (single class III in CM plus MO, single class III in CDH).

6.  For patients with MOH, there is insufficient evidence to support or refute the effectiveness of pregabalin, occipital nerve stimulation, and occipital nerve block.

---

HIT-6: Headache Impact Test-6; VAS: visual analogue scale; CDH: chronic daily headache.

# How to Recognize and Decrease Drug-Seeking Behavior

To further characterize the use of narcotics analgesics and potential drug-seeking behavior in the ED, Colman et al. investigated 500 acute migraine headache patient charts that were randomly selected from five Canadian EDs. Medication use was carefully reviewed and analyzed. The majority of patients (59.6 percent) received narcotics as first-line treatment. Factors associated with receiving narcotics as first-line treatment, compared with receiving other first-line treatments, include history of headache ($p < 0.001$), any medication allergy ($p = 0.003$), self-administration of anti-headache medication prior to ED presentation ($p < 0.001$), and arrival to the ED on the weekend, any time on Saturday and Sunday ($p = 0.016$). Those who received narcotics as a first-line agent were more likely to have received an anti-emetic in their treatment ($p < 0.001$) and they were less likely to have received other treatments including non-narcotic analgesics, non-steroidal anti-inflammatory drugs, dihydroergotamine, or corticosteroids (all $p < 0.005$). Time spent in the ED was significantly shorter for those who received narcotic analgesics as a first-line agent compared with those who did not ($p < 0.001$). However, those who received first-line narcotics were significantly more likely to return to the same ED with a headache within seven days of the original visit ($p = 0.011$). While this study did not control for underlying disease severity, these data suggest that treating acute migraine headache with narcotics may result in worsening of the headache post-ED discharge [51].

Providing an opioid prescribing guideline in the ED may be effective in lowering the chance of abuse or generating MOH. Del Portal et al. reported the impact of providing physicians with an opioid prescribing guideline in the acute care setting for patients with non-cancerous pain including dental, neck/back, or chronic pain. Among the included

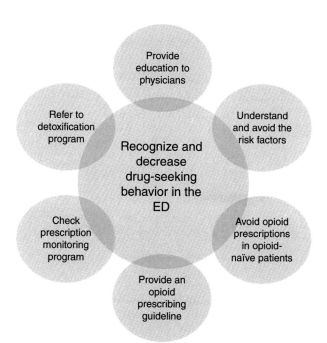

13,187 patient visits, the rate of opioid prescribing decreased significantly from 52.7 percent before the guideline to 29.8 percent immediately after its introduction, and to 33.8 percent at an interval of 12–18 months later. Of note, the decrease in opioid prescriptions was observed in all of these diagnosis groups and in all age groups. This guideline was 100 percent endorsed by all 31 survey-responders (eligible attending physicians) [52]. Highlights from the guideline include: (1) patients with chronic non-cancer pain should not receive injections of narcotic analgesics in the ED; (2) patients with suspected addictive behavior will be referred to the Psychiatric Crisis Response Center or other detoxification resources, if available; (3) patients identified with multiple ED visits for pain, problematic or dishonest behavior (abusive, altering prescriptions, false reports), or use of multiple hospitals for pain will be reviewed by the ED physician leadership team, which is authorized to send a certified letter stating the patient will no longer be provided narcotics in the ED [52]. Although this study did not specifically include patients with headache, decreasing opioid prescriptions when treating other pain conditions may decrease the incidence of MOH.

Avoiding opioid prescriptions in otherwise opioid-naïve patients is crucial to decrease the risk of creating opioid dependence and drug-seeking behavior. One retrospective cohort study reported the risk of recurrent opioid use after receipt of an ED opioid prescription. In total, 4801 patients discharged from an academic ED with an acute painful condition were studied during a five-month period and data were linked to Colorado's prescription drug monitoring program. Recurrence was defined as filling an opioid prescription within 60 days before or after the first anniversary of the ED visit. Almost 38 percent of previous opioid-naïve patients (299 of 775) that received and filled an opioid prescription went on to recurrent use [53]. The initiation of opioid use in acute care setting should be judiciously evaluated.

Providing education to providers may also be useful in decreasing opioid prescriptions. A survey done in patients attending a tertiary care headache center reported that among the 218 patients (83.9 percent of them diagnosed with migraine) who completed the survey, more than half reported having been prescribed an opioid (54.8 percent) or a barbiturate (56.7 percent). According to the report, the most frequent first prescribers for opioids and barbiturates were ED physicians and general neurologists, respectively [54].

Finally, when drug-seeking behavior is a concern, available prescription monitoring programs should be checked. Patients with drug-seeking behavior need referral to a detoxification program. Emergency physicians should avoid writing opioid prescriptions. In Figure 10.2

we summarize the key points to recognize and decrease drug-seeking behavior in the ED.

## Conclusion

It is important to recognize patients that have MOH in order to provide appropriate treatments for headache, and to avoid perpetuating the patient's medication overuse. In general, ED treatment of patients with frequent headaches should not include narcotics or butalbital-containing medications, as they are associated with the highest risk of developing MOH as well as creating drug-seeking behavior. Proper follow-up should be arranged prior to discharge from the ED.

## References

1. Headache Classification Subcommittee of the International Headache Society. The International Classification of Headache Disorders, 2nd edition. *Cephalalgia*. 2004;24(Suppl. 1):9–160.

2. Silberstein S, Olesen J, Bousser M-G, et al. The International Classification of Headache Disorders, 2nd edition (ICHD-II): revision of criteria for 8.2 medication-overuse headache. *Cephalalgia*. 2005;25(6):460–5.

3. Headache Classification Committee, Olesen J, Bousser M-G, et al. New appendix criteria open for a broader concept of chronic migraine. *Cephalalgia*. 2006;26(6):742–6.

4. Headache Classification Committee of the International Headache Society (IHS). The International Classification of Headache Disorders, 3rd edition (beta version). *Cephalalgia*. 2013;33(9):629–808.

5. Chiang CC, Schwedt TJ, Wang SJ, Dodick DW. Treatment of medication-overuse headache: a systematic review. *Cephalalgia*. 2016;36(4):371–86.

6. Wang SJ, Fuh JL. Medication overuse headache in Taiwan. *Cephalalgia*. 2008;28(11):1240–2.

7. Katsarava Z, Diener HC. Medication overuse headache in Germany. *Cephalalgia*. 2008;28(11):1221–2.

8. Becker WJ, Purdy RA. Medication overuse headache in Canada. *Cephalalgia*. 2008;28(11):1218–20.

9. Pascual J, Mateos V, Gracia M, Láinez JM. Medication overuse headache in Spain. *Cephalalgia*. 2008;28(11):1234–6.

10. Ravishankar K. Medication overuse headache in India. *Cephalalgia*. 2008;28(11):1223–6.

11. Jensen R, Bendtsen L. Medication overuse headache in Scandinavia. *Cephalalgia*. 2008;28(11):1237–9.

12. Kanki R, Nagaseki Y, Sakai F. Medication-overuse headache in Japan. *Cephalalgia*. 2008;28(11):1227–8.

13. Castillo J, Muñoz P, Guitera V, Pascual J. Epidemiology of chronic daily headache in the general population. *Headache*. 1999;39(3):190–6.

14. Scher AI, Stewart WF, Liberman J, Lipton RB. Prevalence of frequent headache in a population sample. *Headache*. 1998;38(7):497–506.

15. Green AL, Gu P, De Felice M, et al. Increased susceptibility to cortical spreading depression in an animal model of medication-overuse headache. *Cephalalgia*. 2014;34(8):594–604.

16. Meng ID, Dodick D, Ossipov MH, Porreca F. Pathophysiology of medication overuse headache: insights and hypotheses from preclinical studies. *Cephalalgia*. 2011;31(7): 851–60.

17. Le Bars D, Dickenson AH, Besson JM. Diffuse noxious inhibitory controls (DNIC): I. Effects on dorsal horn convergent neurones in the rat. *Pain*. 1979;6(3):283–304.

18. Okada-Ogawa A, Porreca F, Meng ID. Sustained morphine-induced sensitization and loss of diffuse noxious inhibitory controls in dura-sensitive medullary dorsal horn neurons. *J Neurosci*. 2009;29(50):15828–35.

19. Munksgaard SB, Bendtsen L, Jensen RH. Modulation of central sensitisation by detoxification in MOH: results of a 12-month detoxification study. *Cephalalgia*. 2013;33(7):444–53.

20. Grazzi L, Chiapparini L, Ferraro S, et al. Chronic migraine with medication overuse pre–post withdrawal of symptomatic medication: clinical results and FMRI correlations. *Headache*. 2010;50(6):998–1004.

21. Bigal ME, Lipton RB. Excessive acute migraine medication use and migraine progression. *Neurology*. 2008;71(22):1821–8.

22. Meskunas CA, Tepper SJ, Rapoport AM, Sheftell FD, Bigal ME. Medications associated with probable medication overuse headache reported in a tertiary care headache center over a 15-year period. *Headache*. 2006;46(5):766–72.

23. Jensen R, Zeeberg P, Dehlendorff C, Olesen J. Predictors of outcome of the treatment programme in a multidisciplinary headache centre. *Cephalalgia*. 2010;30(10):1214–24.

24. Relja G, Granato A, Bratina A, Antonello RM, Zorzon M. Outcome of medication overuse headache after abrupt in-patient withdrawal. *Cephalalgia*. 2006;26(5):589–95.

25. Katsarava Z, Muessig M, Dzagnidze A, et al. Medication overuse headache: rates and predictors for relapse in a 4-year prospective study. 2005;25(1):12–15.

26. Zeeberg P, Olesen J, Jensen R. Probable medication-overuse headache: the effect of a 2-month drug-free period. *Neurology*. 2006;66(12):1894–8.

27. Munksgaard SB, Bendtsen L, Jensen RH. Treatment-resistant medication overuse headache can be cured. *Headache*. 2012;52(7):1120–9.

28. Relja G, Granato A, Bratina A, Antonello RM, Zorzon M. Outcome of medication overuse headache after abrupt in-patient withdrawal. *Cephalalgia*. 2006;26(5):589–95.

29. Katsarava Z, Limmroth V, Finke M, Diener HC, Fritsche G. Rates and predictors for relapse in medication overuse headache: a 1-year prospective study. *Neurology*. 2003;60(10):1682–3.

30. Zidverc-Trajkovic J, Pekmezovic T, Jovanovic Z, et al. Medication overuse headache: clinical features predicting treatment outcome at 1-year follow-up. *Cephalalgia*. 2007;27(11):1219–25.

31. Fontanillas N, Colás R, Muñoz P, Oterino A, Pascual J. Long-term evolution of chronic daily headache with medication overuse in the general population. *Headache*. 2010;50(6):981–8.

32. Sances G, Ghiotto N, Galli F, et al. Risk factors in medication-overuse headache: a 1-year follow-up study (care II protocol). *Cephalalgia*. 2010;30(3):329–36.

33. Zeeberg P, Olesen J, Jensen R. Discontinuation of medication overuse in headache patients: recovery of therapeutic responsiveness. *Cephalalgia*. 2006;26(10):1192–8.

34. Lake AE, Saper JR, Hamel RL. Comprehensive inpatient treatment of refractory chronic daily headache. *Headache*. 2009;49(4):555–62.

35. Bøe MG, Mygland Å, Salvesen R. Prednisolone does not reduce withdrawal headache: a randomized, double-blind study. *Neurology*. 2007;69(1):26–31.

36. Pageler L, Katsarava Z, Diener HC, Limmroth V. Prednisone vs. placebo in withdrawal therapy following medication overuse headache. *Cephalalgia*. 2008;28(2):152–6.

37. Krymchantowski AV, Barbosa JS. Prednisone as initial treatment of analgesic-induced daily headache. *Cephalalgia*. 2000;20(2):107–13.

38. Evers S, Jensen R, European Federation of Neurological Societies. Treatment of medication overuse headache: guideline of the EFNS headache panel. *Eur J Neurol*. 2011;18(9):1115–21.

39. Garza I, Schwedt TJ. *Medication Overuse Headache: Treatment and Prognosis*. 10th ed. Waltham: UpToDate; 2012.

40. Dodick DW, Silberstein SD. How clinicians can detect, prevent and treat medication overuse headache. *Cephalalgia*. 2008;28(11):1207–17.

41. Bigal ME, Lipton RB. Modifiable risk factors for migraine progression. *Headache*. 2006;46(9):1334–43.

42. Aurora SK, Winner P, Freeman MC, et al. OnabotulinumtoxinA for treatment of chronic migraine: pooled analyses of the 56-week PREEMPT clinical program. *Headache*. 2011;51(9):1358–73.

43. Silberstein S, Lipton R, Dodick D, et al. Topiramate treatment of chronic migraine: a randomized, placebo-controlled trial of quality of life and other efficacy measures. 2009;49(8):1153–62.

44. AAN (American Academy of Neurology). *Clinical Practice Guideline Process Manual*, 2011 ed. St. Paul, MN: The American Academy of Neurology; 2011.

45. Tassorelli C, Jensen R, Allena M, et al. A consensus protocol for the management of medication-overuse headache: evaluation in a multicentric, multinational study. *Cephalalgia*. 2014;34(9):645–55.

46. Dodick DW, Turkel CC, DeGryse RE, et al. OnabotulinumtoxinA for treatment of chronic migraine: pooled results from the double-blind, randomized, placebo-controlled phases of the PREEMPT clinical program. *Headache*. 2010;50(6):921–36.

47. Silberstein SD, Blumenfeld AM, Cady RK, et al. OnabotulinumtoxinA for treatment of chronic migraine: PREEMPT 24-week pooled subgroup analysis of patients who had acute headache medication overuse at baseline. *J Neurol Sci*. 2013;331(1–2):48–56.

48. Silberstein SD, Lipton RB, Dodick DW, et al. Efficacy and safety of topiramate for the treatment of chronic migraine: a randomized, double-blind, placebo-controlled trial. 2007;47(2):170–80.

49. Diener HC, Dodick DW, Aurora SK, et al. OnabotulinumtoxinA for treatment of chronic migraine: results from the double-blind, randomized, placebo-controlled phase of the PREEMPT 2 trial. *Cephalalgia*. 2010;30(7):804–14.

50. Diener HC, Bussone G, Van Oene JC, et al. Topiramate reduces headache days in chronic migraine: a randomized, double-blind, placebo-controlled study. *Cephalalgia*. 2007;27(7):814–23.

51. Colman I, Rothney A, Wright SC, Zilkalns B, Rowe BH. Use of narcotic analgesics in the emergency department treatment of migraine headache. *Neurology*. 2004;62(10):1695–700.

52. Del Portal DA, Healy ME, Satz WA, McNamara RM. Impact of an opioid prescribing guideline in the acute care setting. *J Emerg Med*. 2016;50(1):21–7.

53. Hoppe JA, Kim H, Heard K. Association of emergency department opioid initiation with recurrent opioid use. *Ann Emerg Med*. 2015;65(5):493–4.

54. Minen MT, Lindberg K, Wells RE, et al. Survey of opioid and barbiturate prescriptions in patients attending a tertiary care headache center. 2015;55(9):1183–91.

**Chapter**

# 11

# Approach to the Pediatric Patient with Headache in the Emergency Department

Serena L. Orr

David Sheridan

## Abstract

Headache is a common presentation in the pediatric emergency department (ED). The majority of pediatric patients presenting to the ED with headache will have a non-life-threatening cause. In order to determine the etiology of the headache, the clinician must take a diligent history and carry out a focused physical exam. Investigations may be required to narrow the differential diagnosis, though in many cases neuroimaging is not required in the acute setting. Headache management will depend on etiology. Although many of the headaches in the pediatric ED are primary headaches, the evidence on how to treat these headaches is limited.

In this chapter, the epidemiology of headache in the pediatric ED will be reviewed. Both detailed and screening approaches to the history and physical exam will be provided. An approach to diagnostic tests and treatment of the primary headaches will be given, incorporating evidence-based recommendations where possible.

## Epidemiology of Pediatric Headache in the ED

Headache is very common in the pediatric population. A recent systematic review of population-based studies showed that the lifetime prevalence of headache among children and adolescents is 58.4 percent [1]. Unsurprisingly given the prevalence, headache is also common in EDs. It accounts for between 0.8 percent and 1.3 percent of all chief complaints in this setting [2–5], with national estimates of over 500,000 pediatric visits a year in the United States [6].

## Epidemiology of Primary vs. Secondary Headaches in the Pediatric ED

Pediatric headache can arise from rare, acute, life-threatening conditions such as bacterial meningitis and brain tumors, or from benign and self-limited disorders like tension-type headache and viral illnesses. As is the case with headaches in adults, it is essential to differentiate primary headaches from secondary headaches when classifying pediatric headaches.

There is significant variability in estimates of headache etiologies in the ED that is likely explained by several factors, two of which predominate: (1) the various locations of the EDs surveyed, reflecting geographic differences in headache pathologies and ED use patterns; (2) differing study methodologies, with the various studies using very different methods to assess diagnoses and differences in inclusion criteria (e.g., some studies excluded post-traumatic headaches). Despite the variability between EDs, one consistent finding is that the majority of pediatric patients presenting to the ED with headache will have a non-life-threatening cause: most commonly a viral illness or primary headache disorder such as migraine (Table 11.1) [2–5,7,8]. Several studies have found that viral illnesses, such as upper respiratory tract infections, account for anywhere from 25 to 60 percent of discharge diagnoses in children and adolescents that presented with headache as their chief complaint. Another important category that requires close outpatient monitoring is post-traumatic headache in the context of acute head injury, such as a concussion, which accounts for up to 20 percent of pediatric ED visits for headache.

Headaches due to secondary causes occur at variable frequencies depending on the ED surveyed and the clinical scenario. For example, the most common form of meningitis encountered in the pediatric population is viral meningitis and can be present in up to 5 percent of headache visits [3,4]. Brain tumors and cerebrovascular disease, including ischemic stroke, hemorrhagic stroke, and cerebral venous sinus thrombosis, are relatively uncommon causes of headache in children and adolescents presenting to the ED,

**Table 11.1** Etiology of headache in the pediatric ED

| Study/parameter | Burton et al., 1997 [3] | Kan et al., 2000 [2] | Lewis and Qureshi, 2000 [7] | Conicella et al., 2008 [5] | Scagni and Pagliero, 2008 [8] | Hsiao et al., 2014 [4] |
|---|---|---|---|---|---|---|
| Location of ED | Miami, Florida, USA | Queens, New York, USA | Norfolk, Virginia, USA | Rome, Italy | Torino, Italy | Kweishan, Taoyuan, Taiwan |
| Number of patients | 288 | 130 | 150 | 432 | 550 | 409 |
| All viral/upper respiratory tract infection (%) | 60 | 29 | 57 | 32 | 38 | 60 |
| Sinusitis (%) | 16 | – | 9 | 12 | – | – |
| All primary headaches (%) | – | 10 | – | 38 | 57 | 28 |
| Migraine (%) | 16 | 9 | 18 | 29 | 5 | 9 |
| Tension-type headache (%) | 5 | 2 | – | 7 | – | – |
| Primary headache not specified (%) | – | – | – | – | 51 | 18 |
| Central nervous system disease[*] (%) | 7 | 45 | – | 6 | 7 | 11 |
| Post-traumatic (%) | 7 | 20 | 1 | 9[**] | Excluded | 2 |
| Meningitis (%) | 5 | 2 | 9 | 2 | 0.4 | 5 |
| Seizures (%) | – | 3 | 1 | 0.3 | 1 | 1 |
| Brain tumor (%) | 0.7 | 2 | 3 | 1 | 0.4 | 1 |
| Cerebrovascular disease[***] (%) | 0.3 | – | 1 | – | 0.5 | 0.5 |
| VP shunt malfunction (%) | 0.3 | 2 | 2 | 1 | 0.4 | 0.5 |
| Other/unclassified (%) | 8 | 33 | 7 | 8 | 4 | 2 |

[*] Defined in a variety of ways (e.g., in [3] defined as serious neurological diseases, in [2] defined as all secondary neurological causes).
[**] Cases of moderate to severe cranial trauma were excluded.
[***] Includes ischemic stroke, ischemic attack, hemorrhagic stroke, and cerebral venous sinus thrombosis.

accounting for 0.4–2.6 percent and 0.3–1.3 percent of all cases, respectively. However, these must be considered in high-risk patients, including sickle cell patients or children with focal neurologic deficits. Mainly seen in pediatric medical centers, patients with ventriculoperitoneal shunt (VP) malfunction can present with headache. In fact, one study showed that the most common presenting symptom of a VP shunt malfunction in children was headache [9].

Primary headaches are also very common in pediatric EDs, accounting for anywhere from 10 to 57 percent of headache visits. Migraine is the most common primary headache disorder encountered in the ED as children and adolescents will present either with their first attack or after home medications have failed to control the pain; children may also not have home abortive medications prescribed to them, which may make them more likely to resort to an ED visit for pain control. As is the case with adults presenting to the ED with primary headache, pediatric patients are commonly discharged with a diagnosis of unspecified primary headache [4,8]. Although this phenomenon is common, it likely leads to a lack of targeted management and perhaps unnecessary investigations, as evidenced by a national study in which approximately one-third of children with headache had a head CT [6].

## Factors Affecting the Frequency of Headache Visits in Pediatric EDs

Factors impacting the prevalence of ED visits for headache have not been well studied, especially in the pediatric population. There does appear to be some degree of seasonal variation in patterns of visits to the ED for pediatric headache. One US study explored a large dataset from the National Hospital Ambulatory Medical Care Survey and found that there were more ED visits for headache in January, and less visits in June, as compared to other months of the year in pediatric patients with presumed primary headache presentations [10]. Another US study that analyzed data from one pediatric ED and excluded most life-threatening secondary headache diagnoses found that there were significantly more visits for headache between September and November, and significantly fewer visits in May and June as compared to the other months of the calendar year. Consistent with these findings, there were significantly fewer pediatric ED visits for headache during the summer months as compared to during the academic year [11], a trend that mirrors the seasonal variation in migraine frequency [12]. The relative increase in headache visits during the academic year is likely multifactorial, relating to factors such as the timing of peak viral season and the impact of academic and psychosocial stressors on patients with primary headaches. For example, often adolescents will experience higher levels of stress and poor sleep during exam periods, which may trigger migraine headaches.

There may also be gender differences impacting ED visits for headache in the pediatric population. Girls may be more likely to present to the ED for headache after the age of 12, whereas boys may be more likely to present under the age of 12 [11]. Unfortunately, there are almost no data available regarding how other demographic factors impact pediatric ED visits for headache.

# Comprehensive History Taking in Pediatric ED Patients with Headache

Below, a detailed approach to history taking and the physical exam for pediatric patients presenting with headache is described. An effort is made to provide a comprehensive overview of the assessment of pediatric headache. In an ED setting, many elements of this assessment will be unnecessary, and the clinician must recognize when particular aspects of the history and exam are required. Immediately after this section, the reader will be provided with a screening assessment appropriate for most patients with headache in the pediatric ED, which can be supplemented with relevant details from the comprehensive assessment where clinically appropriate.

## Headache Characteristics

### Headache Time Course

One of the most important factors in deciphering primary vs. secondary headache etiologies in the

pediatric population is the time course of the headache. It is imperative to inquire about headache onset, frequency, duration, progression of frequency, and intensity over time and predilection for onset at particular times of the day. Children and adolescents presenting to the ED with a serious underlying neurological disease are more likely to describe a headache with an acute or subacute onset (new headache onset within the past two months) [5], often with a worsening course over time [13]. Of particular concern are children who are awaking in the night or early-morning headaches that may be accompanied by vomiting [14]. However, patients with underlying benign secondary causes, like viral illnesses, are also likely to describe an acute headache, and primary headaches often present to the emergency department acutely upon first occurrence. Patients with headache in the context of stroke tend to present in the hyperacute time frame, within hours of symptom onset [15].

Episodic headaches are more likely to be primary in nature, but headaches that occur exclusively in the morning and/or at night should be considered a red flag for increased intracranial pressure [13,16]. Morning headaches can also occur in the context of sleep apnea or sleep bruxism, but this population is less likely to present to the ED. Chronic headaches are more likely to be primary headaches if they occur in isolation of any red flags.

### Headache Location

The location of the headache is particularly relevant, as it can provide clues as to whether the headache is primary or secondary, and in certain cases it can hint at a specific etiology. Patients with underlying intracranial disease may have more difficulty pinpointing a specific location for the pain [5]. It has also been shown that occipital pain in pediatric patients is more likely to be associated with an underlying sinister cause [5,7]. Although pediatric patients with primary headaches will in rare cases describe pain limited to the occiput [17], the ED clinician should consider occipital pain as a red flag in children and adolescents. Pain that is consistently in the distribution of a specific nerve should compel the clinician to consider neuralgia (e.g., trigeminal neuralgia, occipital neuralgia, and cervicogenic headache [17]).

Children and adolescents presenting to the ED with primary headaches are more likely to describe unilateral pain than are patients with secondary headaches [5]. However, the laterality of the headache is

**Table 11.2** ICHD-3 (beta version) diagnostic criteria for pediatric migraine and tension-type headache [17]

| Criterion | Migraine without aura | Migraine with aura | Tension-type headache |
|---|---|---|---|
| A | At least five attacks fulfilling criteria B–D | At least two attacks fulfilling criteria B–D | At least ten attacks fulfilling criteria B–D*** |
| B | Attacks last 2–72 hours if untreated or unsuccessfully treated | One or more of the following fully reversible aura symptoms:<br>• Visual**<br>• Sensory**<br>• Speech and/or language**<br>• Motor<br>• Brainstem<br>• Retinal | Attacks last from 30 minutes to 7 days |
| C | At least two of the following four characteristics are present:<br>• unilateral or bilateral in children and adolescents, most often frontotemporal<br>• pulsating quality<br>• moderate or severe pain intensity<br>• aggravated by or causing avoidance of routine physical activity such as walking or climbing stairs | At least two of the following four characteristics are present:<br>• at least one aura symptom spreads gradually over five minutes or more, and/or two or more symptoms occur in succession<br>• each individual aura symptom lasts 5–60 minutes<br>• at least one aura symptom is unilateral<br>• the aura is accompanied by, or followed within 60 minutes by, a headache | At least two of the following four characteristics are present:<br>• bilateral location<br>• pressing or tightening (non-pulsating) quality<br>• mild or moderate pain intensity<br>• not aggravated by routine physical activity such as walking or climbing stairs |
| D | At least one of the following is present:<br>1. nausea and/or vomiting<br>2. photophobia and phonophobia* | Not better accounted for by another ICHD-3 diagnosis, and transient ischemic attack has been excluded | Both of the following are present:<br>1. no nausea or vomiting<br>2. no more than one of photophobia or phonophobia |
| E | Not better accounted for by another ICHD-3 diagnosis | N/A | Not better accounted for by another ICHD-3 diagnosis |

* Photophobia and phonophobia can be inferred in young children by behavior (e.g., the child goes to lie down in a quiet, dark room during an attack).
** Visual, sensory, and speech and/or language aura symptoms are considered typical aura symptoms, whereas motor, brainstem, and retinal symptoms are more unusual and rare.
*** The frequency varies based on whether the diagnosis is infrequent episodic, frequent episodic, or chronic TTH.

not a reliable variable in differentiating primary and secondary headaches. Although migraine is ordinarily thought of as a unilateral headache, in the pediatric population it is often bilateral, commonly located in the bitemporal or bifrontal areas [17,18]. In addition, children with tension-type headache (TTH) report bilateral locations in the vast majority of cases [17,18].

Table 11.2 lists the International Classification of Headache Disorders, third edition (ICHD-3, beta version) diagnostic criteria for pediatric migraine and TTH. Although the ICHD criteria are considered to be the gold standard for the diagnosis of headache, they can be challenging to apply in the ED setting for a variety of reasons. A recent study carried out in a pediatric ED suggested that the ICHD-2 criteria for pediatric migraine lacked sensitivity,

with only 45 percent of children who were ultimately diagnosed with migraine by a pediatric neurologist meeting criteria at the time of ED presentation. The sensitivity of the ICHD-2 criteria improved to 83 percent when Criterion A (minimal number of attacks) was removed. Nonetheless, in 94 percent of the cases, the ED physician correctly diagnosed migraine in concordance with the pediatric neurologist [19]. The most challenging aspect of applying the ICHD criteria for primary headaches in the ED is therefore related to Criterion A. Thus, although the ICHD should guide the diagnosis of primary headaches in the pediatric ED, the clinician must consider the fact that the criteria will lack sensitivity because many patients will present during their first primary headache episode.

### Pain Intensity

The intensity of the headache pain does not reliably distinguish between primary or secondary headaches, but is a useful historical element to elicit as it may direct your clinical management based on pain response to various medications described later. Patients with life-threatening secondary causes tend to describe high-intensity pain [5,13], as do patients with migraine [5,18]. Mild pain intensity is more likely to occur with non-life-threatening causes of headache, such as some of the non-neurological secondary causes [5] and TTH [17,18].

Headaches that are described as being the "worst in life" may warrant further investigation to a potential secondary cause. Thunderclap headaches, defined as sudden-onset headaches that reach their maximal intensity in under one minute, may be caused by a secondary process, especially vascular diseases such as subarachnoid hemorrhage (SAH) or reversible cerebral vasoconstriction syndrome [17], although these are uncommon in the pediatric population.

### Pain Quality

Pain quality is also a key component of the history taking. Patients with underlying serious secondary causes may have more difficulty describing the pain than patients with more benign causes [5,7], such as underlying viral infections and migraine. Primary headaches vary in terms of their quality, but are most likely to be described as pulsating or constrictive [5,18] (see Figure 11.2).

### Aggravating and Alleviating Factors

The clinician should always inquire about headache triggers and specific factors that cause the headache to worsen, not only for diagnostic purposes, but also for assisting the patient in preventing future attacks. Position can be an important trigger to identify: Headaches caused by increased intracranial pressure tend to begin or worsen upon lying down [13,16], whereas headaches caused by intracranial hypotension [20] or postural orthostatic tachycardia syndrome (POTS) [21] tend to onset or worsen upon standing. Headaches that are provoked by Valsalva, such as bearing down on the toilet or sneezing, can signify increased intracranial pressure. Exercise is a very rare trigger for primary headaches (i.e., primary exercise headache) and generally signifies serious underlying secondary causes, especially of neurovascular nature

[17]. Similarly, illicit drug use, especially with psychostimulants like cocaine, amphetamines, and MDMA, is a concerning trigger for headache and should compel the clinician to consider secondary neurovascular causes. A history of head, neck, and/or spine trauma should be sought in order to rule out post-traumatic headache, cervical artery dissection, intracranial hypotension secondary to a cerebrospinal fluid (CSF) leak or other traumatic causes of headache.

Factors that alleviate the headache should also be sought. It is important to inquire about medications taken for pain relief, both because this may assist the clinician in identifying the headache cause, and because it can impact subsequent treatment decisions. If medications are being self-administered for acute headache relief, it is imperative to inquire about the frequency of use because medication overuse can be an important contributory factor in headache etiology and, if present, needs to be addressed in the management plan. The diagnostic criteria for medication overuse headache stipulate that the patient must be using medications to acutely treat their headache at a minimum frequency of 10–15 days per month, depending on the type of medication being overused, over a three-month period at minimum [17].

## Associated Symptoms

Associated symptoms are key in narrowing the differential diagnosis of headache. One should always inquire about associated neurological symptoms because they constitute red flags in patients presenting to the ED with headache (see Figure 11.1). Blurred vision and ataxia have been shown to occur more frequently in pediatric patients presenting to the ED with increased intracranial pressure (ICP) as compared to those with normal ICP [4]. Children with brain masses, especially supratentorial tumors, commonly report visual disturbances of various forms along with headache [22–24]. Focal neurological deficits and seizures can be seen with masses [22,24], especially with those that are supratentorial in location, or with other supratentorial neurologic diseases such as stroke and intracranial infections. Of note, brain tumors rarely, if ever, present with isolated headache [25]. Seizures, altered level of consciousness, and irritability are red flags for meningitis if the child or adolescent is also febrile [26,27]. An altered level of consciousness is a significant red flag even in the absence of fever. Photophobia and phonophobia are usually associated

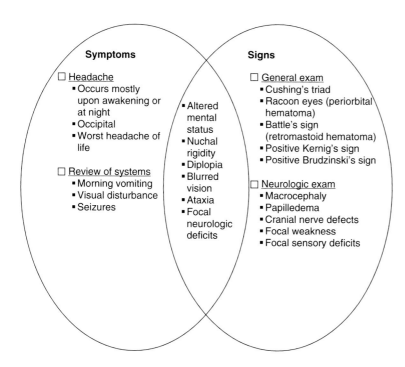

with primary headaches [5,17], but photophobia is also described in patients with meningitis [3]. As a general rule, a child with focal neurologic deficits requires further investigation.

In addition to inquiring about neurological symptoms, it is very important to carry out a full review of systems. Clinicians should always inquire about a history of fever given that it alludes to a secondary cause, namely infectious causes like upper respiratory tract infections or meningitis. If fever is present, symptoms hinting at a specific infectious focus should be sought, and clinicians should be particularly vigilant about identifying historical elements that are congruent with treatable infectious etiologies, such as bacterial meningitis, herpes encephalitis, sinusitis, and streptococcal pharyngitis. Constitutional symptoms may herald the presence of an underlying malignancy. Although emesis is often seen as a red flag and does occur at a relatively high frequency in children presenting with brain tumors [24], it occurs with both primary and secondary headaches presenting to the pediatric ED at similar frequencies [5]. However, a history of early-morning vomiting should be considered a red flag as it is often reported in children with brain tumors, especially among those with infratentorial masses [22].

# The Comprehensive Physical Exam in Pediatric ED Patients with Headache

## The General Physical Exam

The general physical exam adds value to the assessment of the pediatric headache patient given that it provides clues to ruling in or out a secondary headache etiology.

## Vital Signs

Vital signs should be scrutinized for the presence of fever and tachycardia, which can occur with infection. Hypertension is an uncommon cause of pediatric headache in the ED [2,5,8], but blood pressure should always be assessed to rule out this treatable etiology. Many times the hypertension in the pediatric patient is due to pain or anxiety and should be reassessed before investigating for increased intracranial pressure or renal disease. Patients with dizziness or syncope should have orthostatic vitals measured in order to assess for the possibility of POTS. The combination of bradycardia, hypertension, and erratic respirations (i.e., Cushing's triad) is a major red flag for severely elevated ICP in certain patients, such as patients with headache and a ventriculoperitoneal (VP) shunt, altered level of consciousness, or papilledema.

Weight should be measured as it can be relevant in particular situations, namely with suspected idiopathic intracranial hypertension, which is often associated with obesity, or with suspected spontaneous intracranial hypotension, which has a higher incidence among patients with connective tissues disorders like Marfan's syndrome [20], whereby the patient may be tall and thin.

## Head and Neck Exam

The head and neck exam is pertinent where secondary etiologies are suspected. In the patient with periorbital, orbital, or retroorbital headache, the eyes and the periorbital area should be carefully examined for signs of infection, namely local erythema, edema, proptosis, and limited extraocular movements on the affected side, because orbital cellulitis and other infections in the area can present with headache, usually with pain in or around the affected orbit. Autonomic signs, such as conjunctival injection, tearing, and anisocoria should also be sought in these patients because the trigeminal autonomic cephalalgias (i.e., cluster headache, paroxysmal hemicrania, etc.) [17], although rare in the pediatric population, are a diagnostic possibility once secondary etiologies are excluded in patients with severe pain in the supraorbital, orbital, or temporal areas. In patients with recent head trauma, the clinician must search for signs of a basal skull fracture including periorbital hematoma (raccoon eyes), retromastoid hematoma (Battle's sign), CSF otorrhea, or rhinorrhea and epistaxis.

In febrile patients, the tympanic membrane should be examined for signs of acute otitis media, namely bulging, effusion, otorrhea, and erythema. In patients with fever and head pain in the area of the mastoid, the clinician should consider mastoiditis and examine for protrusion of the auricle, local erythema, tenderness, and edema in the skin overlying the mastoid. Because sinusitis is a relatively common cause of pediatric headache in the ED [3,5,7], the face should be palpated for sinus tenderness and the nose examined for purulent discharge in patients with fever and headache. In patients with suspected upper respiratory tract infections, nasal congestion and discharge should be sought in addition to a detailed exam of the oropharynx for tonsillar erythema, exudates, and edema, as well as a neck exam for cervical adenopathy.

In post-traumatic headache, if the cervical spine is stable and has been cleared without concerns for fracture or ligamentous injury, the neck should be examined for signs of cervicogenic headache [17], namely localized pain in the cervical spine or surrounding tissues with provocative range of motion maneuvers or with palpation. In patients with occipital headache and no identified secondary etiology, one can palpate the greater occipital nerve, just lateral and inferior to the external occipital protuberance, for point tenderness, which can be seen in occipital neuralgia [17]. Both patients with cervicogenic headache and occipital neuralgia should be identified if possible as treatment strategies should be targeted (e.g., referral for nerve block).

## Cardiovascular and Respiratory Exams

Cardiac cephalalgia, where headache occurs in the context of myocardial ischemia [17], is rare even in the adult population [28]. However, a cardiac exam may be helpful in assessing select patients with suspected secondary causes of headache. For example, if the clinician suspects headache in the context of stroke, then auscultation for heart murmurs and carotid bruits becomes relevant as these signs may hint at underlying stroke risk factors like congenital heart disease or carotid dissection. However, the practitioner should understand that this is a rare cause of pediatric headache.

The respiratory exam becomes important when the patient presents with fever, headache, and respiratory symptoms, as it is a crucial part of the examination in suspected respiratory tract infections.

## Musculoskeletal and Dermatologic Exams

The musculoskeletal exam is unlikely to assist in narrowing the differential diagnosis in this patient population unless they are complaining of diffuse myalgias that can be seen with viral syndromes and referred to the head musculature. In cases of suspected spontaneous intracranial hypotension, one should search for signs in keeping with diagnostic criteria for connective tissue disorders like Marfan's syndrome and Ehler–Danlos syndrome, such as hypermobile joints.

The dermatologic exam is also unlikely to help pinpoint a specific etiology. Patients with meningitis may present with rash, especially petechiael rash [26], but there should be other clues on the history and physical exam to suggest this diagnostic possibility. Cases with suspected hydrocephalus of unknown etiology should have a dermatologic exam to search for neurocutaneous stigmata, as patients with tuberous sclerosis and neurofibromatosis can present with hydrocephalus.

# The Neurologic Exam

The neurologic exam is crucial to the assessment of the headache patient. Although in most circumstances, a targeted neurologic exam is appropriate, there may be certain pediatric headache patients that warrant a comprehensive neurologic exam in the ED. This can be the most important part of the ED encounter in order to serve as a branch point for primary vs. secondary headache, and should not be overlooked.

## The Mental Status Exam

The age of the patient may limit the clinician's ability to perform a detailed mental status exam. At minimum, one should assess whether the patient appears to be behaving as expected for age and baseline neurocognitive status. Altered level of consciousness is a red flag for serious underlying headache etiologies such as meningitis [26]. Most primary headache disorders will appear in children older than seven years of age, who should be able to answer basic questions. However, due to anxiety in the medical setting, children may be shy and a parent may serve as a great resource to assist the provider in determining whether the child's behavior is usual or not.

## The Cranial Nerve Exam

A cranial nerve exam is essential in the assessment of the pediatric headache patient. Special attention should be paid to the optic nerve, where one should do a careful assessment of the pupils, visual acuity, visual fields, and a careful fundoscopic exam to rule out disk edema or pallor. Disk edema constitutes a significant red flag as it can represent papilledema, which is caused by increased intracranial pressure, usually secondary to a space-occupying lesion or idiopathic intracranial hypertension in the headache patient. Optic disk pallor is also a red flag because it may be secondary to optic atrophy, which can in turn herald an intracranial mass, especially in the setting

of neurofibromatosis and optic nerve gliomas [24] or masses compressing the optic nerve. Where the clinician is not confident in their fundoscopy skills and there is suspicion of an intracranial process, one must consult a colleague who can examine the fundi with confidence. A thorough assessment of eye movements (i.e., oculomotor, trochlear, and abducens nerves) is also required as abnormalities in smooth pursuit, saccades, vergence movements, or the presence of pathological nystagmus not only will compel the clinician to consider neuroimaging but may also assist in precise localization in certain instances.

The remainder of the cranial nerves (i.e., trigeminal, facial, vestibulocochlear, glossopharyngeal, vagus, accessory, and hypoglossal) should be assessed with a screening exam, or more thoroughly if any red flags are present. One can assess the cranial nerves fairly rapidly as such:

- Trigeminal nerve: Assess facial sensation in the $V_1$, $V_2$, and $V_3$ distributions. Assess whether or not the patient can bite down with strength, which involves the innervation of the masseter muscles.
- Facial nerve: Assess facial symmetry in the upper and lower face on inspection of the face at rest and with provocative facial movements. Unilateral upper motor neuron lesions of the facial nerve will yield weakness in only the lower half of the face as the frontalis and orbicularis oculi muscles, which respectively control forehead movement and eyelid closure, receive bilateral innervation from their upper motor neurons.
- Vestibulocochlear nerve: It is difficult to accurately assess the vestibulocochlear nerve. In this setting, a quick hearing screen is sufficient unless there are symptoms consistent with vestibular disease (e.g., vertigo). The clinician can simply rub his or her fingers together at a distance from the patient and assess whether or not the patient can hear the rubbing sound.
- Glossopharyngeal and vagus nerves: The glossopharyngeal and vagus nerves are appropriately assessed together on a screening cranial nerve exam. The clinician illuminates the oropharynx and asks the patient to say "Awe" while watching the movement of the soft palate and uvula, which normally move upwards simultaneously and symmetrically. It is also appropriate to assess a gag reflex if the patient

**117**

has altered mental status and cannot comply with commands.

- Accessory nerve: On a screening exam, the clinician can assess either the trapezius (shoulder elevation) or the sternocleidomastoid (neck rotation) and compare the bulk and strength of the muscles on each side.
- Glossopharyngeal nerve: In this setting, the glossopharyngeal nerve can be quickly examined by asking the patient to protrude their tongue, while observing for tongue deviation.

### The Motor Exam

A screening motor exam should be carried out in pediatric headache patients. Abnormalities in muscle bulk, tone, or power, when compared to the contralateral homologous muscle groups, constitute red flags and require further assessment. Deep tendon reflexes should also be assessed for their presence, magnitude, and symmetry.

### The Sensory Exam

Except in particular circumstances, the sensory exam is unlikely to be of high yield in the assessment of pediatric patients with headache and has limited validity in younger pediatric patients. In the headache patient with ataxia, the clinician should conduct a sensory exam in order to differentiate cerebellar ataxia from sensory ataxia. The Romberg test, where the patient is asked to stand with their feet together and close their eyes, is helpful in this regard as the patient with cerebellar ataxia will have difficulty maintaining this position regardless of visual input, whereas the patient with sensory ataxia will become unsteady only when their eyes are closed and visual input is removed.

### The Coordination Exam

The clinician should carry out a coordination exam, especially because of the fact that infratentorial brain tumors are the most common type of pediatric brain tumor [24] and these patients tend to have cerebellar ataxia. Dysmetria can be highlighted on finger-to-nose or heel-to-shin testing. One can also assess rapid alternating movements in a variety of ways, and lower limb appendicular as well as truncal ataxia will become evident, unless subtle, when observing tandem gait. Subtle ataxia can be elicited with more challenging cerebellar testing, such as with the precision finger tap test, where the patient taps the tip of their index finger against their thumb's interphalangeal joint at a high and consistent frequency [29].

### The Gait Exam

The patient's gait should be observed, especially for ataxia, given the commonality of infratentorial brain tumors in children.

### Signs of Meningism

Headache is a common presenting complaint with meningitis, and for this reason the clinician should assess for meningeal irritation in pediatric patients presenting with headache and fever. Kernig's sign is positive when extension of the knee, while the hip is maintained in 90° of flexion, elicits pain. Brudzinski's sign is positive when the patient's knees flex in response to elevation of the head off the bed while the patient is supine. Although the Kernig and Brudzinski signs are the classical tests for assessment of meningism, they lack sensitivity in assessing pediatric patients with suspected meningitis. In one study carried out among 112 children 16 years and under with suspected meningitis, nuchal rigidity appeared to be a more sensitive sign than the Kernig or Brudzinski signs (65 percent vs. 27 percent and 51 percent, respectively), but had inferior specificity (76 percent vs. 87 percent and 80 percent, respectively) [30] when compared to the gold standard of CSF pleocytosis. It is important to note that the vast majority of cases in this study had aseptic meningitis as opposed to bacterial meningitis. Therefore, if the clinician's pre-test probability of meningitis is high enough, the diagnosis of meningitis should be pursued even if the patient lacks signs of meningeal irritation on exam.

# The Screening History and Physical Exam in Pediatric ED Patients with Headache

The previous section provides a detailed overview of a comprehensive headache history and physical exam for children and adolescents presenting with headache. Many of the elements of the above history and physical exam will not be required for every case of headache presenting to the pediatric ED. Several components of the assessment are, however, necessary in all cases as part of a screening assessment in the ED setting. The screening history and physical exam described below is based on clinical experience, standard clinical practice, as well as recommendations made in the American College of Emergency Physicians Policy for the Initial Approach to Adolescents and

Adults Presenting to the Emergency Department with a Chief Complaint of Headache [31].

## The Screening History in Pediatric ED Patients with Headache

In assessing the child or adolescent with headache, one must determine the headache characteristics: onset, progression, duration, frequency, timing, location, quality, severity, aggravating and alleviating factors, associated symptoms, and whether any aura or prodrome was present. In this process, it is imperative that the clinician identifies headache characteristics that constitute red flags (refer to Figure 11.1). In addition to the red flags that will be elicited from the questions above (e.g., thunderclap onset, occipital location), clinicians should specifically inquire about headaches that are associated with worsening with the Valsalva maneuver. A review of systems should include questions about mental status changes, focal neurologic symptoms, constitutional symptoms, sinus disease, respiratory symptoms, nausea and vomiting (including the timing of the vomiting given that consistent morning vomiting is a red flag). Past medical history should be sought and the clinician should ask about a personal history of primary headache, head trauma, VP shunt, congenital heart disease, hypertension, coagulopathy, immunodeficiency, rheumatologic disease, pregnancy, and substance abuse. A history of current medications should be elicited

and the patient should be questioned about medications taken at home to relieve the pain. The family history can be tailored based on the clinical presentation.

## The Screening Physical Exam in Pediatric ED Patients with Headache

In the ED setting, the aim of the physical exam in children and adolescents presenting with headache is to uncover red flags and clues as to the headache's etiology. Vital signs should be taken with a focus on temperature and blood pressure. A screening general medical exam should include at minimum: (1) a head and neck exam to look for signs of meningism, dental infection, otitis media, upper respiratory tract infection, sinusitis, and stigmata of head trauma; (2) a cardiac exam to rule out heart murmur; and (3) a respiratory exam to search for signs of lower respiratory tract infection.

A screening neurologic exam must be performed. Depending on the history obtained, a more detailed neurologic exam may be necessary. At minimum, each component of the neurologic exam should be assessed in a screening fashion. Mental status can be rapidly assessed through interaction with the patient to determine if their behavior is age-appropriate and to ensure that the level of consciousness is intact. If the patient is verbal, a screening assessment of expressive and receptive language is carried out simply by taking the history. A screening cranial nerve exam is appropriate (Figure 11.2) if no focal deficits are otherwise

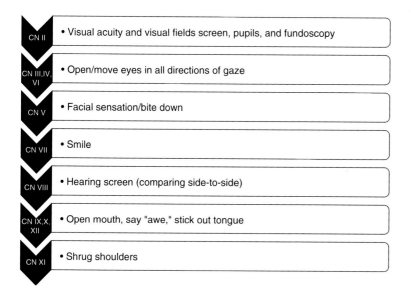

**Figure 11.2** Rapid cranial nerve (CN) exam.

CN II • Visual acuity and visual fields screen, pupils, and fundoscopy

CN III,IV, VI • Open/move eyes in all directions of gaze

CN V • Facial sensation/bite down

CN VII • Smile

CN VIII • Hearing screen (comparing side-to-side)

CN IX,X, XII • Open mouth, say "awe," stick out tongue

CN XI • Shrug shoulders

identified. The motor exam can be done fairly rapidly by comparing the right and left sides of the body in terms of muscle tone, power, and deep tendon reflexes, focusing on any asymmetries. The sensory exam is unreliable in younger children, but a Romberg test can be helpful in differentiating sensory ataxia from cerebellar ataxia. The coordination exam should include a screen for dysmetria with finger–nose testing and assessment of rapid alternating movements. While assessing the gait, the clinician will also be able to identify gait ataxia.

## Diagnostics

A frequent dilemma in the ED is whether a child presenting with headache needs a more extensive workup or can be treated as a primary headache disorder where there are no other etiologies of note. The history and physical exam are the best indicators of an underlying secondary issue. However, overuse and misuse of diagnostic testing is an ongoing problem in the ED. A national study showed that approximately one-third of pediatric patients evaluated in EDs underwent CT imaging [6]. This is concerning as patients with primary headache disorders do not need imaging, and with other etiologies being relatively rare, this trend is exposing a lot of children to ionizing radiation that they most likely do not warrant and increases the risk of malignancy later in life [32]. A lumbar puncture must be considered when central nervous system infections such as encephalitis or meningitis are on the differential diagnosis. The sample should be sent for cell counts, protein, glucose, culture, and specific viral testing depending on the scenario or season (e.g., herpes simplex virus, enterovirus). A lumbar puncture with manometry will also be an essential component of the diagnostic assessment in a patient where idiopathic intracranial hypertension (formerly known as pseudotumor cerebri) is being considered. The decision regarding whether or not to obtain imaging prior to the lumbar puncture is dictated by the history and physical exam. In patients with mental status changes, focal neurologic deficits, vital sign changes consistent with increased intracranial pressure, or disk edema on fundoscopic exam, clinicians should consider imaging prior to the procedure to prevent brain herniation; although this is incredibly rare and limited to case reports [33].

The use and appropriateness of neuroimaging in the acute setting is a frequent area of debate, especially with the advent of newer imaging modalities such as rapid brain magnetic resonance imaging (MRI) and its use in non-VP shunt indications, a practice that is currently uncommon, but associated with growing interest [34]. The most common reason that providers decide to obtain imaging is to rule out a space-occupying lesion. However, imaging in the setting of a normal physical exam is of very low yield [35–37]. The most common brain malignancies in the pediatric population are posterior fossa masses. However, a major limitation of CT is inadequate visualization of the posterior fossa and therefore a negative head CT does not rule out a lesion in this area. Thus, patients with suspected malignancy are better served with an MRI, but these are generally not available emergently. MRIs are also useful as sequences can be added to evaluate the venous and arterial systems in order to rule out vascular malformations or cerebral sinus venous thrombosis. Another significant benefit of this test as compared to CT is the absence of radiation exposure. The strongest indications for considering neuroimaging in the ED include altered mental status, focal neurologic deficits, seizures, or other objective findings of an intracranial lesion.

# Treatment of Primary Headaches in Pediatric ED Patients

## Treatment of Tension-Type Headaches in Pediatric ED Patients

There are no randomized controlled trials (RCTs) assessing interventions for the acute treatment of TTH in pediatric patients presenting to the ED. In fact, there is insufficient evidence to label any medication for acute TTH treatment as evidence-based in the pediatric population.

There is one three-arm RCT that compared the efficacy of solubilized ibuprofen to that of acetaminophen and placebo in a group of patients over the age of 12 with moderate to severe TTH. Patients randomized to solubilized (liquigel) ibuprofen had more rapid pain relief and higher rates of pain freedom within three hours of medication administration as compared to the acetaminophen and placebo groups. However, the number of adolescents in the trial is not reported and it is unclear as to whether there may have been differential efficacy among this subgroup [38].

Several pharmacologic interventions appear to be effective in the acute treatment of TTH in adults.

The European Federation of Neurological Societies (EFNS) released guidelines on the treatment of adult TTH in 2010. The guideline authors concluded that the following medications had level A evidence (established as effective by at least one class I study or two class II studies, defined using EFNS criteria [39]) for efficacy in the treatment of acute TTH in adults: acetaminophen, aspirin, diclofenac, ibuprofen, ketoprofen, and naproxen. Combination medications with caffeine were recommended for use, but only had B level evidence (probably effective based on at least one "convincing" class II study or class III evidence that is "overwhelming") [40]. A variety of other medications, such as chlorpromazine, ketorolac, metamizole, and prochlorperazine, have been assessed for the acute treatment of TTH in adults, but only in limited studies with small sample sizes. A recent systematic review on parenteral treatments for acute TTH in adults only identified eight small studies that met eligibility criteria ($N = 486$ patients in total) and found some, albeit limited, evidence for the efficacy and safety of chlorpromazine, metamizole, and metoclopramide in this setting [41].

Therefore, there is a paucity of data to assist the clinician treating pediatric patients presenting to the ED with TTH. The current approach to treating acute TTH in children derives largely from clinical experience and from the adult literature. Typically, simple analgesic medications administered orally, namely ibuprofen and acetaminophen, are first-line in this setting. Other options include nonsteroidal anti-inflammatory medications other than ibuprofen, such as naproxen and diclofenac.

## Treatment of Pediatric Migraine

The most common primary headaches encountered in the ED are migraine headaches. Therefore, a strong understanding of appropriate acute care is vital. An alarming finding was recently reported in a nationally representative study: approximately 30 percent of children presenting to EDs with headache received opioid medications [6]. The American Academy of Neurology recommends against the use of opioids for treating migraines due to their potential to turn episodic migraine into chronic migraine and the risk of medication overuse headache [42]. In addition, a recent study found that adolescents with headache who had an ED visit in the follow-up period were more likely to use opioids as compared to adolescents

with headache who had not had an ED visit [43]. There are many potential reasons for this association, but it is likely that a proportion of these patients are introduced to opioids in the ED setting and subsequently develop a chronic-use pattern and in some cases opioid abuse. Therefore, ED practitioners must avoid using opioids in migraine patients for the reasons outlined above.

There is a paucity of evidence to guide practitioners in choosing medications to treat migraine in the pediatric ED setting. The best-studied agents in the acute treatment of pediatric migraine include nonsteroidal anti-inflammatories and dopamine antagonists [44,45]. Previous pediatric migraine review papers have provided treatment algorithms that can be useful in the ED [46]. Because of the lack of evidence, there is a significant amount of practice variation from ED to ED in terms of migraine management in children and adolescents [47]. Most providers utilize a cocktail as their first-line treatment, consisting of a nonsteroidal anti-inflammatory such as ketorolac, a dopamine antagonist such as prochlorperazine or metoclopramide, coupled with diphenhydramine to prevent extrapyramidal symptoms/signs, and intravenous fluids [48]. Triptans are one of the few FDA-approved medications for acute pediatric migraine. Their use in the ED setting should be considered based on adult evidence [49] and non-ED-based pediatric evidence [50]. However, in some instances patients with a triptan prescription have already taken a triptan at home and present to the ED beyond the initial hours of the headache, the period during which triptans appear to be the most effective, thus precluding their use [51]. There is no evidence on how to approach the pediatric migraine patient who fails first-line agents. However, new therapies are being investigated for the ED setting, including low-dose propofol, sodium valproate, and magnesium [52–54]. It is important to always avoid opioids in this setting, and to consider admission to hospital when the headache is unrelenting and attempts at first- and second-line therapy are unsuccessful.

## Treatment of Other Primary Headache Disorders in Pediatric ED Patients

The trigeminal autonomic cephalalgias (TACs) are a group of primary headache disorders comprising cluster headache, paroxysmal hemicrania, the short-lasting unilateral neuralgiform headaches, and hemicrania continua [17]. The TACs are exceedingly rare in the pediatric population, and evidence for how to approach acute treatment in this population is severely lacking [55]. Paroxysmal hemicrania and the short-lasting neuralgiform headaches are comprised of very short-lived attacks and do not typically present to the ED requiring acute therapy. The headache of hemicrania continua has a duration of greater than three months by definition [17]. Therefore, patients with suspected hemicrania continua are very unlikely to present to the ED, and if they do they should be referred to a pediatric neurologist. Cluster headache is exquisitely painful and can last up to 180 minutes [17]. There are no controlled studies on the acute treatment of cluster headache in the pediatric population, but case reports have provided preliminary evidence for the efficacy of oxygen, sumatriptan, and aspirin [56]. Because of its established efficacy in the adult literature and its safety, inhalation of high-flow 100 percent oxygen for 15–30 minutes via a non-rebreather mask should be used first-line for pediatric patients presenting to the ED with cluster headache [50]. In addition, patients who present to the ED with suspected TACs should be referred to a pediatric neurologist for further assessment and management.

Other types of primary headaches, such as primary cough headache, primary exercise headache, and nummular headache are rarely seen in the ED. For the most part, they require thorough assessment to rule out secondary causes and referral to pediatric neurology. It is beyond the scope of this text to discuss the management of each of these primary headaches, and evidence for acute therapy in the pediatric population is minimal for most of these disorders.

## Conclusion

Headache is a very common chief complaint in the ED. The majority of children and adolescents presenting to the ED with headache will have a non-life-threatening underlying cause. Primary headaches are common in the ED, and pediatric migraine is the most common of the primary headaches seen in this setting. A targeted history and physical exam is essential in guiding the ED practitioner to an appropriate management plan. Further investigations are indicated in some scenarios, but it is important to use these resources judiciously as they are unnecessary in the majority of cases. There is a severe lack of evidence to guide clinicians in choosing acute pain interventions

for children and adolescents presenting to the ED with primary headaches. Hopefully, future studies will explore acute interventions for pediatric primary headaches in the ED, as this area of research has been neglected thus far.

## References

1. Abu-Arafeh I, Razak S, Sivaraman B, Graham C. Prevalence of headache and migraine in children and adolescents: a systematic review of population-based studies. *Dev Med Child Neurol* 2010;52(12):1088–97.

2. Kan L, Nagelberg J, Maytal J. Headaches in a pediatric emergency department: etiology, imaging, and treatment. *Headache*. 2000;40(1):25–9.

3. Burton LJ, Quinn B, Pratt-Cheney JL, Pourani M. Headache etiology in a pediatric emergency department. *Pediatr Emerg Care*. 1997;13(1):1–4.

4. Hsiao H-J, Huang J-L, Hsia S-H, et al. Headache in the pediatric emergency service: a medical center experience. *Pediatr Neonatol*. 2014;55(3):208–12.

5. Conicella E, Raucci U, Vanacore N, et al. The child with headache in a pediatric emergency department. *Headache*. 2008;48(7):1005–11.

6. Sheridan DC, Meckler GD, Spiro DM, Koch TK, Hansen ML. Diagnostic testing and treatment of pediatric headache in the emergency department. *J Pediatr*. 2013;163(6):1634–7.

7. Lewis DW, Qureshi F. Acute headache in children and adolescents presenting to the emergency department. *Headache*. 2000;40(3):200–3.

8. Scagni P, Pagliero R. Headache in an Italian pediatric emergency department. *J Headache Pain*. 2008;9(2):83–7.

9. Lee TT, Uribe J, Ragheb J, Morrison G, Jagid JR. Unique clinical presentation of pediatric shunt malfunction. *Pediatr Neurosurg*. 1999;30(3):122–6.

10. Kedia S, Ginde A, Grubenhoff J, et al. Monthly variation of United States pediatric headache emergency department visits. *Cephalalgia*. 2014;34(6):473–8.

11. Caperell K, Pitetti R. Seasonal variation of presentation for headache in a pediatric emergency department. *Pediatr Emerg Care*. 2014;30(3):174–6.

12. Soriani S, Fiumana E, Manfredini R, et al. Circadian and seasonal variation of migraine attacks in children. *Headache*. 2006;46(10):1571–4.

13. Lanphear J, Sarnaik S. Presenting symptoms of pediatric brain tumors diagnosed in the emergency department. *Pediatr Emerg Care*. 2014;30(2):77–80.

14. Medina LS, Kuntz KM, Pomeroy S. Children with headache suspected of having a brain tumor: a cost-effectiveness analysis of diagnostic strategies. *Pediatrics.* 2001;108(2):255–63.

15. Yock-Corrales A, Babl FE, Mosley IT, Mackay MT. Can the FAST and ROSIER adult stroke recognition tools be applied to confirmed childhood arterial ischemic stroke? *BMC Pediatr.* 2011;11(1):93.

16. Edgeworth J, Bullock P, Bailey A, Gallagher A, Crouchman M. Why are brain tumours still being missed? *Arch Dis Child.* 1996;74(2):148–51.

17. Headache Classification Committee of the International Headache Society (IHS). The International Classification of Headache Disorders, 3rd edition (beta version). *Cephalalgia.* 2013;33(9):629–808.

18. Pacheva I, Milanov I, Ivanov I, Stefanov R. Evaluation of diagnostic and prognostic value of clinical characteristics of migraine and tension type headache included in the diagnostic criteria for children and adolescents in International Classification of Headache Disorders: second edition. *Int J Clin Pract.* 2012;66(12):1168–77.

19. Trottier ED, Bailey B, Lucas N, Lortie A. Diagnosis of migraine in the pediatric emergency department. *Pediatr Neurol.* 2013;49(1):40–5.

20. Schievink WI, Maya MM, Louy C, Moser FG, Sloninsky L. Spontaneous intracranial hypotension in childhood and adolescence. *J Pediatr.* 2013;163(2):504–10.

21. Heyer GL, Fedak EM, LeGros AL. Symptoms predictive of postural tachycardia syndrome (POTS) in the adolescent headache patient. *Headache.* 2013;53(6):947–53.

22. Reulecke BC, Erker CG, Fiedler BJ, Niederstadt T-U, Kurlemann G. Brain tumors in children: initial symptoms and their influence on the time span between symptom onset and diagnosis. *J Child Neurol.* 2008;23(2):178–83.

23. Ansell P, Johnston T, Simpson J, et al. Brain tumor signs and symptoms: analysis of primary health care records from the UKCCS. *Pediatrics.* 2010;125(1):112–19.

24. Wilne S, Collier J, Kennedy C, et al. Presentation of childhood CNS tumours: a systematic review and meta-analysis. *Lancet Oncol.* 2007;8(8):685–95.

25. Wilne SH, Ferris RC, Nathwani A, Kennedy CR. The presenting features of brain tumours: a review of 200 cases. *Arch Dis Child.* 2006;91(6):502–6.

26. Thompson M, Van den Bruel A, Verbakel J, et al. Systematic review and validation of prediction rules for identifying children with serious infections in emergency departments and urgent-access primary care. *Health Technol Assess Winch Engl.* 2012;16(15):1–100. doi:10.3310/hta16150.

27. Michos AG, Syriopoulou VP, Hadjichristodoulou C, et al. Aseptic meningitis in children: analysis of 506 cases. *PLoS One.* 2007;2(7):e674.

28. Wei J-H, Wang H-F. Cardiac cephalalgia: case reports and review. *Cephalalgia.* 2008;28(8):892–6.

29. Blumenfeld H. An interactive guide to the neurologic examination. Sinaeur Assoc Publ Inc. 2010. Available at: www.neuroexam.com/neuroexam/index.php.

30. Amarilyo G, Alper A, Ben-Tov A, Grisaru-Soen G. Diagnostic accuracy of clinical symptoms and signs in children with meningitis. *Pediatr Emerg Care.* 2011;27(3):196–9. doi:10.1097/PEC.0b013e31820d6543.

31. American College of Emergency Physicians. Clinical policy for the initial approach to adolescents and adults presenting to the emergency department with a chief complaint of headache. *Ann Emerg Med.* 1996;27(6):821–44.

32. Miglioretti DL, Johnson E, Williams A, et al. The use of computed tomography in pediatrics and the associated radiation exposure and estimated cancer risk. *JAMA Pediatr.* 2013;167(8):700–7.

33. Hoffman KR, Chan SW, Hughes AR, Halcrow SJ. Management of cerebellar tonsillar herniation following lumbar puncture in idiopathic intracranial hypertension. *Case Rep Crit Care.* 2015;2015:895035.

34. Thompson EM, Baird LC, Selden NR. Results of a North American survey of rapid-sequence MRI utilization to evaluate cerebral ventricles in children. *J Neurosurg Pediatr.* 2014;13(6):636–40.

35. Dooley JM, Camfield PR, O'Neill M, Vohra A. The value of CT scans for children with headaches. *Can J Neurol Sci.* 1990;17(3):309–10.

36. Maytal J, Bienkowski RS, Patel M, Eviatar L. The value of brain imaging in children with headaches. *Pediatrics.* 1995;96(3 Pt 1):413–16.

37. Medina LS, Pinter JD, Zurakowski D, et al. Children with headache: clinical predictors of surgical space-occupying lesions and the role of neuroimaging. *Radiology.* 1997;202(3):819–24.

38. Packman B, Packman E, Doyle G, et al. Solubilized ibuprofen: evaluation of onset, relief, and safety of a novel formulation in the treatment of episodic tension-type headache. *Headache.* 2000;40(7):561–7.

39. Brainin M, Barnes M, Baron J-C, et al. Guidance for the preparation of neurological management guidelines by EFNS scientific task forces: revised recommendations 2004. *Eur J Neurol.* 2004;11(9):577–81. doi:10.1111/j.1468-1331.2004.00867.x.

40. Bendtsen L, Evers S, Linde M, et al. EFNS guideline on the treatment of tension-type headache: report of an EFNS task force. *Eur J Neurol*. 2010;17(11):1318–25.

41. Weinman D, Nicastro O, Akala O, Friedman BW. Parenteral treatment of episodic tension-type headache: a systematic review. *Headache*. 2014;54(2):260–8.

42. Langer-Gould AM, Anderson WE, Armstrong MJ, et al. The American Academy of Neurology's top five choosing wisely recommendations. *Neurology*. 2013;81(11):1004–11.

43. DeVries A, Koch T, Wall E, et al. Opioid use among adolescent patients treated for headache. *J Adolesc Health*. 2014;55(1):128–33.

44. Brousseau DC, Duffy SJ, Anderson AC, Linakis JG. Treatment of pediatric migraine headaches: a randomized, double-blind trial of prochlorperazine versus ketorolac. *Ann Emerg Med*. 2004;43(2):256–62.

45. Trottier ED, Bailey B, Dauphin-Pierre S, Gravel J. Clinical outcomes of children treated with intravenous prochlorperazine for migraine in a pediatric emergency department. *J Emerg Med*. 2010;39(2):166–73.

46. Sheridan DC, Spiro DM, Meckler GD. Pediatric migraine: abortive management in the emergency department. *Headache*. 2014;54(2):235–45.

47. Richer L, Graham L, Klassen T, Rowe B. Emergency department management of acute migraine in children in Canada: a practice variation study. *Headache*. 2007;47(5):703–10.

48. Leung S, Bulloch B, Young C, Yonker M, Hostetler M. Effectiveness of standardized combination therapy for migraine treatment in the pediatric emergency department. *Headache*. 2013;53(3):491–7.

49. Orr SL, Aubé M, Becker WJ, et al. Canadian Headache Society systematic review and recommendations on the treatment of migraine pain in emergency settings. *Cephalalgia*. 2014;35(3):271–84.

50. Evers S. The efficacy of triptans in childhood and adolescence migraine. *Curr Pain Headache Rep*. 2013;17(7):342.

51. D'Amico D, Moschiano F, Bussone G. Early treatment of migraine attacks with triptans: a strategy to enhance outcomes and patient satisfaction? *Expert Rev Neurother*. 2006;6:1087–97.

52. Sheridan DC, Spiro DM, Nguyen T, Koch TK, Meckler GD. Low-dose propofol for the abortive treatment of pediatric migraine in the emergency department. *Pediatr Emerg Care*. 2012;28(12):1293–6.

53. Gertsch E, Loharuka S, Wolter-Warmerdam K, et al. Intravenous magnesium as acute treatment for headaches: a pediatric case series. *J Emerg Med*. 2014;46(2):308–12.

54. Sheridan D, Sun B, O'Brien P, Hansen M. Intravenous sodium valproate for acute pediatric headache. *J Emerg Med*. 2015;49(4):541–5.

55. Lambru G, Matharu M. Management of trigeminal autonomic cephalalgias in children and adolescents. *Curr Pain Headache Rep*. 2013;17(4):323.

56. Antonaci F, Alfei E, Piazza F, De Cillis I, Balottin U. Therapy-resistant cluster headache in childhood: case report and literature review. *Cephalalgia*. 2010;30(2):233–8.

# Chapter 12

# Approach to Pregnant or Lactating Patients with Headache in the Emergency Department

Sylvia Lucas
Esther Rawner

## Abstract

Most pregnant women with migraine improve during pregnancy, though migraine can resume following delivery and during breastfeeding. Since many women limit their exposure to drugs during pregnancy or breastfeeding, a migraine may be undertreated, become severe, refractory, and result in the need for an emergency department (ED) visit during this period. As with non-pregnant women, early management requires differentiation between primary and secondary headache, and though most headaches evaluated in the ED are migraines, some patients will need imaging or specialty consultation for this determination. Drug safety during pregnancy and lactation will limit the use of some drugs used in the treatment of migraine. Medications for acute treatment of refractory migraine in pregnant or lactating women are discussed and include dopamine antagonists, nonsteroidal anti-inflammatory medications, magnesium, opioids, triptans, and corticosteroids. Recommendations for medication use are made on the basis of risk of the drug to a pregnant woman or nursing infant and evidence for efficacy in the ED population.

## Natural History of Primary Headaches During Pregnancy and Postpartum

The peak prevalence of migraine occurs during a woman's reproductive years, with approximately one in five women experiencing episodic moderate to severe headache [1]. Migraine frequency typically decreases early in pregnancy, with approximately half of pregnant women with migraine improving during the first trimester and up to 87 percent during the third trimester [2,3]. Only 3–7 percent of women note the onset of new migraine during pregnancy, typically occurring during the first trimester [4,5].

Despite improvement during pregnancy, migraines usually recur after delivery. At least half of women experience recurrence of migraine attacks within the first month after delivery and at least two-thirds by six months. Until six months after delivery, women who are breastfeeding have a lower recurrence rate than if bottle-feeding [3].

Though improvement is likely to happen over the course of the first trimester, migraine does occur during early pregnancy, when fetal exposure to drugs during organogenesis may carry higher risk. Most women, after knowing of their pregnancy, attempt to minimize their exposure to medication or other potentially harmful substances such as alcohol, nicotine, and caffeine. They may go without any treatment at all for migraine or use non-pharmacologic treatment such as ice and sleep, or simple analgesics such as acetaminophen. Pregnant women with severe migraine come to the ED or urgent care center for the same reasons as those who are not pregnant. However, they may not have attempted treatment at home, given concern about medication use during pregnancy, or may have attempted to self-treat and found their therapy to be ineffective. In general, few ED patients have migraine-specific medications available as usual care. One study showed that up to 31 percent of men and 9 percent of women did not use any medication at all before presenting to an ED for headache [6]. In patients who come to the ED, pain may be severe or prolonged, unusual symptoms such as new aura or different pain characteristics that are frightening may be present, or vomiting may be so severe and refractory that the patient's usual medication cannot be absorbed. Hypovolemia, lightheadedness, or anorexia may be present. Patients may be so ill with a migraine attack that they are concerned for the health of their fetus. An ancillary benefit of seeking treatment is the resulting ease of mind regarding the health of the pregnancy.

General management of headache in the ED begins with triage, followed by clinician evaluation [7]. This is often an unpleasant experience for a patient in severe pain that may worsen with movement, who may be vomiting, and whose pain is significantly worsened by light and sound. However, the main responsibility of an ED provider is to determine whether a headache is primary or secondary. This may involve taking a history from the patient or accompanying friends or family members, a review of systems assessing possible risk factors for secondary headache such as weakness, diplopia, or paresthesias, review of any available past medical records, vital signs, an examination, and possibly further investigations if the headache is unusual or clinical suspicion is high for a secondary headache. If a woman is pregnant, the evaluation for secondary headaches includes pathology not found in the non-pregnant patient, and medications or procedures that may be used in other contexts may pose risk to the fetus. Approximately 60 percent of pregnancies are unplanned, and although methods of early pregnancy detection for home use are available, it may be several weeks into a pregnancy before its confirmation. Because of this, a pregnancy test should be strongly considered in any woman of reproductive years presenting to the ED with headache.

# Secondary Headaches in Pregnancy

Chapters 3–10 review the differential diagnosis of headache, physical exam findings, and investigations required when patients from the general population come to the ED with headache. Pregnant and early postpartum populations present a unique set of risks. Additionally, patients with primary headache disorders such as migraine may have independent risk factors for vascular complications of pregnancy and the early postpartum period. Conditions that may mimic migraine during pregnancy and postpartum include low-pressure headache following epidural/spinal anesthesia, eclampsia or pre-eclampsia, cerebral venous thrombosis, subarachnoid hemorrhage, pseudotumor cerebri, meningitis, or even brain tumors, particularly those which are stimulated by high progesterone or estrogen levels such as certain meningiomas [8].

Late pregnancy is a hypercoagulable state: fibrinolysis decreases, and platelet aggregability, fibrinogen, Factor 8, and von Willebrand factor increase during the third trimester, with an increased resistance to protein C inhibitor activity and a decrease in protein S concentration [9]. Pregnant women are four times more likely to develop venous thrombotic disease than non-pregnant women [10]. Additionally, the first six weeks postpartum show a 20–80-fold higher risk of venous thrombosis with a peak of 100-fold higher risk in the first week postpartum compared to the risk during pregnancy. Pregnancy-related stroke is most likely to occur during the third trimester and puerperium, with women at highest risk for ischemic stroke in the immediate postpartum period. Hemorrhagic stroke risk is elevated as well. A study of 2850 pregnancy-related discharges which also had a diagnosis of stroke showed that migraine was the medical condition most strongly associated with stroke (OR 16.9 [95 percent CI 9.7–29.5]). Stroke risk increased with age and gestational hypertension [11].

Hypertensive disorders of pregnancy complicate about 1 percent of pregnancies [12]. However, pregnant women with a history of migraine have a higher risk of developing hypertensive disorders, including pre-eclampsia and stroke, than those without migraine [13–15]. Increased risk for hypertension, pre-eclampsia, stroke, myocardial infarction, and pulmonary embolus are seen in women with migraine, with the greatest risk in older women with migraine and overweight women with migraine [13]. In one prospective cohort of 3373 women presenting to prenatal care clinics with no history of pre-gestational hypertension, mean third trimester systolic blood pressure (SBP; Δ 4.08 mmHg 95 percent CI 3.3–4.9), diastolic blood pressure (DBP; Δ 2.39 mmHg 95 percent CI 1.8–3.01), and mean arterial pressure (MAP; Δ 2.95 mmHg 95 percent CI 2.4–3.5) were higher in pregnant patients with a diagnosis of migraine compared to pregnant non-migraineurs. This study also found a 1.53-fold increased odds of pre-eclampsia (95 percent CI 1.09–2.16). However, overweight or obese migraineurs (compared to lean non-migraineurs) had a 6.10-fold increased odds of pre-eclampsia (95 percent CI 3.82–9.75) [16]. These findings are consistent with other reports of a 1.8–2.4-fold increase in risk of pre-eclampsia in migraineurs compared to controls [17,18].

The pregnant woman with a known history of migraine, if presenting to the ED with significant hypertension and headache, may have headache secondary to hypertension or, conversely, the headache may increase blood pressure as is often seen in migraine or other pain conditions. In this situation, careful management of hypertension and headache must be sought as the determination of primary or secondary etiology is being made. Hypertension in pregnancy is somewhat arbitrarily categorized according to severity, with mild hypertension defined as SBP > 140–159 mmHg or DBP > 90–100 mmHg, and severe hypertension defined as SBP > 160 mmHg and DBP > 100 mmHg. Though it is recommended that pregnant women with SBP > 150–160 mmHg and DBP > 100–110 mmHg be treated with medication to lower the pressure [19], because of the possibility that blood pressure is elevated due to pain in this particular population, the clinician can consider giving a pain treatment such as an opioid with mild elevations of blood pressure. If the elevated pressure is severe, giving an opioid is still warranted to treat the pain; however, concurrent treatment of blood pressure is necessary while paying close attention to the evolution of the headache, particularly if there is evidence of renal, central nervous system, hepatic, or other abnormalities. The antihypertensive of choice in the ED is labetalol, an alpha and beta adrenergic blocker. Labetalol can be given IV in 20–40 mg repeat boluses every 10–15 minutes to a maximum of 220 mg, has no known fetal or maternal adverse outcomes when used in pregnancy, and is safe during breastfeeding [20].

If there is clinical suspicion for secondary headache, particularly in the setting of hypertension or abnormal exam findings, initial evaluation would include a complete blood count, comprehensive metabolic panel, urinalysis, 24-hour urine protein assessment, uric acid, LDH, D-dimer, fibrinogen levels, and coagulation studies, though a complete discussion of the work-up of secondary headache is outside the scope of this chapter.

There have only been small retrospective studies of headache diagnosis in pregnant populations presenting to the hospital with headache. In one study of 140 pregnant patients presenting to a single acute care center with headache and receiving neurologic consultation, 56 percent of these women were in their third trimester and 35 percent were diagnosed with secondary headache [21]. In this study, of the 35 percent of patients who were diagnosed with secondary headache, 18 percent presented with hypertensive disorders that included pre-eclampsia, posterior reversible encephalopathy syndrome (PRES), eclampsia, hemolysis with elevated liver enzymes and low platelets (HELLP), arterial hypertension, and reversible cerebral vasoconstrictive syndrome (RCVS). In the remainder of the patients, there were equal diagnoses of cerebral venous thrombosis (CVT), infection, pituitary apoplexy, pneumocephalus, intracranial hemorrhage, and 5 percent had other etiologies.

In another retrospective review of a consecutive case series of 63 pregnant women emergently evaluated for headache, 27 percent of patients had an underlying intracranial etiology for their headache according to emergent neuroimaging. Of these 17 patients who had secondary headache as diagnosed with imaging, four had CVT, four had RCVS, two had idiopathic intracranial hypertension, two had intracranial hemorrhage, and eight had sinusitis. This study was done to investigate demographic and clinical features predictive of intracranial pathologic lesions on neuroimaging studies in pregnant women with emergent headaches and thus only looked at secondary diagnoses in those who had imaging. Key features in the patient history that suggested secondary headache during pregnancy were lack of prior history of headache, prolonged headache lasting longer than 72 hours, and presentation of headache in the third trimester [22].

Certain signs and symptoms may help to differentiate primary from secondary headaches. These signs include hypertension, fever, seizures, altered mental status, and an abnormal neurologic exam. In these two studies, seizure and fever were the only symptoms that presented exclusively in patients with secondary headache who had neuroimaging [21,22]. These studies reported that, in patients with a history of migraine, one feature often associated with secondary headache during pregnancy was a longer duration than the patient's usual headache. Otherwise, in both studies, the primary and secondary headache groups did not differ in presenting headache characteristics. Primary and secondary headaches were similar with regards to intensity of pain, associated phonophobia, nausea, and vomiting, thereby underscoring the need for a judicious assessment and a high clinical suspicion for secondary headaches in this population.

Although an abnormal neurologic exam should compel the clinician to investigate further, it lacks sensitivity. The absence of objective physical findings does

**Table 12.1** Secondary headache etiology in pregnant women presenting to acute care

| All women who received neurologic consultation [21] N = 140 | | All women who received emergent neuroimaging [22] N = 63 | |
| --- | --- | --- | --- |
| Diagnosis | Number (%) | Diagnosis | Number (%) |
| **Primary headache** | **91 (65%)** | **Primary headache** | **46 (73%)** |
| **Secondary headache** | **49 (35%)** | **Secondary headache** | **17 (27%)** |
| Pre-eclampsia | 19 (13.6%) | Sinusitis | 5 (8%) |
| PRES | 6 (4.3%) | Cerebral venous thrombosis | 4 (6%) |
| Pituitary apoplexy | 5 (3.6%) | PRES | 4 (6%) |
| Eclampsia | 4 (2.9%) | Intracranial hemorrhage | 2 (3%) |
| Intercurrent infection | 3 (2.1%) | Pseudotumor | 2 (3%) |
| Pneumocephalus | 3 (2.1%) | | |
| Cerebral venous thrombosis | 2 (1.4%) | | |
| HELLP | 2 (1.4%) | | |
| Ictal headache | 2 (1.4%) | | |
| Intracranial hemorrhage | 2 (1.4%) | | |
| Acute hypertension | 1 (0.7%) | | |
| AVM | 1 (0.7%) | | |
| Moya Moya with stroke | 1 (0.7%) | | |
| Postdural puncture | 1 (0.7%) | | |
| Retropharyngeal abscess | 1 (0.7%) | | |
| RCVS | 1 (0.7%) | | |
| Sickle cell crisis | 1 (0.7%) | | |

Percentages within each study may be greater than 100 percent because of possible multiple diagnoses.
See text for details of study populations.
AVM = arteriovenous malformation
HELLP = hemolysis, elevated liver enzymes, and low platelets
PRES = posterior reversible encephalopathy syndrome
RCVS = reversible cerebral vasoconstriction syndrome

not exclude the possibility of a secondary headache. In the Ramchandren et al. study, of the 17 patients with intracranial pathology on imaging, seven subjects had a normal neurologic exam (in 67 percent of subjects a neurologist was called for examination; the others had a neurologic exam documented by the ED physician). This study also revealed that pregnant patients with an abnormal neurologic exam were 2.7 times as likely to have secondary headache pathology on imaging as compared to pregnant patients with normal neurologic exams [22].

Risks of neuroimaging to a pregnant patient primarily concern fetal exposure to radiation or magnetic field strength, and an appropriate risk versus benefit judgment is necessary for each patient. If she is able to participate in a discussion of risk, informed consent should be obtained. Practice parameters are available from the American College of Radiology (ACR) and the American College of Obstetricians and Gynecologists (ACOG). MRI scans are preferable to CT scans. Overall, with radiation exposure under 5 rads, there is no known in-utero deterministic effect [23]. CT iodinated contrast dye is likely safe in pregnancy, but gadolinium should be avoided during pregnancy unless absolutely necessary [24].

In summary, there is a higher risk of secondary headaches in pregnant and early postpartum patients compared with non-pregnant patients. These populations warrant closer examination and a lower threshold for work-up and diagnosis of secondary headache. In pregnant and early postpartum patients presenting with headache, the clinician must ensure that the work-up is complete and that secondary headache has been ruled out. Clinical suspicion for a secondary headache should be high in the third trimester because primary headaches typically improve but vascular risk increases in the pregnant patient. Even during evaluation, treatment may be instituted with opioids and a dopamine receptor antagonist such as metoclopramide, avoiding medications that are vasoconstrictors such as triptans or NSAIDs.

# General Concepts in the Treatment of the Primary Headaches in the Pregnant or Lactating Patient

There are no evidence-based guidelines for migraine treatment during pregnancy or lactation. Data are limited due to a lack of clinical studies performed in pregnant and lactating women. In some observational reports, multiple drugs have been used during the pregnancy [25,26] or during lactation, further confusing interpretation.

Once it is established that a primary headache is being treated, the principles of ED treatment in the pregnant or lactating patient are similar to those applied to the treatment of non-pregnant or non-lactating patients, except that practitioners must remember they are treating the patient, as well as potentially exposing the fetus to treatment medications. This fact alone makes the judicious choice of medications extremely important, since the goal of making the patient pain-free is paralleled by the goal of doing no harm to the fetus or infant. Additionally, it is important to remember that prolonged severe associated symptoms such as vomiting can have direct negative effects on the fetus. Nausea and vomiting can be as unpleasant and disabling as is pain during a migraine, and possibly more frequent during the first trimester because of pregnancy itself. Most of the following discussion will be focused on treatment of migraine, since this is the most likely primary headache disorder to be treated in the ED setting.

Usually by the time a patient comes to the ED for care of a refractory headache, severe nausea and/or vomiting have occurred as well as reduced oral intake. Given this, the optimal medication delivery route is intravenous (IV), though in certain cases where IV access may be difficult due to hypovolemia, intramuscular or even rectal administration are reasonable alternatives. There is variability in the use of IV fluids (IVF) to treat severe headaches in many EDs,

and one large post-hoc analysis found that IVF did not improve pain outcomes among patients when added to IV metoclopramide [27]. However, IVF may be helpful in migraine treatment even without hypovolemia, though the exact mechanism of improvement is not clear [28]. Future randomized controlled trials are needed to clarify the role of IVF in the acute management of migraine. Despite the lack of data, it is reasonable to administer IVF if the patient is otherwise healthy without any contraindications. Normal saline or Ringer's lactate may be given at a delivery rate up to 1000 cc of fluid volume per hour for two hours. If there is a history of prolonged vomiting, laboratory evaluation of electrolytes is necessary and an electrolyte imbalance such as hypokalemia can be corrected within the IVF. Postural blood pressures can hint at the degree of hypovolemia and guide the clinician in choosing sufficient quantities of IVF. When orthostatic hypotension is present, IVF should be given until postural hypotension is corrected.

Further treatment of refractory migraine is likely to be with parenteral medication. Most patients, if they have tried any medication at all prior to presentation, have taken them at home by the oral route. Pregnant patients may have stopped using migraine-specific therapies that had been effective, given concerns regarding safety during pregnancy, or may have been counseled by their practitioners to avoid their usual migraine medications. They may have waited to come to the ED until pain was quite advanced or nausea or vomiting was present and uncontrolled. As with any severe, prolonged migraine, it is likely that gastroparesis makes any therapy other than parenteral or rectal suboptimal or ineffective, and fast-acting parenteral therapy is desired by both the patient and physician.

ED medication strategies often aim to deliver a combination of medications with different mechanisms of actions, with the intention of improved efficacy. Though there have been many randomized controlled trials on the treatment of migraine in the ED, there are no such trials in the pregnant or lactating patient. In the absence of high-quality data, drugs with high efficacy and the lowest known risk to pregnant or lactating women are optimal.

The treatment opinions discussed in this chapter are solely those of the authors and are distilled in Figure 12.1, with a possible treatment flow for refractory migraine in the pregnant or lactating patient.

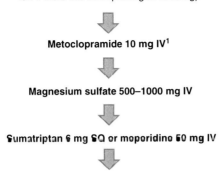

**Intravenous fluids (IVF)**
Normal saline or Ringer's lactate 1–2 liters; high flow rate if hypovolemia present and normal renal function; adjust IVF composition according to electrolyte status (potassium is most likely low if there has been prolonged vomiting)

**Metoclopramide 10 mg IV[1]**

**Magnesium sulfate 500–1000 mg IV**

**Sumatriptan 6 mg SQ or meperidine 50 mg IV**

**Ketorolac 30 mg IV or methylprednisolone 250 mg IV**

**Figure 12.1** Emergency department treatment of refractory migraine in the pregnant or lactating patient. Medications may be given in sequence after IVF have been started, with enough time (e.g., ten minutes) between drugs to evaluate response and possible adverse effects.
[1] Though metoclopramide is likely the best dopamine antagonist to use in pregnant patients, other dopamine receptor antagonists may be used in lactating patients. Since the possibility of side-effects is higher with the more potent dopamine antagonists, diphenhydramine IV 12.5–25 mg can be given prior to use.

## Migraine Treatment of the Pregnant Patient in the ED

### Drug Safety During Pregnancy

Decisions over which medication to use are always made on an individual basis. Because treatment decisions are dependent on what medication a patient has already taken at home and for past migraines, a history of medication use is very important. If drugs have already been used prior to visiting the ED, the use of similar drugs may be indicated or contraindicated based on allowed medication intervals, the maximal daily dose of a medication, or potential drug interactions.

Package inserts for medication will take a precautionary approach for use during pregnancy and suggest that use is not recommended and should only be used "if benefit outweighs risk." Therefore, the majority of drug use during pregnancy is off-label, despite significant potential benefit to a pregnant woman with severe headache in the ED. Documentation of conversations regarding potential risks and side-effects of recommended therapies should be done diligently, although given the severity of headache, the urgency of the situation, and the difficulty of ascertaining risk, admittedly, these conversations are difficult at best.

Since pregnancy is an exclusion criterion in most clinical trials testing new drugs or new drug applications, there are little high-quality data on the safety of a medication during pregnancy or on the potential impact to a fetus. Safety data during pregnancy are derived largely from animal studies, retrospective case reports of women who inadvertently became pregnant during a clinical trial, or from pregnancy registry databases of approved drugs.

There is little information on which to base treatment decisions and the utility of rating scales such as the US Food and Drug Administration (FDA) pregnancy risk rating system is limited. This system assigns medication into one of five categories (A, B, C, D, and X) based on human or animal studies ([29]; see Table 12.2 legend). The usefulness of the rating scale is primarily to avoid category "D" drugs that have shown positive evidence of risk to humans from human or animal studies and category "X" drugs, which are contraindicated during pregnancy. Since there are few category "A" medications (e.g., riboflavin) that have evidence from controlled human studies that there is no associated fetal risk, ordinarily the choice is limited to drugs in category "B" with no evidence of risk in humans but with no controlled human studies and drugs in category "C" where risk to humans has not been ruled out. Since the difference between "no evidence of risk in humans" and "risk to humans has not been ruled out" is a difficult distinction on which to make evidence-based decisions, treatment choices in many cases are based on individual risk–benefit analyses. An additional difficulty is that risk categories may be based on human or on animal risk and therefore difficult to interpret. Lastly, risk is typically based on repetitive use or supra-therapeutic doses in animal studies, which may not be useful when applied to the context of single use or infrequent dosing as is the case for patients in the ED setting.

## Avoid Teratogenic Drugs

There is no consensus on a single method of assessing drug risk in pregnant women. Historically, the placenta was thought to serve as a barrier that would protect the fetus from the potentially harmful effects of drugs. However, the thalidomide disaster, with observed congenital malformation rates in the 20–30 percent range, demonstrated that exposure of the fetus at a critical time in its development resulted in severe limb defects and organ dysgenesis [30]. A teratogen is any agent that can induce or increase the incidence of a congenital malformation, affecting either fetal morphology or function. Fewer than 30 drugs have been recognized as human teratogens and most of these drugs are not typically used in the acute treatment of primary headache disorders. Some drugs can have morphologic or functional effects at critical times of fetal development. For example, nonsteroidal anti-inflammatory drugs (NSAIDs) are to be avoided in the third trimester as inhibition of prostaglandin synthesis may contribute to premature closure or constriction of the ductus arteriosus. Though it is unlikely that a single dose of valproic acid would do harm, neural tube defects have been reported and this potential teratogen is to be avoided during pregnancy, particularly since risk is high as compared to relatively low efficacy for the treatment of acute migraine [31]. At later stages of pregnancy, exposure to anticholinergic drugs can cause neonatal meconium ileus, and psychoactive drugs such as barbiturates, opioids, or benzodiazepines, if frequently administered, may cause neonatal abstinence syndrome [30]. This is important to consider when selecting potential discharge medications. Because of the known teratogenicity of these drugs, they have been placed in FDA category "D."

It is of great importance to be aware of category "X" drugs in treating women with migraine

who are pregnant so that they can be avoided. Dihydroergotamine (DHE), a parenteral migraine-specific medication, should be avoided during pregnancy because it can decrease uterine blood flow, potentially causing fetal hypoxia and growth retardation. More importantly, even with limited or even a single use, it could stimulate uterine contractility and tone, possibly increasing the risk of spontaneous abortion.

## Plasma Level Variability During Pregnancy

In the ED setting, most medication is likely to be administered parenterally, negating oral absorption and bioavailability issues. However, drug distribution may change in pregnancy. The increase in plasma volume seen during pregnancy may increase the fraction of unbound drug in plasma. Effective albumin concentration also decreases during the second trimester, steadily dropping to 70–80 percent of normal values. This will be clinically important if a drug is highly protein bound and total concentrations will significantly underestimate free fraction (e.g., as seen with phenytoin). Renal clearance is increased during pregnancy, so if drugs are primarily renally excreted they may require a dosage adjustment as well [32]. With single use during an ED visit, plasma level variability is unlikely to be of clinical significance, though during labor and delivery, drugs such as fentanyl, midazolam, and bupivacaine are subject to plasma level variability.

## Hepatic Metabolism During Pregnancy

The activity of the CYP enzymes and glucuronidation pathways change during pregnancy. CYP3A4, 2D6, 2A6, 2C9, and uridine 5′-diphosphate glucuronyltransferase (UGT) are increased, whereas CYP1A2 and 2C19 are decreased. This is unlikely to be of clinical significance in the ED setting for single-use medications; however, it is useful to be aware that if a patient is on maintenance or "as needed" (prn) medications while pregnant, drug levels may be altered. For example, one can expect lower drug levels for: eletriptan and verapamil, which are metabolized by the CYP3A4 pathway; metoprolol, fluoxetine, and nortriptyline, which are metabolized by 2D6; and phenytoin, celecoxib, and losartan, which are metabolized by 2C9 pathways. This is pertinent in the ED setting in that the clinician should be aware that suboptimal dosing due to metabolic changes in pregnancy may at least partially explain an exacerbation in the patient's headaches.

# Acute Treatment of Migraine During Pregnancy

The treatment of severe, refractory migraine in the ED usually requires a combination of medications that will work in synergy [28]. For an extensive discussion of acute treatment strategies for migraine in the ED, see Chapter 7. The same principles apply to treatment of a pregnant or lactating woman with the limitation that drugs with the lowest risk to the fetus should be utilized. Combination therapy could include a dopamine antagonist, highly effective for the acute treatment of migraine in the ED setting, the migraine-specific 5-HT 1B/1D agonist sumatriptan, an opioid, or magnesium. Though they do not seem to exhibit significant effectiveness for the acute treatment of migraine, corticosteroids are useful for prolonged, refractory headaches in that they appear to prevent recurrence and reduce the incidence of return visits to the ED (Table 12.2).

**Dopamine Receptor Antagonists.** Dopamine antagonists (DAs) have valuable dual effects in the treatment of refractory migraine. As anti-emetics, they are highly effective for the treatment of nausea and vomiting, as well as in relieving pain. Their target is the dopamine D2 receptor, but they have variable antagonist activity at the H1 histamine site, muscarinic anticholinergic, alpha-adrenergic, and serotonin (5-HT1A and 5-HT2) receptors [33]. The three subclasses of DAs used for the treatment of acute migraine are the phenothiazines (chlorpromazine, prochlorperazine, and promethazine), the butyrophenones (droperidol and haloperidol), and the benzamide metoclopramide. The more affinity the drug has in binding to the D2 receptor, the higher the efficacy; however, side-effects are also likely to be greater. Sedation, akathisia, dystonia and other extrapyramidal symptoms (EPS), hypotension (especially with chlorpromazine), and prolonged QT intervals are common side-effects. Incidence of akathisia can be decreased by slowing down the infusion rate. With metoclopramide, for example, frequency of akathisia was significantly ($p < 0.001$) reduced from 24.7 percent to 5.8 percent when the infusion was given over 2 minutes vs. 15 minutes, respectively [34].

Pretreatment with diphenhydramine can minimize the EPS side-effects [35]. In a systematic review of medications used in the ED setting, prochlorperazine and chlorpromazine were found to have the highest percentages of patients with pain relief (moderate to severe headache pain to mild or no pain after treatment) or pain freedom (moderate to severe headache pain to no pain after treatment) at two hours ([31]; Table 12.2). However, most DAs are Class C drugs within the FDA pregnancy risk rating, with the exception of metoclopramide, which is a Class B drug. Therefore, the recommendation is for metoclopramide to be the DA of choice during pregnancy. Acute dystonic reactions are rarely seen in patients given metoclopramide and may be very distressing. In one ED study, approximately 3 percent of subjects who received 10 mg IV metoclopramide developed an acute dystonic reaction [36]. Diphenhydramine is also a Class B medication and pretreatment with this drug could be considered; however, if metoclopramide is administered over 15 minutes, pretreatment with diphenhydramine is likely unnecessary [37].

**NSAIDs.** Ketorolac is frequently used in the ED setting for refractory headache and is the most commonly used parenteral NSAID in the United States. Though as effective as meperidine for pain relief (Table 12.2), it does not appear to be as effective as the dopamine antagonists. It is a Class C drug in the first and second trimesters, but is considered Class D and contraindicated in the third trimester. Third-trimester use of NSAIDs by inhibition of prostaglandin synthesis may cause oligohydramnios, prolonged labor, or premature closure/constriction of the ductus arteriosus though closure frequently resolves within 24 hours after discontinuation of therapy [38]. Additionally, though previously used in labor and delivery, it is no longer used in this setting because it may adversely affect fetal circulation and inhibit uterine contractions, thereby increasing the risk of hemorrhage. NSAID use in early pregnancy may interfere with implantation, but controversy still exists regarding whether there is an increased risk of miscarriage with NSAID use in early pregnancy. A recent review of over 65,000 women admitted for delivery or spontaneous abortion found that approximately 7 percent had used NSAIDs with no increased risk of spontaneous abortion following NSAID use, with the exception of indomethacin [39]. The recommendation is to limit use to the late first trimester and second trimester and to avoid use after

**Table 12.2** Acute migraine medications for emergency department treatment of the pregnant patient

| Medication | Dose | Pain free[1] | Pain relief[2] | FDA rating[3] pregnancy risk | Cautions |
|---|---|---|---|---|---|
| **High efficacy** | | | | | |
| Prochlorperazine | 5–10 mg IV | 53% | 77% | C | Sedation, akathisia, |
| Chlorpromazine | 2.5–12.5 mg IV | 53% | 65% | C | Dystonia, prolonged QT interval, hypotension, dizziness |
| Metoclopramide | 10 mg IV | 41% | 70% | B | |
| Droperidol | 0.625–2.5 mg IV | 40% | 82% | C | |
| **Moderate efficacy** | | | | | |
| Ketorolac | 30 mg IV | n/a | 60% | C/D (3rd trimester) | Implantation interference in early pregnancy; constriction of ductus arteriosus in late pregnancy |
| Magnesium | 1000 mg IV | 36% | 43% | B | None |
| Meperidine | 50 mg IV | 30% | 58% | C | Sedation, respiratory depression, constipation |
| Sumatriptan | 6 mg SQ | 35% | 78% | C | Paresthesias, chest symptoms |
| **Low efficacy** | | | | | |
| Methylprednisolone | 250 mg IV | May prevent headache recurrence after discharge | | C | Rare avascular hip necrosis; gastritis, insomnia |
| Dexamethasone | 4–12 mg IV | | | C | |

[1] From Figure 2 in Kelley and Tepper's review of ED therapy for acute migraine [31]. These values are from weighted averages of the percentages of patients who were pain-free for medications for which there were two or more randomized trials with the medication used as a single agent.

[2] From Figure 1 in Kelley and Tepper's review of ED therapy for acute migraine [31]. These values are from weighted averages of the percentages of patients who had pain relief for medications for which there were two or more randomized trials with the medication used as a single agent.

[3] FDA risk categories:

Category A: Controlled studies in women fail to demonstrate a risk to the fetus in the first trimester and no evidence of risk in later trimesters, and the possibility of fetal harm appears remote.

Category B: Animal reproductive studies have not demonstrated a fetal risk, but there are no controlled studies in pregnant women; or animal studies have shown an adverse effect (other than fertility) that was not confirmed in controlled studies in women in the first trimester (and there is not evidence of a risk in later trimesters).

Category C: Either studies in animals have shown adverse effects on the fetus and there are no controlled studies in women, or studies in women and animals are not available. Drugs should be given only if the potential benefit justifies the potential risk to the fetus.

Category D: Positive evidence of human fetal risk, but the benefits from use in pregnant women may be acceptable despite the risk (e.g., in a life-threatening situation).

Category X: Studies in animals or human beings have demonstrated fetal abnormalities or there is evidence of fetal risk based on human experience, or both. The risk of use in pregnant women clearly outweighs any possible benefit. The drug is contraindicated in women who are or may become pregnant.

gestational week 32 [40]. Thus, if there are no contraindications to NSAID use, ketorolac may be given in combination with other medication to patients in the late first or second trimesters.

**Magnesium.** Magnesium is an FDA Class B risk drug and use during pregnancy is considered safe. Magnesium has been used extensively during pregnancy for the treatment of pre-eclampsia as an anticonvulsant at a loading dose of 4–5 g followed by doses of up to 1–3 g per hour – enough to significantly increase maternal plasma magnesium concentration above normal. It has an off-label use as a tocolytic to stop preterm labor with a loading dose of 4–6 g IV and maintenance dose of 2–4 g/hr IV for 12–24 hours until contractions stop. These large doses can cause sedation and hypotonia with in-utero exposure; however, the half-life ($T_{1/2}$) of magnesium is less than three hours and single, infrequent IV dosing at the recommended dose of 1–2 g IV for the acute treatment of migraine is not likely to significantly affect fetal physiology [41]. Given its safety and familiarity of use for pregnant women, magnesium is a reasonable treatment option to consider for the acute treatment of migraine in pregnant patients.

**Meperidine.** In general, opioids should be avoided in the treatment of migraine [42]. Meperidine is the most-studied opioid for ED use in this setting and is an FDA Class C risk medication. Side-effects include sedation and respiratory depression. Because of its short $T_{1/2}$ of 3.2 hours and relatively modest efficacy ([31]; Table 12.2), headaches have a high rate of recurrence and if used, for example in situations where triptan medication may already have been used prior to the ED visit, or if the patient is undergoing a workup for possible secondary headache, opioids could be combined with a dopamine antagonist and possibly a corticosteroid in an effort to improve headache management [28].

Repeated doses of meperidine should be avoided, as most opioids rapidly cross the placenta, and fetal/maternal drug ratios may exceed 1.0 after only a couple of hours since maternal metabolism exceeds fetal metabolism of the drug. Highly lipophilic drugs like fentanyl are not recommended because of exceedingly fast placental transfer with detection during early pregnancy in both the placenta and the fetal brain [43].

**Sumatriptan.** Sumatriptan is the only injectable migraine-specific medication in the triptan class and the only migraine-specific medication available outside of Class X. It is a Class C medication that rapidly achieves maximal plasma concentration at 12 minutes and has a $T_{1/2}$ of 1.3 hours. However, the rate of pain freedom at two hours appears to be relatively low at only 35 percent ([31]; Table 12.2). It is well tolerated but may cause "triptan sensations" such as chest, shoulder, or neck tightness, flushing, or tingling sensations. Many practitioners are reticent to use sumatriptan in pregnancy because of its vasoconstrictive properties and labeling indicating that it is contraindicated during pregnancy.

There are no human data to suggest teratogenicity for any of the triptans [44–48]. Data for sumatriptan use is the most extensive because of its longer market presence. Schenker et al. [49] studied sumatriptan transport across the normal term human placenta. Only about 15 percent of a single dose delivered through the maternal surface crossed into the fetal compartment over four hours. Given an average elimination half-life of two hours for sumatriptan, only very small amounts of drug will cross from mother to fetus by passive transport, likely because of its high molecular weight and poor water solubility. Because fetal 5-HT1B/1D receptors develop through the third trimester in human studies, it is not clear whether the triptans could have any possible effect on fetal development [50].

Sixteen years of pregnancy registry data are available for sumatriptan. Final published results of the registry study involve 680 enrolled participants, with 626 exposed to sumatriptan, and the remaining participants exposed to multiple triptans or to the sumatriptan/naproxen combination. The registry detected "no signal" of teratogenicity associated with major birth defects for sumatriptan [25]. Additionally, there was no difference in the proportion of births with defects when exposed to sumatriptan in the first trimester compared to sumatriptan exposures from all trimesters. Despite this reassuring information, the number of pregnancy exposures to date in the registries represents an insufficient sample size to reach any definitive conclusions regarding risk of triptan use during pregnancy.

A population-based, observational, prospective study of 69,929 pregnant women as part of the Norwegian Mother and Child Cohort evaluated risk of congenital malformation and adverse pregnancy outcomes using a standardized questionnaire. 1538 pregnant women, or 2.2 percent of the cohort, used triptans, primarily sumatriptan, during pregnancy. There was no significant association between triptan therapy during the first trimester and major congenital malformations or other adverse outcomes of pregnancy. In the mothers there was a slightly increased risk for atonic uterus and hemorrhage during labor; however, many of the mothers who used triptans during pregnancy also used NSAIDs, paracetamol, and codeine, and results therefore cannot be attributed to isolated triptan use [26].

Given its known efficacy for the acute treatment of migraine and given the promising safety data, sumatriptan is one alternative available to the ED clinician treating pregnant patients with migraine.

**Corticosteroids.** Corticosteroids are primarily used to prevent headache recurrence [51]. In a meta-analysis of seven studies on steroid use as compared to placebo in the ED, dexamethasone IV prevented headache recurrence within 72 hours after discharge from the ED [52]. Though the corticosteroids are considered low risk in pregnancy (FDA risk Class C), there is evidence that they are ineffective for the acute treatment of migraine in the ED [53]. Though unlikely that potential adverse effects such as avascular hip necrosis, severe gastrointestinal upset or ulceration, irritability, or insomnia would occur after a single dose, corticosteroids should be used only for prolonged, refractory migraine.

# Migraine Treatment of the Lactating Patient in the Emergency Department

The safety and recommended use of a drug used during pregnancy does not equate to safety and recommended use during lactation.

The dose of a drug that an infant receives during breastfeeding is dependent on the average plasma concentration of drug in the mother, the amount excreted into breast milk, and the daily volume of milk ingested by the infant [54,55]. The ability of an infant to absorb and eliminate a drug will also determine exposure; the younger the infant, the more likely it is that slower elimination will contribute to adverse events. There is little clinical data available whereby the concentration

of drug in the infant serum is measured while the mother is receiving steady-state concentrations of the same drug – the gold standard method of determining the milk/plasma (M/P) concentration ratio [56]. There are virtually no data on infant serum concentration for single dosing of a drug in the mother.

The physicochemical properties of a drug's lipophilicity, protein binding, and ionization properties determine its excretion into breast milk. Plasma protein binding is the major determinant of transfer of drug into breast milk [57].

In general, after breastfeeding, detectable concentrations of drugs are measured in infants when drugs are <70 percent protein bound in the maternal plasma (30 percent fraction unbound). For drugs >85 percent protein bound, if there is no placental exposure prior to or during delivery, and if mothers have not received excessively high doses during the first week postpartum, breastfeeding will not result in measurable infant concentrations of the drug in question [32,56].

Table 12.3 reviews the same high-, moderate-, and low-efficacy injectable medications as were reviewed in Table 12.2. Maternal protein binding is listed, only as a gauge to approximate excretion into breast milk. However, with single, infrequent dosing, risk would appear to be much less than with frequent and

**Table 12.3** Acute migraine medications for emergency department treatment of the lactating patient

| Medication | Dose | Maternal protein binding | AAP | Hale's lactation risk[1] | Pediatric cautions |
|---|---|---|---|---|---|
| **High efficacy** | | | | | |
| Prochlorperazine | 5–10 mg IV | 90% | Caution | L3 | None reported via milk but observe for possible sedation, hypotension |
| Chlorpromazine | 2.5–12.5 mg IV | 95% | May be of concern | L3 | |
| Metoclopramide | 10 mg IV | 30% | Unknown | L2 | |
| Droperidol | 0.625–2.5 mg IV | >90% | | L3 | |
| **Moderate efficacy** | | | | | |
| Ketorolac | 30 mg IV | 99% | Compatible | L2 | None reported via milk |
| Magnesium | 1000 mg IV | 0% | Compatible | L1 | None reported via milk |
| Meperidine | 50 mg IV | 65–80% | Compatible | L2 (L3 if early postpartum) | Sedation, poor sucking, neurodevelopmental delay |
| Sumatriptan | 6 mg SQ | 14–21% | Compatible | L3 | None |
| **Low efficacy** | | | | | |
| Methylprednisolone | 250 mg IV | 77% | Compatible | L2 | Growth and development may be affected if prolonged therapy in mother |
| Dexamethasone | 4–12 mg IV | 70–77% | Not reviewed | L3 | |

[1] Dr. Hale's lactation risk categories: L1 safest, L2 safer, L3 moderately safe, L4 possibly hazardous, L5 contraindicated.

consistent use postpartum. There are several publications that attempt to stratify risk of drugs to breastfed infants, including the American Academy of Pediatrics (AAP) Committee on Drugs, which rates drugs on compatibility with breastfeeding. Their five-point rating scale rates drugs as (1) contraindicated; (2) requires temporary cessation of breastfeeding; (3) effects unknown but may be of concern; (4) drugs that have been associated with significant effects on some infants and use with caution; and (5) usually compatible [58]. Ratings are available on the AAP policy website [59].

Thomas Hale's publication is an encyclopedia of drug monographs and includes many alternative therapies for a given drug [60]. It lists AAP recommendations for breastfeeding, as well as Dr. Hale's lactation risk categories: L1 safest, L2 safer, L3 moderately safe, L4 possibly hazardous, L5 contraindicated. These categories are based on clinical observation of potential adverse effects of drugs on infants from large numbers of breastfeeding mothers using the drug, or controlled studies demonstrating a possible risk or significant and documented risk. Pharmacokinetic properties of each drug are given if available. For example, magnesium is listed as an L1 medication (safest) with AAP description as "Maternal medication usually compatible with breastfeeding."

Also available with computer access is the National Institute of Health's *LactMed*, with excellent monographs on most medications [61]. Additionally, a comprehensive review on the use of common migraine treatments in breastfeeding women and recommendations for use was published recently [62].

**Dopamine Receptor Antagonists.** Because of the relatively high maternal protein binding of this class of medications, these drugs enter milk in very small amounts. However, neonates are extremely sensitive to the dopamine antagonists and neonatal sedation and lethargy is a risk. These medications should be used with extreme caution in mothers of infants subject to apnea. The most extensive experience with DAs in infants is with metoclopramide, sometimes used clinically in breastfeeding women to stimulate pituitary prolactin release and enhance breast milk production. In these studies on the use of maternal metoclopramide for prolactin stimulation, minimal or undetectable levels of metoclopramide were measured in milk, so there are minimal concerns with the rare use of metoclopramide in lactating patients [63].

**Ketorolac.** Because of the high protein binding of ketorolac, as with all NSAIDs, little drug passes into breast milk. With an adult dose of 30 mg every six hours, at a steady state after 1–2 days, the infant dose was less than 0.2 percent of the daily maternal dose [64]. No pediatric concerns were reported.

**Magnesium.** There is a normal concentrating mechanism for magnesium in human milk. In studies of high doses of magnesium at steady state in pregnant women, the levels of magnesium in milk are approximately twice those of maternal serum magnesium with the milk-to-serum ratio averaging 2.0 [65]. However, with single dosing in the ED and a $T_{1/2}$ of less than three hours, and given the poor oral absorption of magnesium (about 4 percent), it is unlikely that the amount of magnesium in breast milk would be clinically relevant.

**Meperidine.** Significant but small amounts of meperidine are excreted into breast milk with the relative infant dose approximately 1.7 percent of an adult dose. The $T_{1/2}$ for meperidine in neonates is significantly longer than the maternal $T_{1/2}$ (13 hours versus 3.2 hours, respectively). Also, the active metabolite normeperidine has a $T_{1/2}$ of 63 hours in the neonate. With repeated use, both could concentrate in the plasma of a neonate with resulting sedation, poor sucking reflex, and neurobehavioral delay [60].

**Sumatriptan.** Sumatriptan is protein bound between 14–21 percent (package insert). As expected with lower protein binding, sumatriptan has a milk/plasma ratio of 4.9:1, with 0.21 percent of the maternal peak plasma dose measured at eight hours in human breast milk after 6 mg of the subcutaneous dose was given. There are no concerns over significant absorption of sumatriptan through breast milk. In one study of lactating women given a 6 mg SQ injection of sumatriptan, total recovery of drug in milk over eight hours was approximately 3.5 percent of the maternal dose. Given the low oral bioavailability of sumatriptan at 14 percent, the weight-adjusted dose an infant would absorb would be 0.49 percent of the maternal dose [66].

**Corticosteroids.** Though there are no concerns reported through breast milk ingestion with infrequent use, as transfer of steroids into human milk is extremely low, there is concern for infant exposure when the maternal ingestion is prolonged and with high doses; for example, high-dose (1 g) IV pulse steroids for exacerbations of multiple sclerosis. Theoretically, high doses and long duration of any corticosteroid may inhibit epiphyseal bone growth, cause gastric ulcers, glaucoma, and adrenal insufficiency.

**Discharge Medications.** Many patients leave the ED improved, either with significant pain relief or pain-free. However, up to 60 percent of ED patients with treated migraine may experience significant pain 24 hours after discharge [67]. The recurrence of headaches typically happens within 72 hours. Dispensing discharge medications may facilitate the treatment of headaches at home before they become severe, refractory, and are accompanied by nausea and vomiting, thereby avoiding a return to the ED soon after discharge.

Though the ED physician is not likely to be able to discuss discharge medications in detail with patients who may be sedated or exhausted from treatment, a brief written plan may be given to the patient, and follow-up with the primary care provider should be encouraged. Discharge medications may include oral or rectal forms of medications that were given parenterally in the ED, and instructions to treat early may help to prevent recurrence of the severe, refractory headache that sent the patient to the ED in the first place. Therapy should be targeted to headache severity and rate of pain progression. After discharge, for pain that may be mild to moderate and of slow onset, acetaminophen, or NSAIDs during the late first and second trimester of pregnancy may be used. For moderate or escalating pain, opioids, sumatriptan, or other triptans can be taken in moderation in pregnant or lactating patients. Limited amounts of medication should be given to avoid excessive use, particularly in the case of opioids, not only to avoid medication overuse headache, but given the fact that frequent or daily opioid use, especially in mid-to-late pregnancy, increases the risk of fetal mortality and premature labor associated with neonatal opioid withdrawal syndrome [68].

In the case of the breastfeeding patient, the ideal triptan to use is eletriptan, as it has the highest protein binding of all the triptans and the lowest excretion into breast milk. With a milk-to-plasma ratio of 1:4, only 0.02 percent of an 80 mg oral dose was measured in breast milk at 24 hours (package insert).

A dopamine antagonist can be given at discharge in either or both oral and rectal forms, with metoclopramide being the recommended DA for the pregnant or lactating patient. If sedation is to be avoided, ondansetron, a 5-HT3 antagonist, has been studied prospectively and found to be safe for use during pregnancy [69]. It is available as an orally dissolving as well as regular tablet. Additionally, evidence exists for the absence of 5-HT3 receptors in the human umbilical artery at full term. It is an FDA risk Class B drug in pregnancy and an L2 lactation risk according to Dr. Hale's lactation risk categories [60].

# Conclusion

The lack of treatment trials studying the effectiveness and safety of migraine drugs in pregnant and lactating women makes it impossible to suggest a definitive, optimally effective regimen. The recommendations made in this chapter are based on evidence for rescue therapy for acute migraine in the general population, and safety data are taken from the sparse literature available in the pregnant or lactating population. As always, the decision to treat with any medication must weigh the benefit with the risk – in this case risk not only to a patient who can consent to treatment, but also to the one who cannot. In general, single or infrequent use of these IV therapies is probably safe. The use of any risk rating scales is typically based on steady-state use of the medication and not on single use, so can only be seen as a relative guide to safety. While effective ED treatment may provide significant relief to the pregnant or lactating woman, and even avoid serious medical concerns over the fetus with a significantly ill patient, the pregnant or lactating woman with severe headache should ideally have a primary care provider who can formulate a solid and understandable care program.

# References

1. Lipton RB, Bigal ME. The epidemiology of migraine. *Am J Med.* 2005;118(Suppl. 1):3S–10S.

2. Nappi RE, Albani F, Sances G, et al. Headaches during pregnancy. *Curr Pain Headache Rep.* 2011;15:289–94.

3. Hoshiyama E, Tatsumoto M, Iwanami H, et al. Postpartum migraines: a long-term prospective study. *Intern Med.* 2012;51:3119–23.

4. Ertresvag JM, Swart JA, Helde G, et al. Headache and transient neurological symptoms during pregnancy, a prospective cohort. *Acta Neurol Scand.* 2005;111:233–7.

5. Melhado EM, Maciel JA, Guerreiro CM. Headache during gestation: evaluation of 1101 women. *Can J Neurol Sci.* 2007;34:187–92.

6. Fiesseler FW, Riggs RL, Shih R, Richman PB. Do patients with recurrent headaches attempt abortive therapy before their emergency department visit? *J Emerg Med*. 2007;32:245–8.

7. Klapper JA, Stanton JS. Current emergency treatment of severe migraine headaches. *Headache*. 1993;33:560–2.

8. Marcus D. Managing headache during pregnancy and lactation. *Expert Rev Neurotherapeutics*. 2008;8:385–95.

9. Treadwell SD, Thanvi B, Robinson TG. Stroke in pregnancy and the puerperium. *Postgrad Med J*. 2008;84:238–45.

10. Heit J, Kobbervig C, James A, et al. Trends in the incidence of deep vein thrombosis and pulmonary embolism during pregnancy or the puerperium: a 30-year population-based study. *Ann Int Med*. 2005;143:697–706.

11. James AH, Bushnell CD, Jamison MG, Meyers ER. Incidence and risk factors for stroke in pregnancy and the puerperium. *Obstet Gynecol*. 2005;106:506–16.

12. Report of the national high blood pressure education program working group on high blood pressure in pregnancy. *Am J Obstet Gynecol*. 2000;183:S1–S22.

13. Adeney KL, Williams MA. Migraine headaches and preeclampsia: an epidemiologic review. *Headache*. 2006;46:794–803.

14. Bushnell CD, Jamison M, James AH. Migraines during pregnancy linked to stroke and vascular disease in a US population based case control study. *BMJ*. 2009;10:338.

15. Facchinetti F, Allais G, Nappi RE, et al. Migraine is a risk factor of hypertensive disorders in pregnancy: a prospective cohort study. *Cephalalgia*. 2009;29:286–92.

16. Williams MA, Peterlin BL, Gelaye B, et al. Trimester-specific blood pressure levels and hypertensive disorders among pregnant migraineurs. *Headache*. 2011;51:1468–82.

17. Marcoux S, Berube S, Brissan J, Fabia J. History of migraine and risk of pregnancy-induced hypertension. *Epidemiology*. 1992;3:53–6.

18. Adeney KL, Williams MA, Miller RS, et al. Risk of pre-eclampsia in relation to maternal history of migraine headaches. *J Matern Fetal Neonatal Med*. 2005;18:167–72.

19. American College of Obstetricians and Gynecologists. Chronic hypertension in pregnancy: ACOG Practice Bulletin no.125. *Obstet Gynecol*. 2012;119:396–407.

20. Deak TM, Moskovitz JB. Hypertension and pregnancy. *Emerg Med Clin North Am*. 2012;30:903–17.

21. Robbins MS, Farmakidis C, Dayal AK, Lipton RB. Acute headache diagnosis in pregnant women: a hospital-based study. *Neurology*. 2015;85:1024–30.

22. Ramchandren S, Cross BJ, Liebeskind DS. Emergent headaches during pregnancy: correlation between neurologic examination and neuroimaging. *Am J Neuroradiol*. 2007;28:1085–7.

23. ACR-SPR practice parameter for imaging pregnant or potentially pregnant adolescents and women with ionizing radiation. Resolution 39, amended 2014.

24. The American College of Obstetricians and Gynecologists. The American College of Obstetricians and Gynecologists women's health care physicians guidelines for diagnostic imaging during pregnancy and lactation; no. 656, February 2016.

25. Ephross SA, Sinclair SM. Final results from the 16-year sumatriptan, naratriptan, and Treximet pregnancy registry. *Headache*. 2014;54:1158–72.

26. Nezvalova-Henriksen K, Spigset O, Nordeng H. Triptan exposure during pregnancy and the risk of major congenital malformations and adverse pregnancy outcomes: results from the Norwegian mother and child cohort study. *Headache*. 2010;50:563–75.

27. Balbin JEB, Nerenberg R, Baratloo A, Friedman BW. Intravenous fluids for migraine: a post hoc analysis of clinical trial data. *Am J Emerg Med*. 2016;34(4):713–16.

28. Rozen TD. Emergency department and inpatient management of status migrainosus and intractable headache. *Continuum*. 2015;21:1004–17.

29. FDA. Pregnancy categories for prescription drugs. *FDA Drug Bulletin*. 1982;12:24–5.

30. Koren G, Pastuszak A, Ho S. Drugs in pregnancy. *N Engl J Med*. 1998;338:1128–37.

31. Kelley NE, Tepper DE. Rescue therapy for acute migraine: Part 3. Opioids, NSAIDs, steroids, and post-discharge medications. *Headache*. 2012;52:467–82.

32. Anderson G. Using pharmacokinetics to predict effects of pregnancy and maternal–infant transfer of drug during lactation. *Expert Opin Drug Metab Toxicol*. 2006;2:947–60.

33. Peroutka SJ, Snyder SH. Relationship of neuroleptic drug effects at brain dopamine, serotonin, adrenergic and histamine receptors to clinical potency. *Am J Psychiatry*. 1980;137:1518–22.

34. Parlak I, Atilla R, Cicek M, et al. Rate of metoclopramide infusion affects the severity and incidence of akathisia. *Emerg Med J*. 2005;22:621–4.

35. Wijemanne S, Jankovic J, Evans RW. Movement disorders from the use of metoclopramide and other antiemetics in the treatment of migraine. *Headache*. 2016;56:153–61.

36. Cete Y, Dora B, Ertan C, Ozdemir C, Oktay C. A randomized prospective placebo-controlled study of intravenous magnesium sulphate vs. metoclopramide

in the management of acute migraine attacks in the emergency department. *Cephalalgia.* 2005;25:199–204.

37. Friedman BW, Bender B, Davitt M, et al. A randomized trial of diphenhydramine as prophylaxis against metoclopramide-induced akathisia in nauseated emergency department patients. *Ann Emerg Med.* 2009;53:379–85.

38. Momma K, Hagiwara H, Konishi T. Constriction of fetal ductus arteriosus by non-steroidal anti-inflammatory drugs: study of additional 34 drugs. *Prostaglandins.* 1984;28:527–36.

39. Daniel S, Koren G, Lunenfeld E, et al. Fetal exposure of nonsteroidal anti-inflammatory drugs and spontaneous abortions. *CMAJ.* 2014;186:E177–82.

40. Amundsen S, Nordeng H, Nezalova-Henriksen K, Stovner LJ, Spigset O. Pharmacological treatment of migraine during pregnancy and breastfeeding. *Nat Rev Neurol.* 2015;11:209–19.

41. Riaz M, Porat R, Brodsky NL, Hurt H. The effects of maternal magnesium sulfate treatment on newborns: a prospective controlled study. *J Perinatol.* 1998;18:449–54.

42. Langer-Gould AM, Anderson WE, Armstrong MJ et al. The American Academy of Neurology's top five choosing wisely recommendations. *Neurology.* 2013;81(11);1004–11.

43. Cooper J, Jauniaux E, Gulbis B, Quick D, Bromley L. Placental transfer of fentanyl in early human pregnancy and its detection in fetal brain. *Br J Anaesth.* 1999;82:929–31.

44. Soldin OP, Dahlin J, O'Mara DM. Triptans in pregnancy. *Ther Drug Monit.* 2008;30:5–9.

45. Evans EW, Lorbe KC. Use of 5-HT agonists in pregnancy. *Ann Pharmacother.* 2008;42:543–9.

46. Loder E. Safety of sumatriptan in pregnancy: a review of the literature so far. *CNS Drugs.* 2003;17:1–7.

47. O'Quinn S, Ephross SA, Williams V, et al. Pregnancy and perinatal outcomes in migraineurs using sumatriptan: a prospective study. *Arch Gynecol Obstet.* 1999;263:7–12.

48. Shuhaiber S, Pastuszak A, Schick B et al. Pregnancy outcome following first trimester exposure to sumatriptan. *Neurology.* 1998;51:581–3.

49. Schenker S, Yang Y, Perez A, et al. Sumatriptan (Imitrex) transport by the human placenta. *Proc Soc Exp Biol Med.* 1995;210:213–20.

50. Guputa S, Hanff LM, Visser W, et al. Functional reactivity of 5-HT receptors in human umbilical cord and maternal subcutaneous fat arteries after normotensive or pre-eclamptic pregnancy. *J Hypertens.* 2006;24:1345–53.

51. Innes GD, Macphail I, Dillon EC, Metcalfe C, Gao M. Dexamethasone prevents relapse after emergency department treatment of acute migraine: a randomized clinical trial. *CJEM.* 1999;1:26–33.

52. Colman I, Freidman BW, Brown MD, et al. Parenteral dexamethasone for acute severe migraine headache: meta-analysis of randomized controlled trials for preventing recurrence. *BMJ.* 2008;336:1359–61.

53. Orr SL, Aubé M, Becker WJ, et al. Canadian Headache Society systematic review and recommendations on the treatment of migraine pain in emergency settings. *Cephalalgia.* 2015;35:271–84.

54. Begg, EJ, Duffull SB, Hackett LP, et al. Studying drugs in human milk: time to unify the approach. *J Hum Lact.* 2002;18:323–32.

55. Larsen LA, Ito S, Koren G. Prediction of milk/plasma concentration ratio of drugs. *Ann Pharmacother.* 2003;37:1299–300.

56. Atkinson HC, Begg EJ. Prediction of drug distribution into human milk from physicochemical characteristics. *Clin Pharmacokinet.* 1990;18:151–67.

57. Riant P, Urien S, Albengres E, et al. High plasma protein binding as a parameter in the selection of betablockers for lactating women. *Biochem Pharmacol.* 1986;35:4579–81.

58. American Academy of Pediatrics Committee on Drugs. Transfer of drugs and other chemicals into human milk. *Pediatrics.* 2001;108:776–89.

59. http://aappolicy.aappublications.org/cgi/reprint/pediatrics.

60. Hale TW. *Medications and Mothers' Milk.* Amarillo, TX: Hale Publishing; 2008.

61. http://toxnet.nlm.nih.gov/cgi-bin.

62. Hutchinson S, Marmura MJ, Calhoun A, et al. Use of common migraine treatments in breast-feeding women: a summary of recommendations. *Headache.* 2013;53:1–14.

63. Kauppila A, Arvela P, Koivisto M, et al. Metoclopramide and breast feeding: transfer into milk and the newborn. *Eur J Clin Pharmacol.* 1983;25:819–23.

64. Wischnik A, Manth SM, Lloyd J, Bullingham R, Thompson JS. The excretion of ketorolac tromethamine into breastmilk after multiple oral dosing. *Eur J Clin Pharmacol.* 1989;36:521–4.

65. Cruikshank DP, Varner MW, Pitkin RM. Breast milk magnesium and calcium concentrations following magnesium sulfate treatment. *Am J Obstet Gynecol.* 1982;143:685–8.

66. Wojnar-Horton RE, Hackett LP, Yapp P, et al. Distribution and excretion of sumatriptan in human milk. *Br J Clin Pharmacol.* 1996;41:217–21.

67. Trainor A, Milner J. Pain treatment and relief among patients with primary headache subtypes in the ED. *Am J Emerg Med*. 2008;26:1029–34.

68. Broussard CS, Rasmussen SA, Reefhuis J, et al. Maternal treatment with opioid analgesics and risk for birth defects. *Am J Obstet Gynecol*. 2011;204:314.e1–11.

69. Einarson A, Maltepe C, Narioz Y, et al. The safety of ondansetron for nausea and vomiting of pregnancy: a prospective comparative study. *BJOG*. 2004;111:940–3.

# Chapter 13

# Approach to the Elderly Patient with Headache in the Emergency Department

Fabio Frediani

Gennaro Bussone

## Abstract

The approach to the assessment and management of elderly patients presenting to the emergency department (ED) with headache is similar to the general approach to headache in this setting, in that the initial focus should be on differentiating primary vs. secondary headache and initiating an appropriate work-up where necessary. However, the index of suspicion for secondary headaches should be higher in this population, especially in the case of a new headache. Once secondary headache has been ruled out, the choice of pain interventions in this population requires a relatively greater emphasis on medication contraindications, side-effects, and medication interactions, given the general medical profile of the elderly patient. Unfortunately, evidence-based treatment recommendations are precluded by a lack of evidence specific to this population. In this chapter, we provide a general overview of the approach to the elderly patient with headache and a review of common secondary headaches in this population, and we discuss treatment options for primary headaches in the elderly.

## Introduction

The incidence of primary headaches decreases with advanced age and the incidence of secondary headaches rises [1]. Among adults 65 years and older, the prevalence of both migraine and tension-type headache is a fraction of what it is in adults in the fourth and fifth decades of life. Therefore, in the ED setting, one must have a high index of suspicion for secondary headaches, especially when the elderly patient presents with a new headache.

The relative prevalence of primary vs. secondary headaches in the elderly varies depending on the sample of patients studied, and data specific to the ED setting are unavailable. In community-based samples, tension-type headache is more common than migraine in elderly individuals with primary headaches [2–4]. For example, in one community-based study carried out among elderly patients in rural Italy, the one-year prevalence rate for tension-type headache was 44.5 percent, 11.0 percent for migraine, 4.4 percent for chronic daily headache, and 2.2 percent for secondary headache [3]. In a study done in a tertiary care headache unit in Spain, 28.7 percent of patients over 65 years had tension-type headache, 23.8 percent had migraine, and 16 percent were secondary headaches, of which the most common cause identified was medication-induced headache. The authors also identified some cases of headaches that are typically associated with old age, such as hypnic headache, cervicogenic headache, and headaches associated with giant cell arteritis [4].

In assessing the elderly patient, it is therefore important to consider that secondary headaches have a relatively higher incidence as compared to the incidence of secondary headaches in younger individuals and that the distribution of primary headaches is different in this age group.

## History Taking in the Elderly Patient Presenting to the Emergency Department with Headache

The general principles of evaluating patients presenting to the ED with headache are equally applicable to the elderly population. It is important to remember that the physician's most important tool when confronted with headache in the ED is careful history taking [5]. After ensuring that the patient is stable, the physician should proceed with an organized history in order to gather information for making a diagnosis and, more immediately, in order to identify red flags for headache secondary to a potentially serious condition (Box 13.1). It is necessary to establish whether the headache is their "first-ever" or if the patient has

**Box 13.1 Red Flags for Potentially Serious Secondary Headache**

Age >50 years

First- or worst-ever headache

New type of headache/change in symptoms of pre-existing headache

Abrupt onset, may also be severe (thunderclap)

Headache worsens with exertion or change of (head) position

Subacute headache that worsens over day to weeks

Uncontrollable nausea/vomiting

Fever

Neck stiffness

Persistent neurological signs

Altered consciousness, cognitive deficit

**Box 13.2 Questions to Ask the Patient with Headache in the Emergency Department**

Why did this headache bring you to the emergency department?

When did you start having this type of headache?

Have you previously sought medical help for similar headache attacks?

How did the headache start – were you doing anything in particular?

Where exactly is the pain located?

What are the characteristics of the pain?

Do you have other symptoms associated with your headache?

Do you have other health problems?

**Box 13.3  Medications Known to Cause Headache**

Nitrates

Phosphodiesterase inhibitors

Digitalis

Hydralazine

Nifedipine

Dipyridamole

Amiodarone

Lithium

Thyroid hormone replacement

Estrogen

Antihistamines

Selective serotonin reuptake inhibitors

Opioids

Barbiturates

a history of prior headaches. In the former case, a secondary headache must be ruled out. In the latter case, it is important to establish whether the current attack is similar to their past headaches or whether it is substantially different. The characteristics of the pain, mode of onset (sudden, gradual), circumstances of onset (exertion, at rest), progression (improving, worsening), and preceding/associated events (trauma, drug use, exposure to toxins) must be elucidated (see Chapter 3).

Suspicion for a secondary headache is increased if symptoms other than those typically accompanying a primary headache are present. In the elderly population, the index of suspicion for a secondary headache must be higher, even if the phenotype is consistent with migraine or tension-type headache, especially in the absence of a prior history. Even if there is a past history of headache, which one might expect given the very high lifetime prevalence of migraine and tension-type headache in the general population, a high index of suspicion for a secondary headache in an elderly patient presenting to the ED must be present. Although primary headaches can have their onset in old age, this scenario is relatively uncommon and a first-time headache in a patient over the age of 50 is more likely to be a secondary headache.

A list of essential questions to ask the headache patient presenting to the ED is shown in Box 13.2. Furthermore, since most patients turn out to have unremarkable general and neurological examinations, the diagnosis may perhaps be expedited by enquiring why the patient came to the ED and the reason for the visit may prompt further evaluation or treatment. In elderly people, it is important to evaluate the presence of other diseases that can give rise to headache and to take a diligent medication history with the goal of identifying drugs with headache as a potential side-effect (see Box 13.3).

The following cases are typical motivations for seeking ED care for a headache and may help the ED care provider to direct their assessment and management plan:

- Symptoms reported as worrying or never-before-experienced; for example, headache associated with neurological deficit, fever, and cognitive alterations.

- Worst-ever or first-ever headache (*"the first or worst attack syndrome"*).

- Apparently usual headache that has become unbearable with the patient at their "wits' end" (*the last straw syndrome*").
- Apparently usual headache, but lack of response to normally effective treatments.
- Patient presents to the ED because they believe it is the only place where effective treatment can be obtained ("*rely on the ED*").

## The Physical Examination in the Elderly Patient Presenting to the Emergency Department with Headache

As is the case with all headaches in the ED, after history taking, the next priority is the physical examination. Measurement of blood pressure, heart rate, and temperature is followed by general, cardiologic, pulmonary, and neurologic examinations. The carotid arteries should be auscultated. The external auditory canal should be examined for blood arising from trauma or infection. Liquid exuding from the nose or ears may suggest loss of cerebrospinal fluid (CSF). The presence of fever suggests infection or intracranial bleeding. If glaucoma is suspected, ocular tonometry should be performed.

During the neurologic examination, the examiner should assess for an altered level of consciousness, neck stiffness, focal motor or sensory signs, visual field deficits, papilledema, pupillary size and reactivity, ocular motility, pain on palpation of the temporal arteries, and possible trigger points for trigeminal neuralgia.

Several signs are red flags for secondary headache and compel further assessment. A confused mental state or an altered level of consciousness is suggestive of a secondary process, such as meningitis or an expanding intracranial mass. Unilateral mydriasis (pupillary dilatation) can be associated with a variety of serious underlying causes, such as compressive oculomotor neuropathy caused by uncal brain herniation or an aneurysm (especially of the posterior communicating artery). Disk edema on fundoscopic examination in combination with a headache suggests elevated intracranial pressure. Bitemporal hemianopia on visual field examination, in association with a frontally located headache, suggests a suprasellar mass. Any of these findings would indicate the need for further neuroimaging investigation, as would a focal neurological deficit.

Scotomas on visual field examination are a non-specific finding that could be caused by glaucoma, optic neuritis, or an expansive lesion. However, scotomas can also occur during visual aura prior to the onset of migraine, often in association with positive visual phenomena (e.g., a fortification spectrum), but sometimes occur in isolation. Scotomas associated with migraine aura typically expand gradually, which may help to differentiate them from other processes that may have a more acute onset (e.g., transient ischemic attack with amaurosis fugax). Ophthalmoplegia is another important red flag with a multitude of potential causes, such as elevated intracranial pressure (e.g., due to a space-occupying lesion), compression of the oculomotor nerves by an aneurysm or an arteriovenous malformation, brainstem pathology, or cavernous sinus pathology. Horner syndrome may occur in association with cluster headache or paroxysmal hemicrania, but can also occur in association with intracranial or carotid lesions.

The combination of history taking (which will have elicited red flags and reasons for ED presentation) and the clinical examination should be sufficient to point the clinician toward a diagnosis of primary versus secondary headache. In the elderly patient, it is important to remember that age itself is a risk factor for malignant secondary processes [6]. If the patient has primary headache, the next step is to devise a treatment plan (see below). Where secondary headache is suspected, further investigations are necessary.

## Diagnosis of Secondary Headache in the Elderly Patient Presenting to the Emergency Department with Headache

The most common causes of secondary headache in elderly patients are listed in Box 13.4. The differential diagnosis is similar to that in the non-elderly adult, with the exception of giant cell arteritis, which is a disease of later life. The aging body is more prone to pathology of all sorts, including neurovascular insults, bony spinal pathology, and malignancy. Prescription medication is a well-known cause of headache and should be considered in all elderly patients who present to an ED with headache. A list of medications that commonly cause headache is presented in Box 13.3.

**Box 13.4 Causes of Secondary Headache in the Elderly**

Mass lesion
Giant cell arteritis (temporal arteritis)
Subarachnoid hemorrhage
Subdural hematoma
Meningitis/encephalitis
Cerebral abscess
Ischemic stroke
Disorder of ear–nose–throat or eye
Cardiac cephalalgia
Cervicogenic headache

In the ED, pattern recognition may be useful to generate a differential diagnosis [7]. Four common headache presentations are discussed below.

**Scenario 1.** Acute onset ("thunderclap") headache. This presentation, which suggests neurovascular catastrophe, is discussed in Chapter 5. This presentation mandates consideration of intracranial hemorrhage, ischemic stroke, and RCVS.

**Scenario 2.** Headache with fever, altered sensorium, or neck stiffness. This presentation, which suggests CNS infection, is discussed in Chapter 6. Rheumatological processes such as systemic lupus must also be considered in the differential diagnosis. A spinal fluid analysis is usually required to obtain a precise diagnosis.

**Scenario 3.** Gradual onset but persistent headache. The differential diagnosis here is extensive and is discussed in more detail in Chapter 6. Head imaging is required to exclude a mass lesion. In the elderly patient, C-reactive protein and erythrocyte sedimentation rate should be ordered to exclude giant cell arteritis.

**Scenario 4.** Headache that is similar to previous headache attacks with regards to intensity, duration, and associated symptoms. In this situation, the diagnostic hypothesis is that the patient has a primary headache. For these patients, even if they are elderly, diagnostic testing is not warranted acutely.

Unfortunately, pattern recognition is generally of only limited utility in elderly patients with headache.

In non-elderly adults, the incidence of clinically relevant secondary headaches is low and repeated doses of ionizing radiation may lead to downstream sequelae. In elderly headache patients, the frequency of pathological processes presenting with headache is greater, while the downstream consequences of radiation have less time in which to manifest. Therefore, in the elderly patient with headache, the emergency clinician should have a much higher clinical suspicion for secondary processes and, consequently, a lower threshold to order head imaging.

## Diagnosis of Primary Headache in the Elderly Patient Presenting to the Emergency Department with Headache

After a secondary headache has been excluded, the next step is to diagnose the type of primary headache. For this, the International Classification of Headache Disorders may be a useful guide [8]. In the ED, it is most important to apply the first level of the classification, distinguishing among the major categories of primary headaches: migraine, cluster headache, and tension-type headache (Table 13.1).

It is important to remember that uncommon headaches may present in the ED. Migraine with aura can present without pain, making it difficult to distinguish from headache related to a secondary process such as stroke or seizure. Unlike ischemic events, migraine aura without headache has a predominance of visual symptoms, a gradual build-up or expansion of symptoms, a slow progression of visual symptoms throughout the visual fields, a march of sensory symptoms and sequential involvement of one body part and then the other (face then hand, or vice-versa), and an evolution of symptoms from one modality to the next, such as visual followed by sensory and then speech symptoms [9].

Hypnic headaches are a type of primary headache that tend to begin in individuals over the age of 50 years [8] (see Chapter 9 for details on hypnic headaches). Although they are uncommon [4], they have a typical presentation and patients could present to the ED with an undiagnosed hypnic headache. These headaches are recurrent, occur only during sleep, and lead to awakening of the patient. They are frequent, occurring on more than ten days per month for a minimum period of three months, and are not associated with restlessness or cranial autonomic symptoms. Typically, patients report mild to moderate bilateral head pain lasting 15–180 minutes and occurring on a daily basis, though the clinical presentation does

**Table 13.1** Differential diagnosis of the main primary headache types

| Headache | Age of onset, years | Site | Duration | Frequency | Severity | Pain quality | Other characteristics |
| --- | --- | --- | --- | --- | --- | --- | --- |
| **Migraine** | 10–30 | Hemicranium | 4–72 hours | 1–4 per month | Moderate to severe | Pulsating | Nausea, vomiting, photo/phonophobia Aura |
| **Tension-type headache** | 20–50 | Bilateral | 30 min to 7 days | Variable | Mild to moderate | Pressing/tightening | Only one of photophobia or phonophobia (rare) |
| **Cluster headache** | 20–40 | Unilateral, periorbital | 15–180 min | 1–8 per day | Severe | Acute, penetrating | Lacrimation, eye reddening, rhinorrhea, nasal congestion, miosis |
| **Trigeminal neuralgia** | 50–70 | Distribution of trigeminal nerve 2nd and 3rd > 1st | Less than a second to 2 min | Occasional to 100 per day | Excruciating | Paroxysmal, sharp, stabbing | Triggered by innocuous stimuli |

vary [8]. They differ from cluster headache in that they are bilateral, mild to moderate in intensity, and not associated with restlessness, agitation, or cranial autonomic features. Patients presenting with this clinical phenotype should have a work-up for secondary headaches that present with a similar phenotype, such as sleep apnea, nocturnal hypertension, and hypoglycemia [8]. Specific preventive therapies are available, including lithium carbonate and caffeine, but patients with suspected hypnic headache should be referred to a headache specialist.

## Treatment of Primary Headache in the Elderly Patient Presenting to the Emergency Department

Elderly patients are almost always excluded from clinical trials of parenteral migraine therapeutics. Therefore, very limited data exist to determine efficacy and safety in this population. General principles of care are similar to those used in other populations: specifically to provide relief of pain and associated symptoms, allow return to normal function, and minimize adverse medication effects. Elderly migraineurs tend to have higher baseline cardiovascular risk, and greater concomitant use of prescription medications. Treatment selection is therefore not only based on consideration of the general efficacy and safety of the intervention for the specific primary headache, but must also involve

careful consideration of its side-effects in the context of the general health status of the patient and their comorbid health conditions. Given the commonality of polypharmacy in elderly patients, judicious consideration of possible medication interactions is essential in selecting therapy. For these and other reasons, the appropriate ED treatment may not always be those recommendations that are suggested in general treatment guidelines [10,11].

## Approach to Treating Migraine in the Elderly Patient Presenting to the Emergency Department

Although subcutaneous sumatriptan (6 mg) has been shown to be effective in around 87 percent of non-elderly patients with migraine [12], it has never been studied in an elderly population. Therefore, it is unknown whether or not it is efficacious and safe in this population. Use of subcutaneous sumatriptan in the elderly ED population should be limited to those patients who use it regularly.

Similarly, although intravenous dihydroergotamine in association with an anti-emetic (metoclopramide or prochlorperazine) is commonly used for acute migraine [13], cardiovascular concerns make this medication inappropriate for elderly migraineurs.

One-time doses of parenteral nonsteroidal anti-inflammatory drugs (NSAIDs) have a relatively more favorable safety profile in the elderly. Both intravenous (15–30 mg) [14] and intramuscular ketorolac (30–60 mg) [14,15] have been reported to be effective for relieving acute migraine in the ED in general migraine populations. However, the list of associated contraindications must be carefully reviewed when considering the use of ketorolac in elderly patients. For example, it is contraindicated in cases of severe, uncontrolled heart failure, in the setting of active gastric, peptic, or duodenal ulcers, in severe liver impairment, in moderate or severe renal impairment, and in patients with bleeding or coagulation disorders.

Intravenous anti-dopaminergics are used frequently in the emergency department to abort acute migraine, especially in North America [16,17]. These medications are discussed in more detail in Chapter 7. As with the other medication classes discussed above, few data are available to determine efficacy and safety in the elderly population. However, one-time parenteral doses of these medications are generally well tolerated in the elderly and, as in the non-elderly adult population, these medications should be considered first-line therapy, though some data suggest that they are generally less effective and associated with more side-effects as a patient's age increases [18].

Opioids are commonly used in North American EDs to treat migraine [10,19], despite consensus recommendations to avoid their use [20]. In a non-elderly population, meperidine, one of the opioids used most commonly for migraine, had similar efficacy to ketorolac, and was less efficacious than dihydroergotamine and anti-emetics [21]. As with all medications, opioids have to be used with caution in individuals over the age of 65. However, given the general concern about all migraine medications in the elderly, the paucity of safety and efficacy data, and the fact that parenteral opioids are well studied and well tolerated in elderly pain patients in the ED, these medications are a reasonable therapeutic option for elderly migraine patients in the ED.

Corticosteroids are another therapeutic option for acute migraine in the ED. Dexamethasone might be useful for aborting status migrainosus [22,23], though in a recent systematic review the aggregated evidence did not support its efficacy for acute migraine relief in the ED setting [24]. Nonetheless, corticosteroids can be considered for the treatment of elderly patients presenting to the ED with migraine, and in some instances they may be more appropriate from a safety standpoint than some of the other options. However, special attention must be given when considering the use of corticosteroids in patients with diabetes and hypertension, and patients must always be counseled about the rare but serious associated risk of avascular necrosis of the femoral or humeral head(s).

While there is no evidence to support its use as an acute treatment option in the elderly for patients with migraine or cluster headache, occipital nerve blockade with a local anesthetic and corticosteroid is generally considered to be safe, well tolerated, and potentially effective in elderly patients, as it has been shown to be in non-elderly patients.

Because elderly patients presenting to the ED with migraine often experience associated prolonged nausea, vomiting, and anorexia, which may have led to dehydration, it is important to consider whether or not intravenous fluids are required. If dehydration is suspected, intravenous fluids are indicated. In addition, allowing the patient to rest for some time in a quiet, dark room may aid recovery or at least provide comfort to the patient, particularly if photophobia and phonophobia are present.

## Approach to Treating Cluster in the Elderly Patient Presenting to the Emergency Department

The incidence of cluster headache is highest in individuals aged 20–40 years of age [8]. Therefore, it is uncommon for an elderly patient to present to the ED with their first episode of cluster headache.

Subcutaneous sumatriptan (6 mg), an evidence-based treatment for acute cluster in the non-elderly population, should be used very cautiously in elderly patients. Use should be limited to those who have tolerated the medication previously and who are known to not have vascular disease.

Oxygen is also effective provided it is administered at an adequate dose, that is, 100 percent fraction of inspired oxygen (FiO$_2$) at a rate of 12–15 L/min for 10–15 minutes (see Chapter 8). It is easy to administer in the ED, has no side-effects, and rapidly resolves the headache [25]. Oxygen is an excellent alternative to sumatriptan for elderly patients because of its safety profile. No other medication has proven effective, based on high-quality randomized evidence, for aborting ongoing cluster headaches. Other medication options include intravenous or intramuscular

NSAIDs and opioids, but evidence for their efficacy is limited to anecdotal use.

## Approach to Treating Other Primary Headaches in the Elderly Patient Presenting to the Emergency Department

In most circumstances, persons with episodic tension-type headache rarely present to the ED. However, patients with chronic daily headache or with medication overuse headache may view the ED as their last hope of finding a solution to their problem. Such patients are best served by consultation with a headache specialist. Typically they will require both acute and prophylactic approaches, together with the attentive follow-up that can be offered by a headache center.

## Conclusion

Elderly patients presenting to the ED with headache require a different approach as compared to younger patients with headache in this setting. Because the index of suspicion for secondary headache is higher, and because the causes of secondary headache in this population differ, the elderly patient often requires a different work-up. Pain management in this population differs as well. Because of the relative commonality of comorbid chronic health conditions, medical frailty, and the frequency of polypharmacy, the judicious consideration of medication contraindications, potential side-effects, and medication interactions becomes even more paramount in this patient population.

## References

1. Tanganelli P. Secondary headaches in the elderly. *Neurol Sci.* 2010;31(S1):73–6.

2. Benseñor IM, Lotufo PA, Goulart AC, Menezes PR, Scazufca M. The prevalence of headache among elderly in a low-income area of São Paulo, Brazil. *Cephalalgia.* 2007;28:329–33.

3. Prencipe M, Casini AR, Ferretti C, et al. Prevalence of headache in an elderly population: attack frequency, disability, and use of medication. *J Neurol Neurosurg Psychiatry.* 2001;70:377–81.

4. Ruiz M, Pedraza M, Cruz C, et al. Headache in the elderly: a series of 262 patients. *Neurologia.* 2014;29:321–6.

5. Newman LC, Lipton RB, Solomon S. Headache history and neurologic examination. In *Headache Diagnosis and Treatment.* Edited by Tollison CD, Kunkel RS. Baltimore, MA: Williams and Wilkins; 1993, pp. 23–30.

6. Goldstein JN, Camargo CA, Pelletier AJ, Edlow JA. Headache in United States emergency departments. *Cephalalgia.* 2006;26(6):684–90.

7. Cortelli P, Cevoli S, Nonino F, et al. Evidence-based diagnosis of nontraumatic headache in the emergency department: a consensus statement on four clinical scenarios. *Headache.* 2004;44:1–9.

8. Headache Classification Committee of the International Headache Society (IHS). The International Classification of Headache Disorders, 3rd edition (beta version). *Cephalalgia.* 2013;33(9):629–808.

9. Fisher CM. Late-life migraine accompaniments: further experience. *Stroke.* 1986;17(5):1033–42.

10. Vinson DR. Treatment patterns of isolated benign headache in US emergency departments. *Ann Emerg Med.* 2002;39(3):215–22.

11. Minen MT, Tanev K, Friedman BW. Evaluation and treatment of migraine in the emergency department: a review. *Headache.* 2014;54(7):1131–45.

12. Subcutaneous Sumatriptan International Study Group. Treatment of migraine attacks with sumatriptan. *N Engl J Med.* 1991;325:316–21.

13. Kelley NE, Tepper DE. Rescue therapy for acute migraine, part 1: triptans, dihydroergotamine, and magnesium. *Headache.* 2012;52:114–28.

14. Kelley NE, Tepper DE. Rescue therapy for acute migraine, part 3: opioids, NSAIDs, steroids, and post-discharge medications. *Headache.* 2012;52:467–82.

15. Taggart EK, Campbell S, Villa-Roel C, Rowe BH. Ketorolac in the treatment of acute migraine: a systematic review. *Headache.* 2013;53(2):277–87.

16. Kelley NE, Tepper DE. Rescue therapy for acute migraine, part 2: neuroleptics, antihistamines, and others. *Headache.* 2012;52:292–306.

17. Marmura MJ. Use of dopamine antagonists in treatment of migraine. *Curr Treat Opt Neurol.* 2012;14:27–35.

18. Friedman BW, Cisewski DH, Holden L, Bijur PE, Gallagher EJ. Age but not sex is associated with efficacy and adverse events following administration of intravenous migraine medication: an analysis of a clinical trial database. *Headache.* 2015;55(10):1342–55.

19. Colman I, Rothney A, Wright SC, Zilkalns B, Rowe BH. Use of narcotic analgesics in the emergency department treatment of migraine headache. *Neurology.* 2012;62:1695–700.

20. Langer-Gould AM, Anderson WE, Armstrong MJ, et al. The American Academy of Neurology's top five choosing wisely recommendations. *Neurology*. 2013;81:1004–11.

21. Friedman BW, Kapoor A, Friedman MS, Hochberg ML, Rowe BH. The relative efficacy of meperidine for the treatment of acute migraine: a meta-analysis of randomized controlled trials. *Ann Emerg Med*. 2008;52(6):705–13.

22. Friedman BW, Greenwald P, Bania CT, et al. Randomized trial of IV dexamethasone for acute migraine in the emergency department. *Neurology*. 2007;69:2038–44.

23. Colman I, Friedman BW, Brown MD, et al. Parenteral dexamethasone for acute severe migraine headache: meta-analysis of randomised controlled trials for preventing recurrence. *BMJ*. 2008;336(7657):1359–61.

24. Orr SL, Aubé M, Becker WJ, et al. Canadian Headache Society systematic review and recommendations on the treatment of migraine pain in emergency settings. *Cephalalgia*. 2015;35(3):271–84.

25. Cohen AS, Burns B, Goadsby PJ. High-flow oxygen for treatment of cluster headache: a randomized trial. *JAMA*. 2009;302(22):2451–7.

# Preventing Emergency Department Visits in Primary Headache Patients and Prevention of Bounce-Backs to the Emergency Department

Wm. Jeptha Davenport

## Abstract

Acute therapy of primary headaches includes intravenous rehydration, anti-emetics, corticosteroids, nonsteroidal anti-inflammatory drugs, dihydroergotamine, and serotonin 5-HT1B/1D receptor agonists. Different types of primary headaches may respond similarly to these therapies. Many headaches recur not long after treatment in the ED, and the natural history of the primary headaches is such that they will recur in the long term if not within hours to days of discharge. The ED physician must consider the possibility of post-ED headaches for patients presenting to the ED with primary headaches, and provide anticipatory management for these headaches. The appropriate management of primary headache relies on resources outside the ED, developed in collaboration with outpatient headache healthcare providers. This chapter will address post-ED headache management for primary headache patients.

## Introduction

Patients often continue to suffer from headache after the ED visit. The reasons for this are several, and include: (1) persistence of headache despite ED management; (2) recurrence of headache after ED discharge, in particular as it prompts the return of a patient with primary headache recently seen for the same condition in an ED; and (3) subsequent headache attacks that occur in line with the natural history of primary headaches. With respect to headache, traditionally the role of the emergency physician is two-fold: to relieve headache pain and to identify serious and potentially life-threatening causes of headache [1,2]. However, where possible, in patients presenting with primary headaches, it is also important for the ED physician to address persistent/recurrent-ED headaches in an anticipatory manner. In order to properly address persistent/recurrent-ED headaches, it is useful for the emergency physician to consider the overall context within which patients with primary headache disorders are managed.

## Care of the Primary Headache Patient: General Concepts and Framework

The model of primary headache disorders as chronic diseases with episodic manifestations parallels other neurological and non neurological diseases: epilepsy (and seizures) and asthma are mostly managed in the outpatient setting, while the acute manifestations are managed in the ED. As with migraine and the other primary headache disorders, treatment strategies are divided into preventive and acute therapies [3]. In this chapter, the two facets of primary headache disorders, as a chronic phenomenon and as an acute exacerbation, are useful to consider: presentation to an ED is most often linked to the episodic manifestation, but when repeated headache attacks lead to repeated emergency assessment and treatment, the chronic nature of the disease ought to be explored and addressed [4].

## Primary Headache Patients in the Emergency Department

Figure 14.1 represents, in the abstract and not necessarily to scale, the patients nested in a population

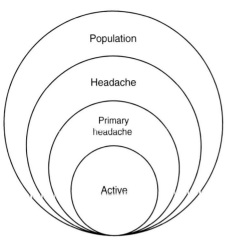

**Figure 14.1** Headache patient types within the population.

experiencing headache. Of this headache population, roughly two-thirds prove to be primary [5]. Of those patients' primary headache disorders, there is a subset whose head pain drives them to alter their behavior in one way or another. This group of active primary headache patients may well seek care in an ED. As explored in depth in Chapter 2, undifferentiated headache may account for 1–4 percent of ED visits in the United States [6–9]. A prevailing sentiment, expressed by patients with recurrent primary headache disorders and their care providers alike, is that the ED is not an ideal venue for episodic or longitudinal primary headache treatment [10]. The assumption rests in part on the definition of primary headache, namely that it is not secondary to a life-threatening process. It also rests on the frequent observation that patients with severe head pain and discomfort frequently seek quiet, dark, non-stimulating environments where their basic needs may be met. While the ED may provide parenteral hydration and analgesia, not commonly available elsewhere, the other environmental conditions sought by the patient with severe head pain may be lacking. The patient with primary headache could be expected to seek emergency care when the pain is novel (for diagnosis at first presentation) or when the pain is overwhelming [11]. In an ideal world, a patient with primary headache would recognize that the headache is part of a larger, self-limited process, and that it is not life-threatening; that the headache would respond to non-pharmacological and pharmacological interventions already at the patient's

disposal; and that refinement of the headache treatment plan could be made with a prompt primary care visit or the implementation of additional, previously acquired self-management skills. In the ideal world, the patient would routinely avoid seeking care through an ED visit, as it would be unnecessary for the patient's best care.

Our world is far from ideal with respect to headache care. Patients and healthcare providers alike often lack an up-to-date understanding of the primary headache disorders [12]. They may fail to recognize primary headache disorders. They may mistake primary headache disorders for other diseases. They may not recognize that migraine and cluster headache require specific treatment. There is often a lack of understanding that primary headaches, like asthma and epilepsy, require ongoing care. Failure to address these issues may result in unnecessary return visits to the ED.

Figure 14.2 illustrates a hypothetical population of patients with primary headache that is active but managed suboptimally. This is contrasted with another hypothetical population of patients with primary headache who are being managed optimally, as displayed in Figure 14.3. When emergency care is sought in this example, it does not lead to a change in patient management – a missed opportunity. A Canadian prospective study suggested that a diagnosis of a primary headache disorder in patients attending EDs was not routinely established, and that physician focus was likely on the exclusion of secondary causes rather than establishing the nature of the primary headache disorder [13]. Patients may seek or be sent for specialist care to explore alternative diagnoses – for example, otolaryngology assessment for vertigo or referred sinus pain; gastroenterology assessment for nausea and vomiting; ophthalmology assessment because of orbital pain or visual obscuration; and so on. Unless these specialists address the primary headache disorder in some fashion, patients continue to suffer from the primary headache disorder, thus placing them at increased risk of a repeat ED visit.

For some patients, the ED is a healthcare safety net. However, research into the reasons for return to an ED in the United States within 30 days of an initial presentation showed that patients typically did have access to a primary care provider, had often already made contact regarding the reason for presentation, and in many cases had healthcare

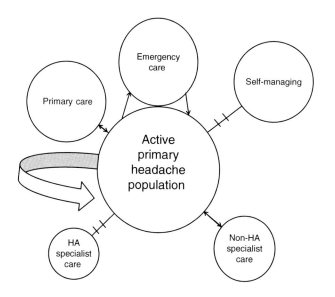

**Figure 14.2** Hypothetical population of active primary headache patients with suboptimal management.

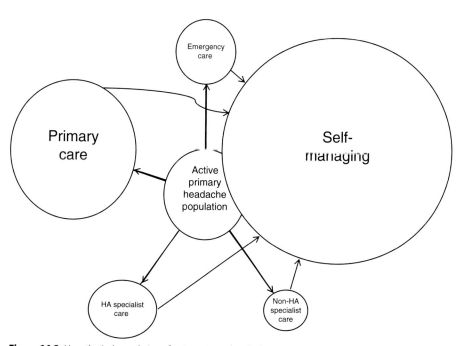

**Figure 14.3** Hypothetical population of active primary headache patients with optimal management.

insurance coverage [14]. Thus, it is important for the clinician to understand the specific issues causing repeat ED visits.

Among patients who account for frequent ED return visits, frequent medication use is reported, suggesting that this subpopulation of patients deserves particular attention [15]. Expanding upon the dual role of adequate analgesia and exclusion of secondary causes, headache care in the ED could be extended to include patient education, prescriptions for acute therapy, and referral to non-emergency headache care resources [16], all of which are strategies that may help to reduce the incidence of post-ED headaches.

## Preventing Headache After ED Discharge

In the days following an ED visit for acute headache, 49 percent of patients report headache [17]. Nearly one-third of migraine patients and 19 percent of patients with tension-type headache report a moderate or severe headache within 24 hours of ED discharge [18]. Often, patients are functionally impaired by these post-ED headaches. As highlighted in the introduction, post-ED headaches have three forms, which will be addressed below: (1) headache persistence (resistance to treatment); (2) headache recurrence; and (3) new primary headache attack.

## Preventing Headache Persistence After ED Discharge

Eliminating headache during the ED visit is ideal. However, persisting headache is common and significant: in a prospective observational cohort study in an urban US ED, 70 percent of patients visiting the ED with primary headache reported persistent headache 24 hours after ED discharge; in nearly half of these, the headache was moderate or severe, and in more than half of these, the headache limited usual activities [19]. In a randomized, double-blind, placebo-controlled multicenter trial testing interventions for acute migraine in the ED, the control arm showed that only 19 percent of patients were persistently pain-free at 24 hours [20]. Unlike many other outpatient settings with relatively brief visits, ED treatment of headache allows for serial application of additional treatments when initial treatment fails. Within the

limits of patient tolerance for extended time and treatment attempts, an in-ED pain score of zero is the target.

Whether a headache resolves in the ED but recurs quickly, or resolves and only later returns in a pattern of primary headache attacks, or never truly disappears, may be significant in evaluating best treatment. In the larger scope of future research studies to address headache after ED discharge, consensus on outcome measures, including timing and duration of headache resolution, as well as minimal clinically important differences, is needed [21].

## Preventing Acute Headache Recurrence

### Definitions Pertaining to Headache Recurrence

The variety of labels attached to a recurrent ED visit for the same or similar problem indicates there is not consensus on terminology. "Recidivism" [22] connotes a faulty lapse into poor behavior at best and criminality at worst, despite the neutral etymology of (a patient) "falling back" (into an ED). Such a term is problematic for another reason, as patients are properly and routinely instructed to return to the ED in the event of worsening or unanticipated sequelae [2]. "Repeater" [15] and "bounce-backs" [14] are terms which also seem to pass judgment upon a patient, as if in a refereed sport. "Unplanned return visits" [23] as a term places no blame on the patient but excludes expected return or contingency-based return, strictly speaking. "ED return rate" [24] has a statistical ring. "Revisits" [23] is a short term and an uncommon turn for a noun in English (so perhaps suited for medicalization), but it is also rather broad. In this chapter, under the different rubrics as set out by their respective authors of reference, the "return visit to ED defined as an unscheduled visit for worsening symptoms" [21] is addressed.

### The Commonality of Headache Recurrence

The phenomenon of headache recurrence is substantial in absolute numbers. From the perspective of an individual treating emergency physician, estimates of treatment efficacy are often inflated, since routine data collection ceases at discharge. Follow-up studies find frequent headache recurrence and continued impairment of function in the days after ED discharge [25,26]. The fourth most common cause of all unplanned revisits within 72 hours in a retrospective analysis from a secondary teaching referral hospital in Taiwan was headache, at 2.1 percent (following abdominal pain [12.9 percent], fever [12.6 percent], and vertigo [4.5 percent]) [23]. In an ED-based prospective observational study of patients with primary headache disorders, headache recurrence was found to be common: almost one-third of migraine patients, one-fifth of tension-type headache patients, and over one-quarter of other headache patients had moderate or severe head pain within 24 hours of discharge from the ED [18]. In the next section the prevention of post-discharge headache is addressed.

## Preventing Post-Discharge Headache in Adults

### Pharmacological Interventions for the Prevention of Acute Migraine Recurrence

The first step in preventing post-ED headache is to be sure that the acute headache was adequately treated. Recurrence of acute pain in general and headache pain in particular is common in the ED. The practitioner may be distracted by the need to exclude

secondary causes of headache and thereby not focus on pain management. Alternatively, the acute abortive agent chosen may be suboptimal or ineffective for that particular patient. As a first step, practitioners should effectively treat the acute migraine pain using sequential evidence-based therapies. The ED practitioner in the United States has 20 parenteral medications from which to choose, from half as many general drug categories (e.g., anti-emetic, neuroleptic, benzodiazepine, triptan, etc.) [6,21]. Treatment may be sequential, with various evidence-based therapies used sequentially until the headache has dissipated; alternatively, the practitioner may use combination therapy with multiple evidence-based therapies at the same time.

There is no acute migraine therapy that completely eliminates the potential for post-ED headache recurrence. Some acute therapeutics are notorious for post-ED recurrent headaches. In a multicenter, ED-based study, two-thirds of patients randomized to subcutaneous sumatriptan experienced post-discharge headache recurrence [27]. In addition, it has been difficult to accurately pre-identify just which patients will be likely to have headache recurrence after sumatriptan [28]. Post-ED headache has been reported only intermittently in ED-based studies. Rates of post-ED headache and return visits to the ED by medication type are listed in Table 14.1.

**Table 14.1** Acute migraine recurrence data by intervention

| Intervention | Return visits | Post-ED headache |
|---|---|---|
| Dihydroergotamine SC | 0% return visits within 24 h; 2% admitted to hospital [29] | 17.7% at 24 h [30]<br>5% no relief at 24 h [29] |
| Sumatriptan SC | | 45.0% at 24 h [30]; 47% by 24 h [28] |
| Sumatriptan PO | | 50% by 48 h, moderate or severe [31] |
| Normal saline IV | | Headache freedom same as without [32] |
| Prochlorperazine IV | 0% return visits within 24 h; 2% admitted to hospital [29] | 5% no relief at 24 h [29]<br>45% headache within 5 days [33] |
| Metoclopramide IV | | 43% 24 h recurrence vs. 52% placebo, not statistically significant [34] |
| Diclofenac IM | | 63.3% pain-free at 24 h vs. 46.7% placebo (migraine without aura)<br>83.3% pain-free at 24 h vs. 73.3% placebo (migraine with aura) [35] |
| Dexamethasone IV | Repeat physician visit decreased at 9% vs. 29% for placebo, from 48 to 72 h [36] | Recurrence decreased at 24–72 h (meta-analysis: RR = 0.68, CI: 0.49, 0.96; I2 = 63%); recurrence at 7 days and at 30 days, not clinically significantly different (single study each); as reported in [21] |

### Corticosteroids for Preventing Migraine Recurrence

Mounting evidence has led to the conclusion that as adjuvant treatment to migraine care, corticosteroid use tempers recurrent headaches, so that they are milder and more responsive to subsequent therapies [37–39]. In a systematic review from the introduction of corticosteroid use through 2014, parenteral dexamethasone was the most common corticosteroid tested to prevent headache recurrence, with a range of doses of 4–24 mg at a single median dose of 10 mg [37]. Other corticosteroids analyzed, in decreasing order of use, were prednisolone (oral, with six-day taper), prednisolone (oral, 150 mg), and, in roughly equal amounts, cortisone (oral, 50 mg), oral dexamethasone (single dose or taper), other prednisolone dosing (single dose or taper, doses 20–150 mg), and methylprednisolone (parenteral, 500 mg) [37]. Adverse effects occurring more often than placebo included restlessness, paresthesias, and flushing, when specified [39]. The sum of the literature suggests an absolute risk reduction of 11 percent (number needed to treat of 9) and a 26 percent relative risk reduction for headache recurrence within 72 hours [37]. Overall, as adjuvant therapy, for limited use, and in patients at higher risk of recurrence, parenteral dexamethasone in a single dose of 10 mg can be recommended.

### Corticosteroids for Cluster Headache

Acute cluster rarely lasts longer than three hours. An emergency clinician may be tempted to consider the dissipation of an acute cluster headache to be a success. However, cluster headache will almost inevitably occur again after ED discharge. These patients cannot be discharged without addressing this fact. Corticosteroids are not necessarily or even typically acute therapy for cluster headache (i.e., for a single attack, for which the acute therapies, discussed in Chapter 8, are preferred). However, corticosteroids do have an established place in what has been called transitional therapy, to decrease the likelihood of future attacks. For this reason they are an important tool in the hands of the emergency physician who is discharging a patient with frequent episodic cluster headaches. The available usual routes are: (1) oral (prednisone, roughly 1 mg/kg in a single daily dose, repeated daily for four days, for example, then tapered off in 5 mg decrements per day); and (2) a single or repeated occipital nerve block ipsilateral to the pain

using methylprednisolone (or similar in doses equivalent to) 40–80 mg [40].

### Take-Home Prescriptions as a Strategy for Managing Acute Migraine Recurrence

Beyond prescribing interventions in the ED that can prevent acute migraine recurrence, the ED physician may also choose to send the patient home with a prescription for an acute therapy to be used if the migraine recurs in the 48 hours following discharge. In a randomized, double-blind efficacy trial which measured primary headache recurrence after ED discharge, both naproxen (500 mg) and sumatriptan (100 mg) were satisfactory, and equally well tolerated. It was also noted, in this study, that both migraine headache episodes and other, non-migraine primary headache episodes responded to the nonsteroidal anti-inflammatory drug and to the serotonin 5-HT1B/1D receptor agonist [31].

## Preventing Post-Discharge Headache in Children

In a retrospective chart review of children with status migrainosus discharged from an urban pediatric teaching hospital ED, 11.2 percent returned within a month of treatment [41] (It should be noted that one exclusion criteria was presentation with status migrainosus within six months prior, meaning that in theory patients most likely to return may not have become part of the study cohort). At the time of the study, a protocol in place directed that IV metoclopramide be given, with the option to repeat doses or to add chlorpromazine in the event of first-dose failure. Children who returned to the ED were statistically more likely to have received brain imaging, to have had a follow-up visit with another physician pre-booked, and to have migraine equivalents (in children, episodic neurological symptoms similar in tempo and severity to migraine attacks in adults, but lacking characteristic head pain). These could have been causative factors or instead associated factors more closely related to initial headache severity; an answer was not discernible. Also, 42.9 percent of the children who "bounced back" once did so again. The type of acute therapy used was uniform for the cohort, which precluded efficacy testing. However, whether or not preventive treatment was given to the child did not seem to influence rates of return [41]. In a different retrospective chart review at another urban teaching pediatric hospital, corticosteroid administration was not associated with significant differences in headache recurrence rates after presentation with intractable migraine. In the same study, outpatient treatment was more likely than inpatient treatment in cases of recurrence, as was male gender and a diagnosis of chronic migraine rather than episodic migraine [42].

Children presenting to the ED with headache receive different treatment depending on whether the ED is a pediatric emergency department or a general ED [43]. Randomized controlled trial evidence for best management of pediatric headache in the ED is scarce [43,44]. Nevertheless, retrospective data suggest that a small proportion of children (5.5 percent) presenting to an ED with migraine return within three days, that prochlorperazine seems superior to metoclopramide, and that both appeared to be better than diphenhydramine [45]. In the United Kingdom, pizotifen is used to prevent migraine recurrence in the pediatric population and is felt to be safe, but is untested by randomized controlled trial evidence in this population [44]. In a retrospective chart review in a US pediatric ED, although a standardized combination therapy (intravenous fluid bolus, ketorolac, prochlorperazine or metoclopramide, and diphenhydramine) reduced pain scores, length of ED stay, and rates of hospital admission, this therapy did not reduce rates of return to the ED [24].

## Preventing Repeated Attacks of Cluster Headache

In addition to considering corticosteroids as a transitional therapy (see above), another useful transitional therapy is dihydroergotamine, which can also be used as an acute therapy for cluster headache. At discharge from the ED, a patient in the midst of episodic cluster attacks may do well to continue this transitional therapy, especially if it has been successful acutely, on a regular basis – for example, taking a prescription for 1 mg subcutaneously twice daily for one week (along with cautions about possible vasoconstriction). This transitional therapy allows for bridging until the effect of preventive therapy takes effect, usually either verapamil or lithium. Of these two preventives, lithium may become effective within one week of the initial dosing of 300 mg twice daily. Verapamil, typically first-line as a preventive, requires more in the way of upward titration and is necessarily slower to reach target dosing [32]. Both typically will require monitoring of some

kind (leukocyte counts, renal and thyroid function, and serum levels for lithium, and electrocardiograms for verapamil) after the patient has been discharged from the ED.

## Preventing Acute Recurrence of Tension-Type Headache

Tension-type headache does not commonly lead to ED visits; when it does, it is likely severe or otherwise disconcerting to the patient. For practical reasons, tension-type headache is frequently managed alongside other similar but less diagnostically defined (but still benign) headache types. In a randomized double-blind study of patients presenting to an urban teaching hospital ED with non-migraine, non-cluster primary headaches, 47 percent receiving IV ketorolac and 35 percent receiving IV metoclopramide plus diphenhydramine required analgesic medication within 24 hours of ED discharge [46]. This need for further analgesia is in keeping with rates of recurrent head pain noted for other primary headache types. As a group of headaches that are not especially frequent in the ED, a means of reducing tension-type recurrence is less obvious. The clinician should reassure the patient and provide a description of the expected natural history of tension-type headache, appropriate treatment, adequate analgesia for future attacks [16], and cautions regarding medication overuse.

## Preventing Future Primary Headache Attacks in the Longer Term

One goal for the care of primary headache in the emergency setting is to decrease the likelihood of future headaches [47]. It is well-established that ED migraine patients are under-identified and often not formally diagnosed during their ED visit, and migraine-specific treatment is not necessarily offered at the visit or by prescription [13,48]. Attention to diagnosis and appropriate discharge prescriptions may decrease the likelihood of future visits.

Frequent acute medication use is associated with increased headache frequency. For example, although opioids are frequently used to treat headache acutely [49], patients exposed to opioids on more than about eight days per month risk progression of high-frequency episodic migraine to chronic migraine [50]. Patients exposed to barbiturates on more than five days per month risk progression [50]. NSAIDs and triptans may be associated with headache progression when used more than 10–14 days per month [50]. These associations are thought to be causal in at least some individuals, and both causation (i.e., medication overuse causes chronic headache) and reverse causation (i.e., frequent headache leads to frequent medication use) are likely operating [50]. Despite potential pitfalls with repeated use of opioids in primary headache patients, their use in US EDs increased from 2001 through 2010 [49]. A retrospective study found an association between initial opioid use and longer length of stay in the ED [51]. Another study found that when opioids were used, there was an increase in return visits within one week of ED discharge [52]. Again, certainty in interpretation is elusive here, and more study would be welcome. Nonetheless, it is important to understand the risk associated with overuse of acute medications, given that liberal prescription of outpatient acute therapies without appropriate counseling could play a part in headache chronification and more frequent headache attacks.

It is not clear if headache-specific education can be delivered in the ED to create a lasting effect. Education should be tailored to individual patients. Important teaching points include that acute treatment is available and recommended for use early in the self-management of migraine. ED-based educational interventions focusing on self-management strategies have not been studied in randomized trials. While it may be assumed that ED-based patient education would lead to beneficial changes in behavior, this is not necessarily so [53]. Or, it may be so, but difficult to demonstrate: In a randomized controlled trial of an educational intervention as part of a comprehensive migraine intervention in a US ED, substantially more patients in the treatment arm did subsequently use migraine-specific acute therapy but did not show significant improvements in the HIT-6 score (a measure of headache impact) one-month post-intervention; all patients receiving the intervention found it helpful or very helpful [54].

Although unplanned return visits to the ED by patients who received a diagnosis of primary headache could be interpreted as failures in care, an alternative explanation allows for humility and patient-focused care by viewing such visits as an opportunity to reassess diagnostic accuracy, to tailor management, to educate, and to improve patient outcomes [23]. "[R]evisits are a safeguard against misdiagnoses and insecurities" [23]. At some level, the early recurrence

of headache, the failure to control future attacks, and repeat visits are emblematic of the lack of treatments that are specific for the disorder, robust in efficacy, and proven by evidence. Clearly, much more research and treatment advances are needed to enable physicians the opportunity to deliver the most effective therapy.

## Conclusion

Emergency physicians must be attuned to the likelihood of headache during the days and weeks after an ED visit for acute headache. Appropriate strategies to address post-ED headache include: (1) effective initial therapy; (2) ED-based parenteral therapies proven to decrease headache recurrence, including corticosteroids for migraine and verapamil for cluster; (3) providing the patient with appropriate expectations about the expected course of the acute headache and the means to treat headache recurrence and future headaches during the days and weeks following the ED visit; and (4) helping patients to understand the natural history of primary headache disorders and what resources are available to help them treat their underlying headache disorder.

## References

1. Schaffer JT, Hunter BR, Ball KM, Weaver CS. Noninvasive sphenopalatine ganglion block for acute headache in the emergency department: a randomized placebo-controlled trial. *Ann Emerg Med.* 2015;65(5):503–10.

2. Swadron SP. Pitfalls in the management of headache in the emergency department. *Emerg Med Clin North Am.* 2010;28(1):127–47.

3. Halm EA, Mora P, Leventhal H. No symptoms, no asthma: the acute episodic disease belief is associated with poor self-managment among inner-city adults with persistent asthma. *Chest.* 2006;129(3):573–80.

4. Pringsheim T, Davenport WJ, Becker WJ. Prophylaxis of migraine headache. *CMAJ.* 2010;182(7):E269–76.

5. Davenport R. Acute headache in the emergency department. *J Neurol Neurosurg Psychiatry.* 2002;72(Suppl. II):ii33–7.

6. Vinson DR. Treatment patterns of isolated benign headache in US emergency departments. *Ann Emerg Med.* 2002;39(3):215–22.

7. Lucado J, Paez K, Elixhauser A. Headaches in US Hospitals and Emergency Departments, 2008: Statistical Brief #111. *Healthcare Cost and Utilization Project (HCUP) Statistical Briefs.* 2011;24:1–12.

8. Fiesseler FW, Riggs RL, Shih R, Richman PB. Do patients with recurrent headaches attempt abortive therapy before their emergency department visit? *J Emerg Med*. 2007;32(3):245–8.

9. Bellolio MF, Hess EP, Gilani WI, et al. External validation of the Ottawa subarachnoid hemorrhage clinical decision rule in patients with acute headache. *Am J Emerg Med*. 2015;33(2):244–9.

10. Rozen TD. Emergency department and inpatient management of status migrainosus and intractable headache. *Continuum*. 2015;21(4):1004–17.

11. Minen MT, Loder E, Friedman B. Factors associated with emergency department visits for migraine: an observational study. *Headache*. 2014;54(10):1611–18.

12. Peters M, Jenkinson C, Perera S, et al. Quality in the provision of headache care: 2. Defining quality and its indicators. *J Headache Pain*. 2012;13(6):449–57.

13. Nijjar SS, Pink L, Gordon AS. Examination of migraine management in emergency departments. *Pain Res Manage*. 2011;16(3):183–6.

14. Moskovitz JB, Ginsberg Z. Emergency department bouncebacks: is lack of primary care access the primary cause? *J Emerg Med*. 2015;49(1):70–7.

15. Maizels M. Health resource utilization of the emergency department headache "repeater." *Headache*. 2002;42:747–53.

16. Friedman BW, Grosberg BM. Diagnosis and management of the primary headache disorders in the emergency department setting. *Emerg Med Clin North Am*. 2009;27(1):71–87.

17. Ducharme J, Beveridge RC, Lee JS, Beaulieu S. Emergency management of migraine: is the headache really over? *Acad Emerg Med*. 1998;5:899–905.

18. Friedman BW, Hochberg ML, Esses D, et al. Recurrence of primary headache disorders after emergency department discharge: frequency and predictors of poor pain and functional outcomes. *Ann Emerg Med*. 2008;52(6):696–704.

19. Friedman BW, Hochberg M, Esses D, et al. Pain and functional outcomes of patients with primary headache disorder discharged from the emergency department (abstract). *Acad Emerg Med*. 2006;13(5 Suppl. 1):S18.

20. Friedman BW, Greenwald P, Bania TC, et al. Randomized trial of IV dexamethasone for acute migraine in the emergency department. *Neurology*. 2007;69:2038–44.

21. Sumamo Schellenberg E, Dryden DM, Pasichnyk D, et al. *Acute Migraine Treatment in Emergency Settings. Comparative Effectiveness Review No. 84.* Rockville, MD: Agency for Healthcare Research and Quality; 2012. Available at: www.effectivehealthcare.gov/reports/final.cfm.

22. Kelley NE, Tepper DE. Rescue therapy for acute migraine, part 3: opioids, NSAIDs, steroids, and post-discharge medications. *Headache*. 2012;52(3):467–82.

23. Wu C-L, Wang F-T, Chiang Y-C, et al. Unplanned emergency department revisits within 72 hours to a secondary teaching referral hospital in Taiwan. *J Emerg Med*. 2010;38(4):512–17.

24. Leung S, Bulloch B, Young C, Yonker M, Hostetler M. Effectiveness of standardized combination therapy for migraine treatment in the pediatric emergency department. *Headache*. 2013;53(3):491–7.

25. Blumenthal HJ, Weisz MA, Kelly KM, Mayer RL, Blonsky J. Treatment of primary headache in the emergency department. *Headache*. 2003;43:1026–31.

26. Mellick LB, Mellick GA. Treatment of primary headache in the emergency department. *Headache*. 2004;44(8):840–1.

27. Akpunonu BE, Mutgi AB, Federman DJ, et al. Subcutaneous sumatriptan for treatment of acute migraine in patients admitted to the emergency department: a multicenter study. *Ann Emerg Med*. 1995;25(4):464–9.

28. Visser WH, Jaspers NMWH, de Vriend RHM, Ferrari MD. Risk factors for recurrence after sumatriptan: a study in 366 migraine patients. *Cephalalgia*. 1996;16:264–9.

29. Callaham M, Raskin N. A controlled study of dihydroergotamine in the treatment of acute migraine headache. *Headache*. 1986;26:168–71.

30. Winner P, Ricalde O, Le Force B, Saper J, Margul B. A double-blind study of subcutaneous dihydroergotamine vs subcutaneous sumatriptan in the treatment of acute migraine. *Arch Neurol*. 1996;53:180–4.

31. Friedman BW, Solorzano C, Esses D, et al. Treating headache recurrence after emergency department discharge: a randomized controlled trial of naproxen versus sumatriptan. *Ann Emerg Med*. 2010;56(1):7–17.

32. Balbin JEB, Nerenberg R, Baratloo A, Friedman BW. Intravenous fluids for migraine: a post hoc analysis of clinical trial data. *Am J Emerg Med*. 2016;34(4):713–16.

33. Callan JE, Kostic MA, Bachrach EA, Rieg TS. Prochlorperazine vs. promethazine for headache treatment in the emergency department: a randomized controlled trial. *J Emerg Med*. 2008;35(3):247–53.

34. Cete Y, Dora B, Ertan C, Ozdemir C, Oktay C. A randomized prospective placebo-controlled study of intravenous magnesium sulphate vs. metoclopramide in the management of acute migraine attacks in the Emergency Department. *Cephalalgia*. 2005;25(3):199–204.

35. Bigal ME, Bordini CA, Speciali JG. Diclofenaco intramuscular no tratamento agudo da migrânea: um estudo duplo cego placebo controlado. *Arq Neuropsiquiatr.* 2002;60(2-B):410–15.

36. Baden EY, Hunter CJ. Intravenous dexamethasone to prevent the recurrence of benign headache after discharge from the emergency department: a randomized, double-blind, placebo-controlled clinical trial. *CJEM.* 2006;8(6):393 400.

37. Woldeamanuel Y, Rapoport A, Cowan R. The place of corticosteroids in migraine attack management: a 65-year systematic review with pooled analysis and critical appraisal. *Cephalalgia.* 2015;35(11):996–1024.

38. Colman I, Friedman BW, Brown MD, et al. Parenteral dexamethasone for acute severe migraine headache: meta-analysis of randomised controlled trials for preventing recurrence. *BMJ.* 2008;336(7657):1359–61.

39. Singh A, Alter HJ, Zaia B. Does the addition of dexamethasone to standard therapy for acute migraine headache decrease the incidence of recurrent headache for patients treated in the emergency department? A meta-analysis and systematic review of the literature. *Acad Emerg Med.* 2008;15(12):1223–33.

40. Becker WJ. Cluster headache: conventional pharmacological management. *Headache.* 2013;53(7):1191–6.

41. Legault G, Eisman H, Shevell MI. Treatment of pediatric status migrainosus: can we prevent the "bounce back"? *J Child Neurol.* 2011;26(8):949–55.

42. Cobb-Pitstick KM, Hershey AD, O'Brien HL, et al. Factors influencing migraine recurrence after infusion and inpatient migraine treatment in children and adolescents. *Headache.* 2015;55(10):1397–403.

43. Richer L, Graham L, Klassen T, Rowe B. Emergency department management of acute migraine in children in Canada: a practice variation study. *Headache.* 2007;47(5):703–10.

44. National Institute for Health and Care Excellence. *Diagnosis and Management of Headache in Young People and Adults.* London: NICE; 2012. Available at: www.nice.org.uk/CG150.

45. Bachur RG, Monuteaux MC, Neuman MI. A comparison of acute treatment regimens for migraine in the emergency department. *Pediatrics.* 2015;135(2):232–8.

46. Friedman BW, Adewunmi V, Campbell C, et al. A randomized trial of intravenous ketorolac versus intravenous metoclopramide plus diphenhydramine for tension-type and all nonmigraine, noncluster recurrent headaches. *Ann Emerg Med.* 2013;62(4):311–18.

17. Becker WJ, Krysciu RJ. Treatment of migraine: a headache for the emergency department. *Neurology.* 2007;69(22):2034–5.

48. Gupta MX, Silberstein SD, Young WB, et al. Less is not more: underutilization of headache medications in a university hospital emergency department. *Headache.* 2007;47(8):1125–33.

49. Mazer-Amirshahi M, Dewey K, Mullins PM, et al. Trends in opioid analgesic use for headaches in US emergency departments. *Am J Emerg Med.* 2014;32(9):1068–73.

50. Bigal ME, Lipton RB. Excessive acute migraine medication use and migraine progression. *Neurology.* 2008;71:1821–8.

51. McCarthy LH, Cowan RP. Comparison of parenteral treatments of acute primary headache in a large academic emergency department cohort. *Cephalalgia.* 2014;35(9):807–15.

52. Colman I, Rothney A, Wright S, Zilkalns B, Rowe BH. Use of narcotic analgesics in the emergency department treatment of migraine headache. *Neurology.* 2004;62(10):1695–700.

53. Gross A, Forget M, St George K, et al. Patient education for neck pain. *Cochrane Database Syst Rev.* 2012;3:CD005106.

54. Friedman BW, Solorzano C, Norton J, et al. A randomized controlled trial of a comprehensive migraine intervention prior to discharge from an emergency department. *Acad Emerg Med.* 2012;19(10):1151–17.

# Index

Locators in **bold** refer to tables; those in *italic* to figures
ED = Emergency Department

accessory nerve assessment 23
acetaminophen 55
acetylsalicylic acid 75
acute headache
  pregnancy 132–35
  trauma patients 52
acute sinusitis **29–30**, 82
adult ED
  headache prevalence 6–8
  prevention of ED visits 153–54
age of the patient 4–5, 15, 17. *See also*
  elderly patients; pediatrics
air pollution, headache
  prevalence 5
American Academy of Neurology
  Choosing Wisely
  recommendations 2
  Classification of Evidence
  Matrix for Therapeutic
  Questions 105–6
American College of Emergency
  Physicians (ACEP) 28, 43
American College of
  Radiology (ACR)
  appropriateness criteria 28, 38
  Choosing Wisely list 37–38
American Headache Society;
  Choosing Wisely campaign 37
American Migraine Prevalence and
  Prevention Study (AMPP) 8–9,
  65–66
analgesics (simple), medication
  overuse headache 101–2. *See also*
  acetaminophen; NSAIDs; etc.
aneurysm 33, 47
angiography, aneurysm 33
anxiety, patient 37, 68
aortic dissection **46**
arteriovenous malformations 44
arteritis. *See* giant cell arteritis
aura, migraine 16–17, 68
autonomic dysreflexia 60

bacterial meningitis. *See* meningitis
blood pressure, high/low 19,
  55–58. *See also* intracranial
  hypertension/hypotension
  pediatrics 115–16
  pregnancy 126–27
blood tests 26–27, 96
bounce-backs 152. *See also* prevention
  of ED visits
brain tumor. *See* malignancy
Brazil, headache prevalence 4
breast cancer metastases 50–51

C-reactive protein (CRP)
  arteritis 58
  laboratory tests 26–27
caffeine, hypnic headache 95
calcitonin gene-related peptide
  (CGRP) 101
calcium-channel blockers 85
Call Fleming syndrome. *See* reversible
  cerebral vasoconstriction
  syndrome
Canada
  headache prevalence 5
  migraine management 2
Canadian CT Head Rule 54
carbon monoxide poisoning 18,
  **29–30**, 60
cardiovascular exam 116
carotid artery dissection (CAD)
  **44–46**, 82
central retinal artery occlusion
  20–21
cerebral venous sinus
  thrombosis **45–46**
cerebrospinal fluid (CSF) analysis 27
cerebrovascular disease **111**
cerebrovascular exam 20
cervicogenic headache 59
Chiari malformations 58
chlorpromazine
  lactation **135–36**
  pregnancy **132–33**
Choosing Wisely campaign
  (AHS) 37

Choosing Wisely recommendations,
  (AAN) 2
Classification of Evidence Matrix
  for Therapeutic Questions
  (AAN) 105–6
clinical decision rules
  neuroimaging 31–32
  trauma patients 54
cluster headaches **80–81**. *See
  also* trigeminal autonomic
  cephalalgias
  diagnosis 82, 84
  differential diagnosis **83–84**
  economic burden 11
  elderly patients 146–47
  frequency of ED visits 9
  headache prevalence **7**
  history taking 16
  pediatrics 121–22
  physical exam 20
  post-discharge prevention 154–55
  treatment 84–85
combination agents, migraine 75–76
computed tomography (CT)
  scanning 28
  aneurysm 33
  cost of headache care 9
  dural sinus thrombosis 31
  initial investigations 35
  subarachnoid hemorrhage 1, 31,
  **33–34**, 46–47
  trauma patients 54
consultations to specialists,
  cost 9–10
cortical spreading depression
  (CSD) 100–1
corticosteroids. *See also*
  dexamethasone;
  methylprednisolone;
  prednisone; etc.
  cluster headaches 85
  elderly patients 146
  lactation 136–37
  meningitis 55
  post-discharge 154
  pregnancy 133–35

cost of headache care 1. *See also* economic burden
  epidemiology 9–10
  migraine 66–67
  neuroimaging 36
  strategies to reduce 11–12
cough headache 89–90
cranial nerve exam 22–23, 317.40117–20
CRP. *See* C-reactive protein
cryptococcal meningitis 27
*Cryptococcus neoformans* 54–55
CT scans. *See* computed tomography scanning

data, physical exam 1
decision rules. *See* clinical decision rules
dehydration, laboratory tests 26. *See also* IV fluids
demographics, prevalence of headache 4–5
dental caries, physical exam 19
dermatologic exam 116–17
dexamethasone
  elderly patients 146
  lactation **135–36**
  migraine 73, 77
  pregnancy 133–35
diagnosis (general information) 1
diagnostic criteria
  cluster headaches 82
  cough headache 89
  exercise headache 90
  hypnic headache 94
  medication overuse headache 99–100
  migraine 16, 68
  new daily persistent headache 95
  pediatrics **113**
  post-traumatic headache 52
  sexual activity-induced headache 91
  thunderclap headache 93
  trigeminal autonomic cephalalgias 80, 82
differential diagnosis 1
  cough headache 88–90
  elderly patients 143–45
  history taking 17
  hypnic headache 95
  laboratory tests 27
  migraine 68–71
  neuroimaging 28–31
  new daily persistent headache 96
  pediatrics 114–15
  physical exam 18
  pregnancy 127
  subarachnoid hemorrhage 33
  tension-type headaches 70–71

thunderclap headache 44–46, 93–94
trigeminal autonomic cephalalgias 82–84
dihydroergotamine (DHE). *See* ergotamines
diphenhydramine 74
diplopia, assessment 22
dopamine receptor antagonists
  elderly patients 146
  lactation **135–36**
  migraine 73
  post-traumatic headache 54
  pregnancy **132–33**
droperidol
  lactation **135–36**
  pregnancy **133**
drug seeking behavior 106–8. *See also* medication overuse headache
dural sinus thrombosis 29–31

eclampsia 17
economic burden 10–11. *See also* cost of headache care
EFNS. *See* European Federation of Neurological Societies
elderly patients 141, 147
  cluster headaches 146–47
  diagnosis 143–45
  epidemiology 141
  history taking 141–43
  migraine 145–46
  physical exam 143
  treatment 145
eletriptan
  lactation 137
  pregnancy 131
*Enterovirus* 54–55
environmental factors, headache 5
epidemiology 1, 12
  cost of headache care 9–10, 66–67
  economic burden 10–11
  elderly patients 141
  frequency of ED visits 8–9, 180.5065–67
  headache prevalence 4–8
  medication overuse headache 99–100
  migraine 65–68
  pediatrics 110–12
  pregnancy 125–26
  primary headache **89–88**
  strategies to reduce resource utilization 11–12. *See also* prevention of ED visits
  tension-type headaches 69
ergotamines
  elderly patients 145–46

medication overuse headache 101–2
  migraine 75
erythrocyte sedimentation rate (ESR) 26–27
etiology of headache
  elderly patients 144
  headache prevalence 6–8
  pediatrics **111**
  pregnancy **128**
European Federation of Neurological Societies (EFNS)
  medication overuse headache 104
  tension-type headaches 71, 121
evidence-based therapies 2. *See also* guidelines
exercise headache 89–91
  history taking 18
  pediatrics 114
  thunderclap headache 93
eye disorders 59
eye exam 20–21
eye movement assessment 22

facial nerve/weakness 23
family history taking 15, 18
fracture, skull/vertebral 52
frequency of ED visits. *See also* epidemiology
  pediatrics 111–12
  primary headache 8–9, 180.5065–67

gait assessment 24, 118
gender differences
  frequency of ED visits 67
  inpatient admissions 10
  pediatrics 111–12
  prevalence of headache 4–5
general medical exam. *See* physical exam
giant cell arteritis 58–59
  migraine 68
  neuroimaging **29–30**
  physical exam 19
  thunderclap headache **46**
Glasgow Coma Scale **21–22**
glaucoma 59, 68
glossopharyngeal nerve assessment 23
Greece, headache prevalence 4
guidelines 1
  medication overuse headache 104–6
  neuroimaging in patients with non-acute headache 28
  strategies to reduce resource utilization 11
  tension-type headaches 121

head and neck exam 19–20, 116
headache not otherwise
    specified 7–8
hemicrania continua (HC) 86,
    121–22. See also paroxysmal
    hemicrania
hepatic metabolism,
    pregnancy 131–32
herpes encephalitis 54–55
history taking 1, 15, 24
    elderly patients 141–43
    pediatrics 112–15
    primary headaches 16
    red flags 18
    secondary headaches 16–18
    Horner syndrome 20, 38
hydrocephalus **44**, **46**
hypertension/hypotension. See
    blood pressure, high/low;
    intracranial hypertension/
    hypotension
hypnic headache 84, **89–88**, 94–95,
    144–45
hypoglossal nerve assessment 23

idiopathic intracranial hypertension.
    See intracranial hypertension
ID-Migraine™ instrument 69
income. See socioeconomic status
individual differences, headache
    prevalence 4–5
indomethacin
    cough headache 90
    exercise headache 91
    hypnic headache 95
    infection 16–17, 54–55. See also
        meningitis
    laboratory tests 26–27
    migraine 68
    pediatrics **111**, 114
    vital signs 19
inflammation, systemic 26–27
infratentorial tumor-related
    headaches 50
inpatient headache admission
    costs 10
insurance status, and frequency of ED
    visits 66
intermittent headaches, history
    taking 17
internal carotid artery dissection 82
International Burden of Migraine
    (IBMS) study 65
International Classification of
    Headache Disorders 1. See also
    diagnostic criteria
international comparisons
    frequency of ED visits 8
    prevalence of headache 4

International Headache Society 68,
    73
intracranial hematoma 52
intracranial hemorrhage
    migraine 68
    neuroimaging 33
    thunderclap headache
        44, **46**
intracranial hypertension,
    neuroimaging **29–30**,
    55–56
intracranial hypotension 56–58
    history taking 17–18
    neuroimaging **29–30**
    thunderclap headache 45–46
intracranial pressure (ICP), cough
    headache 88
investigations 26–27, 39. See also
    neuroimaging; physical exam
intravenous (IV) fluids
    elderly patients 146
    migraine 73–74
    pregnancy 129
Italy, prevalence of headache 4

Jacod syndrome 51

ketonuria, laboratory tests 26
ketorolac
    elderly patients 145–46
    lactation **135–36**
    pregnancy 132–33

laboratory tests 26–27
lactation, migraine treatment
    **135–37**
last straw syndrome 143
lithium
    cluster headaches 85
    hypnic headache 95
location, headache 43,
    112–13
low-pressure headaches 56–58. See
    also blood pressure, high/low
lumbar puncture 35–36
    infection 55
    neuroimaging 36, 55
    new daily persistent headache
        96
    pediatrics 120
    post-puncture headache 56–58
    subarachnoid hemorrhage 1
    thunderclap headache 47
lung cancer metastases 50–51
Lyme neuroborreliosis 27, 54–55

magnesium 75
    lactation **135–36**
    pregnancy 133–34

magnetic resonance imaging (MRI) 28
    aneurysm 33
    brain metastases 50–51
    cost of headache care 9
    new daily persistent headache 96
    subarachnoid hemorrhage 31,
        34–35
malignancy 143.10050–53. See also
    metastases
    history taking 17
    migraine 68
    neuroimaging 38
    pediatrics **111**, 114
management, ongoing 150–52.
    See also prevention of ED visits
medical information exchange 11
medication, headache caused by 50,
    142. See also below
    elderly patients 142, 145
    pregnancy 17
medication to treat headache
    infection headaches 55
    in lactation 135–37
    low-pressure headaches 57
    pediatrics 120–22
    post-discharge **153–55**
    post-traumatic headache 54
    in pregnancy 125–26,
        129–31
medication overuse headache (MOH)
    60, 99, 108
    algorithm 103–2
    Classification of Evidence
        Matrix 105–6
    diagnosis/ diagnostic criteria 99–100,
        102
    drug-seeking behavior 106–8
    epidemiology 99–100
    headache prevalence 5
    medication causing 101–2
    pathophysiology 100–1
    pediatrics 114
    prevention of ED visits 155–56
    treatment 102–5
medicolegal liability, neuroimaging
    indications 37
melanoma metastases 50–51
meningitis 54–55
    laboratory tests 27
    pediatrics **111**, 118
    physical exam 19–20
mental status exam 21–22, 117
meperidine
    lactation **135–36**
    pregnancy 133–34
metastases 50–51. See also malignancy
    history taking 17
    neuroimaging 38
    thunderclap headache 44

methylprednisolone, lactation **135–36**
metoclopramide
    lactation **135–36**
    migraine 74, 76
    pregnancy **133**
migraine
    cost of headache care 10
    diagnosis 68–69
    differential diagnosis **83**
    elderly patients 145–46
    epidemiology 5, 7–8,
        65–68
    evidence-based therapies 2
    history taking 16
    lactation **135–37**
    medication overuse 105
    neuroimaging **29–30**
    opioids 2
    pediatrics **111, 113**, 121
    post-discharge **153–54**
    pregnancy 125–27, 129–37
    strategies to reduce resource
        utilization 11
    and tension-type headaches
        69–72
    trauma patients 52–53
    treatment 72–77
MOH. *See* medication overuse
    headache
motor symptoms 23–24, 118
MRI. *See* magnetic resonance
    imaging
musculoskeletal exam 116–17

narcotics analgesics 106
national variations, US prevalence of
    headache 4
neck
    exam 19–20, 116
    pain 59
*Neisseria meningitidis* 54–55
nerve blocks, occipital 85, 146
neuroimaging 27–28. *See also*
        computed tomography; magnetic
        resonance
    aneurysm 33
    clinical decision rules 31–32
    cost of headache care 9
    differential diagnosis 28–31
    dural sinus thrombosis 31
    further investigations 35–36
    indications 37–38
    initial investigations 35
    lumbar puncture 36, 55
    malignancy 38
    neurological conditions **29–30**
    pediatrics 120

pregnancy 35, 128
red flags 32–33
sinus headache 38–39
subarachnoid hemorrhage 28–31,
    **33–34**, 46–47
tests available 28
thunderclap headache 46–47
trauma patients 36–37, 53–54
trigeminal autonomic
    cephalalgias 82–83
neuroleptic medication, migraine 74
neurologic exam, pediatrics
    117–18
neurological symptoms
    history taking 15–16, 18
    malignancy 50–51
    neuroimaging **29–30**
    pediatrics **111**, 114–15
    physical exam 20–24
    secondary headaches 17, 53
neuronal nitric oxide synthase
    (nNOS) 101
new daily persistent headache
    (NDPH) **89–88**, 95–97
New Orleans criteria, post-traumatic
    headache 54
nonsteroidal anti-inflammatories
    (NSAIDs) 55. *See also*
        acetylsalicylic acid; ketorolac; etc.
    elderly patients 145–46
    medication overuse
        headache 101–2
    migraine 74
    post-traumatic headache 54
    pregnancy 131–33
    tension-type headaches 71–72

occipital condyle syndrome 51
olfactory nerve assessment 22
ophthalmologic exam. *See* eye exam
opioids
    elderly patients 146
    headache prevalence 5
    medication overuse headache
        101–2, 106–7
    migraine 2, 66, 75
    pediatrics 121
    pregnancy 134
    strategies to reduce resource
        utilization 11
optic nerve assessment 22
orbital apex/Jacod syndrome 51
oxygen, elderly patients 146–47

pain intensity, pediatrics 113–14
pain quality, pediatrics 114
papilledema, physical exam 20
parasellar syndrome 51

paroxysmal hemicrania (PH) **80–81**,
    85, 121–22
patient expectations 2
pediatrics 110, 122
    cranial nerve exam 317.40117–20
    diagnostic criteria **113**
    epidemiology 110–12
    etiology of headache **111**
    headache prevalence 6–8
    history taking 112–15
    malignancy 50
    medication to treat 120–22
    meningitis 118
    migraine **113**, 121
    neuroimaging 120
    physical exam 115–18
    post-discharge 154–55
    red flags 112, 114–15, 119
    screening overview 118–20
    tension-type headaches **113**,
        120–21
    trigeminal autonomic
        cephalalgias 121–22
persistent headache, trauma
    patients 52
PH. *See* paroxysmal hemicrania
physical exam 1, 18–19, 24
    elderly patients 143
    head and neck 19–20
    motor symptoms 23–24
    neurological 20–24
    ophthalmologic 20–21
    pediatrics 115–18
    sensory screening 24
    vital signs 19
physical exertion triggers. *See* exercise
    headache
pituitary apoplexy **29–30**, 51, 53
pituitary tumors 51–52
polypharmacy, elderly patients 145.
    *See also* medication overuse
    headache
post-discharge prevention 152–55
post-dural puncture headache
    56–58
post-traumatic headache 51–54
    neuroimaging 36–37
    pediatrics **111**, 116
posterior reversible encephalopathy
    syndrome (PRES) 17
    differential diagnosis 93–94
    neuroimaging **29–30**
    thunderclap headache **45–46**
postural component, symptoms
    17–18, 114
prednisone, cluster headaches 85
pre-eclampsia/eclampsia 17
pregnancy 125, 137

etiology of headache **128**
laboratory tests 26
lactation **135–37**
medication use 125–26,
   129–31
migraine 125–27, 129–37
natural history 125–26
neuroimaging 35
secondary headaches 17,
   126–29
treatment principles 129
PRES. *See* posterior reversible
   encephalopathy syndrome
prevalence of headache in ED visits
   4–8. *See also* epidemiology
preventative medication,
   migraine 11
prevention of ED visits 156
headache persistence 152
headache recurrence 152–55
long-term strategies 155–56
ongoing management 150–52
patient types 150
primary headaches 149–52
primary (idiopathic) stabbing
   headache 61
primary angiitis of the central nervous
   system (PACNS) 93–94
primary headaches 1, 88, 97. *See also*
   hypnic headache; migraine;
   tension-type headaches;
   thunderclap headache
cough headache 89–90
diagnosis 80–81
elderly patients 144–45
epidemiology 27.306–11,
   **89–88**
exercise headache 90–91
history taking 16
new daily persistent
   headache 95–97
pediatrics 110–11
prevention of ED visits 149–52
sexual activity-induced headache
   **89–88**, 91–93
prochlorperazine 76
lactation **135–36**
pregnancy **132–33**
promethazine, in pregnancy 132
propofol 75
psychiatric comorbidities 11,
   66, 68
radiation-induced headache 50

radiation risks, neuroimaging 9, 27,
   36, 120
RCVS. *See* reversible cerebral
   vasoconstriction syndrome

recurrences
migraine 76–77
post-discharge prevention 152–55
red flags 1
cough headache 88
elderly patients 142
medication overuse headache 102
migraine 68
neuroimaging 32–33
pediatrics 112, 114–15, 119
sexual activity-induced
   headache 92
SNOOP mnemonic 18
thunderclap headache 43
relapses. *See* recurrences
renal cell cancer metastases 50–51
respiratory exam, pediatrics 116
return visits 152. *See also* prevention
   of ED visits
reversible cerebral vasoconstriction
   syndrome (RCVS) 92–94
neuroimaging **29–30**
thunderclap headache **45–46**
Romberg test 24
rules. *See* clinical decision rules

SAH. *See* subarachnoid hemorrhage
seasonal variations, headaches 5–6,
   111–12
secondary headaches 1, 50, 61.
   *See also* giant cell arteritis;
   malignancy; post-traumatic
   headache; trigeminal neuralgia
autonomic dysreflexia 60
blood pressure 55–58
cervicogenic headache 59
Chiari malformations 58
differential diagnosis 69
elderly patients 143–44
eye disorders 59
history taking 16–18
infection 54–55
pediatrics 110–11
pregnancy 126–29
prevalence 6–8
substance use/withdrawal 60, 114
seizures 19, **111**
sensory screening 24, 118
sexual activity-induced headache
   **89–88**, 91–93
sinus headache 38–39
sinusitis
neuroimaging **29–30**, 82
pediatrics **111**, 116
physical exam 19
SNOOP mnemonic, red flags 18
socioeconomic status, patient 5, 66
specific gravity, tests 26

Standardized Mini-Mental State
   Examination 21
stress 93, 111–12
stroke
neuroimaging **29–30**
pregnancy 126
thunderclap headache **44**
subarachnoid hemorrhage (SAH) 1
history taking 17–18
laboratory tests 27
lumbar puncture 35–36
migraine 68
neuroimaging 28–31, **33–34**,
   46–47
sexual activity-induced
   headache 92
thunderclap headache **43–44**, **46**,
   93
substance use/withdrawal headaches
   60, 114. *See also* medication
   overuse headache
sudden-onset severe headaches 17–18
sumatriptan
cluster headaches 84–85
elderly patients 145–47
lactation **135–36**
medication overuse
   headache 100–1
pregnancy 133–34
SUNCT (short unilateral
   neuralgiform headache with
   conjunctival injection and
   tearing) **80–81**, 86
systemic inflammation 26–27
systematic symptoms, history taking
   15–18
systemic vasculitis **58–59**

TAC. *See* trigeminal autonomic
   cephalalgias
take-home prescriptions 154
temozolomide 50
temporal arteritis. *See* giant cell
   arteritis
temporomandibular joint disorders 19
tension-type headaches. *See also*
   sexual activity-induced headache
diagnosis of exclusion 69–70
diagnostic criteria **70**
epidemiology 7–9, 11, 69
history taking 16
and migraine 69–72
neuroimaging **29–30**
pediatrics **111**, **113**, 120–21
post-discharge 155
trauma patients 52
treatment 71–72
teratogenic drugs, in pregnancy 131

thrombophilia, laboratory tests 27
thunderclap headache 43–44, 47–48
    associated symptoms 46
    differential diagnosis 44–46
    epidemiology **89–88**
    further investigations 47
    lumbar puncture 47
    neuroimaging 36, 46–47
    physical exam 18
    primary 93–94
    subarachnoid hemorrhage
        33, 43
time course of the headache,
    pediatrics 112
TN. See trigeminal neuralgia
Tolosa Hunt syndrome (THS)
    ophthalmoplegia 22
transient ischemic attack (TIA) 17
traumatic brain injury 52–53. *See also*
    post-traumatic headache
trigeminal autonomic cephalalgias
    (TACs) **80–81**, 86. *See also*
    cluster headaches; hemicrania
    continua; paroxysmal
    hemicrania; SUNCT
    diagnosis 80–82, 84
    differential diagnosis 82–84

neuroimaging 82–83
    pediatrics 121–22
    treatment 84–85
trigeminal nerve assessment 22
trigeminal neuralgia (TN) 60–61,
    **83–84**
triggers
    history taking 15, 18
    pediatrics 114
triptans. *See also* sumatriptan etc.
    medication overuse headache
        101–2
    migraine 11, 66, 70, 193.14072–74
    post-traumatic headache 51

UK, prevalence of headache 4
urine tests 26
US Headache Consortium
    evidence-based guidelines for
    neuroimaging in patients with
    non-acute headache 28
US, prevalence of headache 4

VAD. *See* vertebral artery dissection
vagus nerve assessment 23
Valsalva maneuvers 50
    cough headache 89–90

thunderclap headache 93
vascular imaging 36, 44. *See also*
    angiography
vasculitis 58–59. *See also* giant cell
    arteritis
venous thrombosis, pregnancy 126.
    *See also* stroke
ventriculoperitoneal (VP)
        shunt malfunction,
        pediatrics **111**
verapamil, cluster headaches 85
vertebral artery dissection (VAD)
        **44–46**
vestibulocochlear nerve assessment 23
viral meningitis 55
vital signs
    pediatrics 115–16
    physical exam 19
VP shunt. *See*
        ventriculoperitoneal shunt

Westergren erythrocyte sedimentation
    rate, arteritis 58
white matter abnormalities, trauma
    patients 53

xanthochromia 27, 47

Printed in the United States
by Baker & Taylor Publisher Services